PROFESSIONALIZATION OF NURSING

Current Issues and Trends

PROFESSIONALIZATION OF NURSING
Current Issues and Trends

Second Edition

Margaret M. Moloney
Ph.D., R.N., F.A.A.N.

J. B. Lippincott Company
Philadelphia
New York   London   Hagerstown

Editor: David P. Carroll
Editorial Assistant: Amy Stonehouse
Production Supervisor: Robert D. Bartleson
Production: Editorial Services of New England, Inc.
Compositor: Circle Graphics
Printer/Binder: R. R. Donnelley & Sons

Second Edition

6   5   4   3   2   1

Library of Congress Cataloging-in-Publication Data
Moloney, Margaret M.
    Professionalization of nursing : current issues and trends /
Margaret M. Moloney.—2nd ed.
        p.   cm.
    Includes bibliographical references and index.
    ISBN 0-397-54842-7
    1. Nursing—Practice.   2. Nursing—Study and teaching.   I. Title.
    [DNLM: 1. Education, Nursing—trends.   2. Nursing—trends.
    3. Professional Competence. WY 16 M728p]
    RT86.7.M65 1992
    610.73—dc20
    DNLM/DLC
    for Library of Congress   91-19707
                                                                    CIP
ISBN: 0-397-54842-7

To
Nurses
Worldwide
who continually strive to exemplify
humanistic caring attitudes and professionalism
in their teaching and clinical practice

Preface

To say that the nursing profession in the 1990s is on the move and making great strides toward gaining self-assurance and professionalism has never been more accurate. Unity among nurses is evident despite considerable diversity in their views. Issues and trends observable in today's health care climate indicate the potential strength that over 2,000,000 nurses wield in efforts to assure a better health care environment for our nation.

Public opinion is calling attention to aspects of health care that reflect values and humanitarian concerns as a result of witnessing the devastating effects of AIDS, drug and alcohol abuse, an aging population, and the growing numbers of homeless and disenfranchised people. These public health problems challenging our nation require nursing expertise and intervention for their solutions. Nursing, in its present position of advocating social change and endeavoring to use its resources in resolving health and welfare issues, is providing a new and better image for the American public. Whether nurses will continue to retain this image remains to be seen.

Considerable progress has been made in restructuring nursing services within many hospitals. However, as the chief providers of care in these settings, nurses wield little power in formulating health care policies. On the other hand, nurses have a power source in their relationship with patients that has increased as nursing practice moves from institutions to community settings such as homes and to other job opportunities outside of hospitals. With a shift in health care from institutions to the community, organization of nursing care is being patterned on newer professional practice models of health care.

In preparing the second edition of this book, I noted that many of the issues and trends presented in the original text were not only right on target but continue to concern nurses, the nursing profession, and the public. For example, results of recent surveys on the nursing shortage that continues into the 1990s reflect several of the underlying issues and trends presented in this book. My beliefs, that nurses need to be informed about the meaning of professionalism and the personal commitment it requires in order to enhance their own professional growth and that of the nursing profession, have not changed. The challenge to the nursing profession to set new goals for its education and practice is being supported and developed from within its ranks. Progress to date indicates that many nurses are striving to reach their professional goals as reflected in trends presented in this revised text. And yet, other nurses remain unconvinced about their professional future and the need to strive for professionalism. Moreover, many health care institutions are providing only minimal evidence that professionalism for nursing is one of their main goals.

The purpose of this book is to create for nurses a clearer awareness and understanding of nursing as a profession by examining the meaning of profession and the extent to which nursing is developing its scientific knowledge base and controlling its education and practice. The challenge to nurses is to reach agreement on their claim to expertise. Although many similarities with the previous edition exist, there are several significant changes made in this new edition. An expanded discussion on the U.S. health care system and nursing's key role in effecting change through cost-effective consumer-oriented outcome measures should provide an opportunity for nurses to debate about these issues. Also, a timely and informative new chapter on the nursing shortage describes factors affecting supply and demand for nurses, reasons for nurses' discontent, and strategies to remedy the shortage.

The final chapter on a futuristic view of nursing in the 1990s and beyond has been greatly expanded. Perspectives of the health care system of the future, such as a shift from hospital to community-based care, restructuring nursing care in hospitals and community agencies, and the cost-effectiveness of health care services provided by nurses, are presented. In addition, economic reforms for nursing, educational preparation for nursing that includes new curricular patterns of caring, increased nurse autonomy, and an improved public image provide nurses with substantive material for additional debate.

Although many nursing books describe the practice of nursing, few have considered the concept of autonomous nursing practice as a means to advance professionalism. Undoubtedly, where autonomous practice is allowed, nurses are demonstrating a high degree of professionalism. I believe this book is unique in its approach to viewing *autonomy* from both a nursing-education and nursing-practice viewpoint. Other topics presented, for example, are a scientific theory base to increase nursing's professionalism, expanded roles for nursing, managed care, nursing centers, and restructuring the health care system. All of these topics add strength to the unique aspects of this second edition.

As in the previous edition, this book is divided into six parts which identify and examine the most critical issues and trends in contemporary nursing. Part I focuses on an introduction to the professionalism of nursing. Chapter 1 presents an overview of the development of professions. Part II presents perspectives on the professionalism of nursing. Chapter 2 examines the evolution of nursing as a profession. Chapter 3 describes the development of a scientific knowledge base for nursing practice. Part III focuses on the nursing shortage. In Chapter 4, a comprehensive overview of key issues involving the nursing shortage is presented. Part IV introduces the concept of control of professional nursing education. Chapter 5 provides an overview of the status of nursing education at all levels. In Chapter 6, selected issues in nursing education are examined. Chapter 7 emphasizes related issues in nursing education. Chapter 8 is concerned with faculty governance in bureaucratic organizations in relation to the concepts of autonomy, authority, and accountability. Part V focuses on *control* of professional nursing practice. Chapter 9 deals with evolving roles in nursing practice, and Chapter 10 addresses economic issues affecting such practice. In Chapter 11, the topics of governance and self-regulation of nursing practice are considered in relation to autonomy and authority. Chapter 12 describes the status of accountability and responsibility for patient care. Part VI examines the strategies needed to advance the professionalization of nursing, both present and future. Chapter 13 explores the concepts of power and motivation. Chapter 14 focuses on a vision of the future of nursing based on strategies requiring significant changes that can be attained by the late 1990s. This chapter concludes on a positive note indicating that nursing will attain *full* professional status and deserve to be ranked among other prestigious health professions. Finally, a summary of key points is presented at the end of each chapter.

This book is intended for undergraduate and graduate nursing students, nurses involved in continuing education programs, and nursing educators at all levels. Moreover, it can serve as an excellent resource for clinical specialists, administrators, researchers, and all nurses engaged in professional nursing practice. In this second edition, bibliographical references and suggested readings are extensive and have been updated throughout the text. I would emphasize that Chapter 1 has not been changed. It provides the necessary background for understanding the meaning of profession and professionalism and thus sets the tone for all remaining chapters.

I am grateful to those who have expressed appreciation for the previous edition and have shared their insights on issues and trends. A special word of thanks is extended to Judith Cronin-Powers and Nancy Reeves for their superb secretarial assistance. Gratitude is also expressed to my sister, Mary Ellen, my Community, and to many colleagues and friends who provided continued encouragement and support during the preparation of this second edition. Finally, special appreciation is extended to J. B. Lippincott, a division of Wolters-Kluwer Company, and to David P. Carroll, senior editor of the Nursing Division, for his excellent assistance and cooperation as this second edition became a reality.

If its contents serve to motivate nurses to continue to commit themselves to the pursuit of authentic professionalization, it will have accomplished its goal.

Margaret M. Moloney
Ph.D., R.N., F.A.A.N.

Contents

INTRODUCTION TO THE PROFESSIONALIZATION OF NURSING

I

Overview of the Development of Profession

1

INTRODUCTION

Whether nursing in our society can be characterized as having full professional status is a question that has been debated since the turn of the century. Describing the nursing scene at that period, Isabel Hampton Robb, one of the great nursing leaders of her time, observed that "medicine has taken the decision out of our hands, and has made trained nursing a profession, but how soon we shall attain to the full profession level depends upon ourselves entirely . . . "[1] It seems ironic, but if Robb were to evaluate the nursing scene over nine decades later, she might conclude that her observation is as pertinent today as in 1900. Although nurses have enjoyed being called professional, "as much from courtesy as tradition," full professional status for nursing is claimed by few today.[2]

Nurses have assumed the title of professional, but they are often unaware of the meaning of profession or the problems involved in achieving professionalism. They lack a "professional identity."[3] If nursing has not been successful to date in reaching a high level of professionalism, perhaps one of the reasons might be nurses' inability to reach agreement on the definition of profession and the responsibilities required of professionals. These issues are important in understanding the evolution of nursing over the past century and the efforts made to achieve professionalization of its members.

3

The question of why nursing has not achieved full professional status, having a recognizable body of knowledge and a monopoly over its services, after delivering nursing services for over a century and discussing the problems of professionalism for a decade or more, is a ponderous one.[4] Observation of contemporary professional nursing reveals that many nurses are not committed to nursing as a self-regulating profession, "for . . . true professionalism is not about being well paid or climbing the hierarchical tree . . . [but] about controlling one's own practice and making one's own decisions."[5] Many occupational groups include members who are reluctant to accept their individual responsibilities. Nursing is no exception; a significant number of practicing nurses demonstrate an unwillingness to assume responsibility for their actions while simultaneously decrying their lack of professional autonomy. Some nurses not only are unwilling to assume responsibility for their practice but also are unwilling to demonstrate commitment to their professional development or to work toward control over their practice.

Much of the controversy surrounding nursing's professional status is due to an inadequate interpretation of the definition of profession. Although most nurses view themselves as professionals, nursing has yet to meet the two main criteria of profession: autonomy and control of nursing education and practice. As a result, debate over the controversial issue of nursing's full professional status continues. Indeed, over a quarter of a century has passed since Martha Rogers, an esteemed nurse leader and educator, aptly pointed out that "a philosophy of nursing as a learned profession demands a major reorientation for the bulk of nurses [and] . . . loose usage of the prestigious word 'professional' must give way to more precise definition."[6] Thus, it seems appropriate at the outset to examine the meaning of "profession," "professionalism," and "professionalization" as defined by social scientists over the past few decades.

Numerous authors have attempted to define "profession" and to evaluate which occupations have successfully achieved professional status. According to some sociologists, there exists a tendency for occupations to seek professionalism but only a few ever attain it. Perhaps there are no more than 30 or 40 that have achieved *full* professional status, depending on how many specialty groups within a given field are included in the rankings.[7]

The professions of medicine, law, the ministry, and university teaching have been well established since the Middle Ages. Architecture, dentistry, and some branches of engineering were professionalized by the early nineteenth century. Several scientific and engineering fields along with certified public accountants have been professionalized more recently.[8] However, some occupations are still in the process—social work, school teaching, librarianship, nursing, and pharmacy. Traditionally, the concept of profession has "become an ideology, not only an image which consciously inspires collective or individual efforts, [but having] a predominantly ideological [function] justifying inequality of status and closure of access in the occupational order."[9] In other words, the "ideal" profession presupposes that its members are ranked higher in status than others and can boast of selecting only the most highly qualified candidates.

DEFINITION OF PROFESSION

Carr-Saunders and P. A. Wilson, in their pioneer study on professions published in 1933, categorized them by the amount of knowledge in which each laid claim to professional status. Those disciplines whose knowledge demanded rigorous, *lengthy* study in the basic sciences and humanities were ranked as professions. Those with lesser knowledge requiring shorter periods of study were classified as near-professions or marginal ones.[10]

In 1953, Morris L. Cogan offered a definition of profession based on an understanding of the theoretical underpinnings of some specific knowledge area and its accompanying abilities, which are applied to man's welfare.[11] In his view, a profession has an ethical obligation to provide altruistic service to its clients. This same view was expressed by Robert Habenstein, when he observed that "to some, what is symbolized is the idea of altruism, i.e., selfless laboring in the service of mankind . . . [while] . . . to others 'profession' symbolizes technical competence."[12] Interestingly enough, the concept of "altruistic service" is sometimes attacked in feminist literature. It is viewed historically as being detrimental to nursing's professional advancement.

According to some sociologists, "profession" signifies a relatively high social status or ranking. Professions are close to the top of prestige ratings for occupations.[13, 14] Studies show that the public ranks professions at the top of prestigious occupations, and professionals are better satisfied with the rewards of their work than are members of other occupations.[15] For almost a century, nursing's attempts to be recognized as a legitimate, full profession have been observed. Although there are numerous occupations claiming to be professions, recognition of this status may not have been granted by society at large.[16] For too long, nurses have equated licensure with professionalism. Society, however, extends prestige and status to those whose education reflects a long and intensive period of study. Inability to achieve the most *important* criteria for professionals, i.e. standardization of education and control over practice, should not imply that these criteria are irrelevant, unnecessary, or to be disregarded by the membership.

EDUCATION—THE ESSENCE
OF A LEGITIMATE PROFESSION

High status, authority, and prestige are criteria that courts attribute to professions. From a legal standpoint, courts have traditionally emphasized "a rigorous and systematic educational program" for entry into the field.[17] Nursing has achieved licensing laws, a professional association, code of ethics, research and theory development, and a commitment to social values. And yet, nursing *still* lacks high social status and what the courts consider the essence of professionalism—a *standardized* system of education that all recognized professions have achieved.[18] As a result, "nursing's present educational system comes off looking second-rate, deprives nursing of full professional status and creates significant legal handicaps."[19] Nursing has a tendency to either ignore or compromise on this most important criteria for professions with the belief that achieving power more than compensates for other deficiencies.[20]

Another proponent of *knowledge* as a basis for judging true professionalism is H. S. Becker, who defined "professions" as "occupations which possess a monopoly of some esoteric and difficult body of knowledge . . . [and] . . . consist, not of technical skills and the fruits of practical experience, but, rather, of abstract principles arrived at by scientific research and logical analysis."[21] A similar train of thought was expressed by Wilbur Moore in 1970, in referring to "profession" as an occupation whose members create and utilize systematic knowledge in solving individual client's problems or problems of groups of clients.[22] Each of these definitions of profession stresses *knowledge* as a requirement. Other authors apply the term "profession" to an *ideal* type of occupational institution, identified by characteristics that distinguish one occupation from another.[23] Characteristics of professions continue to be utilized by social scientists in evaluating professional status, and power—how it is achieved and retained—has begun to occupy the interest of contemporary sociologists.

In addition to defining a profession in terms of a sound knowledge base, autonomy and social prestige or status are characteristics mentioned by other authors. For example, at the beginning of the last decade, Eliot Friedson, a sociologist, defined profession by stating, "when a number of people perform the same activity and develop common methods which are passed on to new recruits and come to be conventional, we may say that the workers have been organized into an occupational group, or an occupation . . . [and] . . . in the most general classification, a profession is an occupation."[24] However, Friedson distinguished between profession and occupation by pointing out that the greatest distinction is in "legitimate autonomy" as it gives the profession "the right to control its own work."[25] This special status is sustained by promoting a high level of trustworthiness for its members and their devotion to society's need, for which they are granted power and prestige.[26, 27]

Although nursing has increased public awareness of its mission and enjoys public trust, the image of nurses as the physician's handmaid continues to permeate the public view. Changing this public image to include the concept of nursing's autonomy, a distinct body of knowledge, and equal status with other professional groups is the challenge that nurses are concentrating on in the 1990s.

Some of the reasons why certain occupations have achieved full professional status are their importance to society, esteem for the prolonged training, knowledge, and skills that they require, and respect resulting from their professionalism. Such attitudes toward an occupation do not occur suddenly but rather develop over time. They result, historically, from an occupational group's efforts to become distinctive from others, to develop standards of education and practice, to regulate members' conduct, and to further their base of knowledge.[28] Ranked as ideal types of occupations, medicine and law have been the recipients of power, increased income, and prestige. However, their success is the result of a complex struggle that occurs among all the occupations. Occupations that have succeeded in the struggle to obtain professionalism demonstrate a vested interest in drawing a line between professionals and nonprofessionals.[29]

PROFESSIONALISM DEFINED

The term "professionalism" is not referred to as frequently as "profession" in literature. It has been defined as a "set of attributes" among the characteristics of professionals. Many members of other occupational groups, such as nursing, reflect the same professional attitudes as those of the medical profession.[30] Attitudes such as commitment to one's work and an orientation toward service rather than personal profit are often observed among professional workers. In referring to attitudinal variables, other authors mention the "practitioner's sense of calling and self-regulation by colleagues," or peer review.[31] Upon entering a profession, one becomes committed to the development of characteristic attitudes and responses, even to donning an acceptable attire such as the nurse's uniform that distinguishes the nurse from other occupational workers.

THE CONCEPT OF PROFESSIONALIZATION

"Professionalization" encompasses the extent to which the characteristics of the learned, ideal professions have been acquired by occupations. It is described as "a dynamic process whereby many occupations can be observed to change certain crucial characteristics in the direction of 'profession.' " But this process cannot describe the *realities* of any one occupation.[32] Moreover, professionalization is viewed as "an exchange process between society and an occupational group striving for professional status."[33] In discussing the relationship between professionalism and professionalization, many occupations expressing the ideology of professionalism may not, in fact, be advanced regarding the process of professionalization.[34] Depending on one's viewpoint, this may be true of nursing; Some nurses who speak the language of professionalism retreat when the price to be paid involves sacrifice and commitment.

CHARACTERISTICS OF A PROFESSION

In order to examine the extent to which nursing has progressed in the process of professionalization, a review of the common characteristics essential to a profession is presented here. This review should clarify the reasons for the so-called irreconcilable differences that currently exist in nursing over the profession/nonprofession issue.

By the turn of the century, the study of professions received considerable emphasis and priority among various occupational groups. In 1915, Abraham Flexner identified specific characteristics to describe the ideal profession, based on his observations of the ministry, law, and medicine. He was convinced that these three occupations qualified as professions but that social work definitely did not. Even up to the present period, these criteria continue to form the basis for judging whether or not an occupation has achieved full professional status.

Flexner's six characteristics of a profession are as follows:

1. It is basically intellectual, carrying with it high responsibility.
2. It is learned in nature, because it is based on a body of knowledge.
3. It is practical rather than theoretical.
4. Its technique can be taught through educational discipline.
5. It is well organized internally.
6. It is motivated by altruism.[35]

It is noteworthy that Flexner listed intellectual endeavor as the first criterion, viewing it as the *core* of the professions. That he valued the importance of learning is noted in the following statement:

> How are we to distinguish professions that belong to universities from vocations that do not belong to them? The criteria are not difficult to discern. Professions are, as a matter of history—and very rightly—'learned

professions'; there are no unlearned professions; unlearned professions—a contradiction in terms—would be vocations, callings, or occupations.[36]

From the Middle Ages to the present century, universities have standardized education and served as watchdogs for preventing inroads by those lacking university preparation. It should be mentioned that medical schools had great difficulty gaining acceptance into universities. Surgery, in particular, was regarded as a technical field.

The significant question to ask about occupations, however, is not whether or not they are professions but to what extent they exhibit the characteristics of professions.[37] As an occupation comes close to professionalism, certain internal structural changes occur and the member's relationship to society is changed.[38] Moreover, changes in its education, practice, research, and legislative activities become apparent. Physical scientists, social scientists, lawyers, engineers, doctors, and architects are considered professional groups.[39] This distinction is based on two characteristics of scientists and professionals, namely, considerable technical expertise and holding fast to professional norms rather than to those of an organization.[40]

It has been asserted that there is a continuum of professionalism upon which the professions and the semi-professions are identified. In the semi-professions, a predominance of females are employed in bureaucratic institutions (nurses and teachers). Since the more traditional professions have only recently allowed women to enroll, it is easily recognized why women were found primarily in nursing and school teaching. Although men are found in these fields, they are considered "female" occupations. In institutions employing nurses and school teachers, the bureaucratic structures have not been conducive to fostering professionalism among their employees. True professionals are seldom subject to supervision as are semi-professionals. Other characteristics of semi-professions are a shorter period of training, a less legitimate status, a less specialized body of knowledge, a less established right to privileged communication, and less autonomy from controls than the established professions.[41]

SUMMARY

This chapter began with a discussion of nursing's progress as a profession and the reasons why, to date, it has not achieved *full* professional status. Several external factors that have impeded nursing's advancement as a profession are the public's poor image of nurses, lack of autonomy, power, a standardized system of education, and inadequate leadership in health care matters. Nurses can advance toward full professionalism if they thoroughly understand the definition and meaning of profession and their responsibilities for achieving full professional status.

Several opinions and theories about profession were presented, along with descriptions of characteristics of professions. Definitions of profession and professionalism emphasized altruistic service, prestige, competence, and the importance of the profession's service to society. The concept of professionalization as a process, indicating the extent to which professional characteristics are acquired, was also presented.

The prestige and high social status awarded professions was highlighted, and it was observed that a firm knowledge base and autonomy headed the list of characteristics consistently emphasized by the majority of the authors. The importance of maintaining trust between the professional and the client was stressed because the public withdraws esteem and the right to self-control from a profession when it observes that self-interest supersedes altruistic interests.

Some authors believe that nursing remains a semi-profession. In other words, it lacks the main characteristics of a profession: an authentic *knowledge base* and *autonomy* or control over its education and practice. These two characteristics form the basis for the remaining parts of this book as we trace nursing's progress in the professionalization process.

REFERENCES

1. Robb, I. "A General Review of Nursing Forces," in L. Flanagan, *One Strong Voice: The Story of the American Nurses Association.* Kansas City: American Nurses Association, 1975, 326.
2. Gamer, M. "The Ideology of Professionalism," *Nursing Outlook* 27:2 (February, 1979), 108.
3. Lewis, E. "The Professionally Uncommitted" (editorial), *Nursing Outlook* 29:5 (May, 1979), 323.
4. Cohen, H. *The Nurse's Quest for a Professional Identity.* Menlo Park, Calif.: Addison-Wesley, 1981, 3.
5. Iveson-Iveson, J. "Professing Self-Control," *Nursing Mirror* 153:15 (April 9, 1981), 37.
6. Rogers, M. *Reveille in Nursing.* Philadelphia: F. A. Davis, 1964, 10.
7. Wilensky, H. "The Dynamics of Professionalism: The Case of Hospital Administration," *Hospital Administration* 7 (Spring, 1962), 12.
8. Goode, W. "The Theoretical Limits of Professionalization," in A. E. Etzioni, (ed.), *The Semi-Professions and Their Organizations: Teachers, Nurses, Social Workers.* New York: The Free Press, 1969, 280.
9. Larson, M. *The Rise of Professionalism.* Berkeley, Calif.: University of California Press, 1977, xviii.
10. Carr-Saunders, A. and Wilson, P. *The Professions.* Oxford: Clarendon Press, 1933.

11. Cogan, M. "Toward a Definition of Profession," *Harvard Educational Review* 23 (1953), 49.
12. Habenstein, K. "Critique of 'Profession' as a Sociological Category," *Sociological Quarterly* 4 (1963), 293.
13. *Ibid.*, 294.
14. Hughes, E. "Professions," in K. S. Lynn and the editors of Daedalus, *The Professions in America*. Boston: Houghton Mifflin, 1965, 3.
15. Barber, B. "Some Problems in the Sociology of the Professions," in K. S. Lynn and the editors of Daedalus, *The Professions in America*. Boston: Houghton Mifflin, 1965, 19.
16. Beletz, E. "Professionalization—A License Is Not Enough," in N. Chaska, (ed.), *The Nursing Profession: Turning Points*. St. Louis: C. V. Mosby, 1990, 16.
17. Segal, E. "Is Nursing a Profession?" *Nursing '85* 15:6 (June, 1985), 43.
18. *Ibid.*
19. *Ibid.*
20. Beletz, "Professionalization—A License Is Not Enough," 16.
21. Becker, H. "The Nature of a Profession," in *Education for the Professions: The Sixty-First Yearbook of the National Society for the Study of Education, Pt. II.* Chicago: University of Chicago Press, 1962, 35.
22. Moore, W. *The Professions: Roles and Rules.* New York: Russell Sage Foundation, 1970, 53–54.
23. Vollmer, H. and Mills, D. *Professionalization.* Englewood Cliffs, N. J.: Prentice-Hall, 1966, 2.
24. Freidson, E. *Profession of Medicine.* New York: Dodd, Mead and Co., 1970, 71–72.
25. *Ibid.*
26. *Ibid.*, xvii.
27. Larson, M. *Rise of Professionalism.* x.
28. National Manpower Council. *A Policy for Scientific and Professional Manpower.* New York: Columbia University Press, 1953, 38–39.
29. Goode, W. "Encroachment, Charlatanism, and the Emerging Profession: Psychology, Sociology, and Medicine," *American Sociological Review* 25 (December, 1960), 902.
30. Freidson, E. *Profession of Medicine.* 70.
31. Olesen, V. and Whittaker, E. *The Silent Dialogue.* San Francisco: Jossey-Bass, 1968, 185.
32. Vollmer H. and Mills, D. *Professionalization*, vii–viii.
33. Aaronson, L. "A Challenge for Nursing: Re-viewing a Historic Competition," *Nursing Outlook* 37:6 (November–December, 1989), 274.
34. Vollmer and Mills, *Professionalization*, vii–viii.
35. Flexner, A. "Is Social Work a Profession?" in *Proceedings of the National Conference of Charities and Corrections.* Chicago: Hildermann Printing Co., 1915, 578–581.
36. Flexner, A. *Universities: American, English, German.* New York: Oxford University Press, 1930, 29.
37. Hughes, E. "Professions," 3.
38. Gross, E. *Work and Society.* New York: Thomas Y. Crowell Co., 1958, 77.

39. Kast, F. and Rosenzweig, J. *Organization and Management.* New York: McGraw Hill, 1970.
40. *Ibid.,* 500.
41. Etzioni, A. (ed.), *The Semi-Professions and Their Organizations: Teachers, Nurses, Social Workers.* New York: The Free Press, 1969, vii.

SUGGESTED READINGS

Barber, B. "Control and Responsibility in the Powerful Professions," *Political Science Quarterly,* Winter, 1978.

Ben-David, J. "Science as a Profession and Scientific Professionalism," in J. J. Loubser (ed.), *Exploration in General Theory in the Social Sciences: Essays in Honor of Talcott Parsons.* New York: The Free Press, 1976.

Carr-Saunders, A. M. *Professions: Their Organization and Place in Society.* Oxford: The Clarendon Press, 1928.

Cheek, N. H., Jr. *The Professions: A Paradigmatic Approach.* New York: New York State School of Labor and Industrial Relations, 1965.

Cogan, M. L. "The Problem of Defining a Profession," in *The Annual of American Academy of Political and Social Science* 297 (1955), 105–111.

Habenstein, K. W. "A Critique of 'Profession' as a Sociological Category," *Sociological Quarterly* 4 (1963), 291–300.

Kleingartner, A. *Professionalism and Salaried Worker Organization.* Madison, Wis.: University of Wisconsin, Industrial Relations Research Institute, 1967.

McGlothlin, W. J. *The Professional Schools.* New York: Center for Applied Research, 1964.

Parsons, T. "Professions," in *The International Encyclopedia of the Social Sciences.* Vol. 12. New York: Macmillan, 1968.

Schein, E. H. *Professional Education.* New York: McGraw-Hill, 1972.

Starr, P. *The Social Transformation of American Medicine.* New York: Basic Books, 1982.

Thomas L. *The Youngest Science: Notes of a Medicine Watcher.* New York: Viking Press, 1983.

Tyler, R. W. "Distinctive Attributes of Education for the Professions," *Social Work Journal* 33 (April, 1952), 55–62.

U.S. Office of Education. Lloyd E. Blauch (ed.), *Education for the Professions.* Washington, D.C.: U.S. Government Printing Office, 1955.

PERSPECTIVES ON THE PROFESSIONALIZATION OF NURSING

II

Evolution of Nursing as a Profession

2

INTRODUCTION

Public expectations at all levels of health care delivery have changed. As the health care delivery system undergoes a major transformation, nurses are beginning to play a more important role in reshaping the profession. Perhaps at no other time has the nursing profession more to gain than in the decade of the 1990s. Many opportunities exist in both the legislative and regulatory arenas.

Significant changes in the organization and financing of health care systems are beginning to have a substantial impact on the directions the nursing profession should take to solidify its future. "The shifting focus of care into the community and proliferation of alternative delivery systems, the 'graying of America,' and the movement from infectious to chronic illness as the nation's most pressing health problem, are other influences reshaping the care marketplace and providing a wealth of opportunities for nurses who adapt to and act on the changes."[1] To accommodate these societal changes, restructuring of curricula in nursing education programs is occurring to guarantee that quality preparation of nursing leaders will enable nursing to meet the public demands for high standards of health care for the future.

As the health care system evolves, nursing education and nursing practice are experiencing increased pressure to implement change. With the movement of patient care from tertiary settings to the home and community, nursing is in an excellent position to provide service to the growing number of aged underserved and uninsured in this country, those people unable to afford the present illness-directed health delivery system. Evolution of new models of nursing care to accommodate the shift from institution to the community are a high priority on nursing's present agenda.

Health care spending reached $600 billion and consumed 11.5 percent of the G.N.P. in 1989, according to a Commerce Department Report that predicted a "total tab of $661 billion in 1990.[2] ". . . We as a nation spent 40% more per capita than any other developed nation, and yet, we have 37 million individuals in the nation who lack access to health care."[3] Through the efforts of nursing's professional organizations, problems of the aged, indigent, AIDS or HIV virus epidemic, drug and alcohol abuse, and the prevalence of chronic illness, are uppermost in the minds of nursing leaders who recognize nursing's responsibility to assume a position of power in developing health care reform measures.

THE PROCESS OF PROFESSIONALIZATION

The process of professionalization has generally been described as a series of stages, characterized by changes in the structure of the occupation as it strives to achieve professional status. The sociologist H. L. Wilensky, in questioning whether a comparison of the relatively few occupations that are recognized as professions would reveal anything about this process of professionalization, observed that there is a progression of events or steps that the established professions have completed in their move toward professionalism.[4]

> There is a typical process by which the established professions have arrived: men begin doing the work full time and stake out a jurisdiction; the early masters of the technique or adherents of the movement become concerned about standards of training and practice and set up a training school, which, if not lodged in universities at the start, makes academic connections within two or three decades; the teachers and activists then achieve success in promoting more effective organization, first local, then national. . . . Toward the end, legal protection appears; at the end, a formal code of ethics is adopted.[5]

Natural History of Professionalization

The "natural history" of professionalization is observed in the chronological arrangement of events occurring throughout these various stages. Table 2-1 presents a comparison of the natural history of profes-

Table 2-1. The process of professionalization

Profession	Became full-time occupation	First training school	First university school	First national professional association	First state license law	Formal code of ethics
Law	17th century	1784	1817	1878	1732	1908
Medicine	1700	1765	1779	1847	Before 1780	1912
School teaching	17th century	1823	1879	1857	1781	1929
Librarianship	1732	1887	1897	1876	Before 1919	1938
Nursing	17th century	1861	1909	1897	1903	1950
Social work	1898	1898	1904	1874	1940	1948

Modified from Wilensky, H. L. "The Professionalization of Everyone?" *American Journal of Sociology* 70:2 (September, 1964), p. 143. Reprinted by permission of the University of Chicago Press. Copyright © 1964. University of Chicago Press.

sionalization of selected professions and occupations in the process of becoming professionalized. It reveals the sequence of events that has characterized the development of professions in this country.

In examining Table 2-1, it is readily observed that medicine, nursing, librarianship, law, school teaching, and social work show great differences in the dates in which their first training and university schools were established and when their first national professional associations were organized. Social work, school teaching, nursing, and librarianship, contrary to the older professions of medicine and law, organized their first national professional associations before establishing university schools.

Wilensky elaborates further on this point by stating that a "clue to the obstacles to any marked growth of professionalism is in the difference between the process by which the established professions have achieved their position and the process pursued by occupations aspiring to professional status."[6] He adds that "in the recent history of professionalism, the organization push comes before a solid technical and institutional base is formed; the professional association, for instance, typically precedes university-based training schools, and the whole effort seems more an opportunistic struggle for the rewards of monopoly than a natural history of professionalism."[7] It is worthy of note that in occupations where professionalization has gone farthest, a training school is typically not established.[8]

Continuum of Professionalism

In evaluating occupations involved in the process of professionalization, it is helpful to consider them as identifiable along a continuum of professionalism, ranging from those possessing none of the attributes of profession at one end to those having all of the characteristics previously presented, the full-fledged professions, at the other end. An occupation judged to be a semi-profession would be located somewhere along the middle of the continuum of professionalism because its professional characteristics are not fully developed. For example, a theoretical knowledge base or code of ethics may be lacking or somewhat unclear, its professional association may lack strength in numbers, and the power base may be so limited as to prevent sufficient control over its members through the supervision of work.

Using the concept of a continuum, it is possible to determine how professionalized an occupational group has become in various identifiable behaviors. In adopting this approach, the dichotomy between professional and nonprofessional is avoided in favor of less rigid variations. In relation to the characteristics by which a profession can be judged, there may be variations at different times. Certain characteristics may develop more rapidly than others. Occupations may rank higher in one characteristic and lower in another as they continue to implement the process of professionalization.

Nursing's Position on the Occupation-Profession Continuum

Nursing in the United States has pursued the goal of professionalism over the past century. During this time period, sociologists continued to classify nursing as a semi-profession, a marginal profession, or an emerging profession.[9-13] Although it has not met with much success in being recognized as a *full* profession, it has made remarkable progress within the past 10 to 15 years. For example, tremendous improvements have occurred in schools of nursing, in scholarly research productivity, in state nursing boards, and in the educational preparation of nursing service administrators. A growing self-confidence based on an appreciation of self-worth has become evident among nurses in more recent years. Moreover, great strides have been made in national and state accreditation of nursing education programs. When they begin seeking employment, nursing graduates are better prepared to use negotiating skills learned through assertiveness training.

Despite this progress, society has yet to recognize nursing's technical competence. It still needs to be persuaded that nursing has met the characteristics of a full profession and is capable of assuming the responsibilities and obligations of professionals. As nursing continues to refine and improve its professional characteristics in implementing the process of professionalization, a look at nursing's position on the occupation-profession continuum will assist nurses in setting priorities for the achievement of this goal. Answers to the question, "How far has nursing progressed in acquiring and improving its professional characteristics?" can be found using a continuum model.

R. M. Pavalko, a sociologist interested in the study of professions, constructed an occupation-profession model consisting of eight dimensions, with occupations at one end of the continuum and professions at the other.[14] By inserting an additional column for nursing it is possible to determine the extent to which nursing has advanced toward the professional pole in each of these dimensions (see Table 2-2).

The data in Table 2-2 show that when nursing is compared with professions in general, it has scored very well on relevance to social values, a service motivation, and a code of ethics. However, nursing's theory is still in the process of being developed and refined; its education is still not

Table 2-2. Position of nursing on the occupation-profession model

Dimension	Occupation	Nursing	Profession
1. Theory	Absent	Present (limited)	Present
2. Relevance to social values	Not relevant	Relevant	Relevant
3. Training period	Short, not specialized	Varied in length; some specialization	Long and specialized
4. Motivation	Self-interest	Service	Service
5. Autonomy	Absent	Incomplete	Complete
6. Commitment	Short-term	Varies; relatively short	Long-term
7. Sense of community	Low	Minimal	High
8. Code of ethics	Undeveloped	Highly developed	Highly developed

Adapted from Pavalko, R. M. *Sociology of Occupations and Professions*. F. E. Peacock Publishers, Inc., Itasca, Ill., 1971, Diagram 2, p. 26. Reprinted by permission of the publisher.

standardized with university preparation as a minimum requirement; control over its practice is limited; many of its members are not wholly committed to their work; and a sense of community and cohesion has yet to be fully realized. Because some of nursing's professional characteristics are not as highly developed as in the learned professions, it continues to rank just slightly above the midpoint on the Pavalko continuum. In addition to having made progress on some of these dimensions, nursing has accomplished legislation protecting practitioners and clients by means of nurse practice acts. Nurses have also organized a professional association.

Although nursing has made substantial progress to date in achieving professionalism, two characteristics for which nursing exhibits relatively limited evidence are (1) a theoretical knowledge base and (2) control over its education and practice. Mary Conway, former Dean of the School of Nursing at the Medical College of Georgia, Augusta, observed that nursing's "most demanding task—is that of expediting the development of its knowledge base."[15] According to Margretta Styles, prominent nurse leader, former dean, and educator, "nursing has scored moderately well" in achieving professional characteristics, with the exception of "the standards relating to a scientific knowledge base and to self-control," adding that "controversy still simmers and erupts over these two issues."[16] The beliefs expressed by these two leaders reflect those of many highly skilled professional practitioners and nurse educators throughout the country who recognize nursing's lack of autonomy and a somewhat meager scientific knowledge base for practice.

Collective Action Required

If the professionalization of nursing is ever to occur, recognizing that professions are continually engaged in this process, it will have to happen through the *collective* action of many individual nurses. Individuals on their own can do little to influence or strengthen a profession, yet collectively each individual's contribution is felt. Lewis, former editor of *Nursing Outlook*, in referring to the need for collectivity, expressed a genuine concern:

> [W]hat troubles me today is the magnitude and impact of our problems, on the one hand, and the relatively small number of nurses taking part in the deliberations and decisions, on the other. Such issues as entry into practice, collective bargaining, and the credentialing recommendations must be resolved by the professional organization, yet the percentage of nurses in this country who are members of it is very small indeed.[17]

Although the American Nurses Association (ANA), established in 1897, has continued to represent the goals, needs, and concerns of nurses nationwide, its strength is lessened by the low rate of membership and the internal conflicts generated by many diversified subgroups and specialty groups. A survey of ANA membership in 1988 revealed that of approximately 2,033,032 registered nurses in the United States, 627,035 were employed and only 195,500 nurse members belonged to the association through the federation of constituent state nurses' associations.[18] (A federation model was adopted at the ANA Convention of the House of Delegates in 1982.)

A comparison of the figures just reported clearly identifies nursing's shortcomings in striving for a cohesive professional association. A decline in ANA membership has been occurring for the past several years; in fact, many nurses felt their needs were not being met by the ANA. The proliferation of national special interest groups, currently numbering over 50 and drawing their members from among nurses, accounts for part of that decline. Although it is encouraging to realize that the knowledge base of nursing is growing, as evidenced by these numerous subassociations, little cohesion will occur unless special efforts are exerted to unite these diversified groups. Unfortunately, many nurses who choose not to join the ANA are profiting by the productive activity undertaken by the association to improve the education, economic status, and work environments of practicing nurses throughout the country. By not joining the ANA, paying dues, or contributing time and talents to increase the association's power and influence, these nurses profit from the benefits obtained without contributing to the organization. In industrial unions the opposite can occur, because organizational membership in some states is mandatory, and all workers are obliged to support the unions that bargain for improved salaries and other fringe benefits.

In an effort to provide a means of reaching agreement on "issues of common concern to the nursing profession and to promote concerted action on these issues," the ANA sponsored the first meeting of the Nursing Organization Liaison Forum (NOLF) for this purpose.[19] It was suggested that this forum "could provide an arena for the development of consensus around such issues as federal funding for nursing education and research; access of patient population to quality health care services, including nursing services; and the role of the government in meeting basic human needs [and] protecting the environment and public health."[20] Such forum activity is designed to allay the fears of some nurse members who believe there is the possibility that nursing in this country may have as spokespersons the million voices of individual nurses, or the "fragmented voices" of various specialty groups, rather than that of "a single, forceful voice."[21]

COMMISSION ON ORGANIZATIONAL ASSESSMENT (COAR)

The ANA Board of Directors established the Commission on Organizational Assessment (COAR) in December 1987 to conduct a national study of its professional association in order to strengthen it. This two year study involved input from state nurses associations and other nursing groups that responded to a national nursing survey addressing issues and interrelated problems confronting the association. Margretta Styles, Chairperson of the twenty-three member Commission, stated that "in a brief period of time and with limited resources, COAR has assessed and surveyed the profession, both internal and external to ANA through a process of greater breadth and magnitude, than ever used before . . . COAR sounds the drum beat for progress."[22]

In June 1989 the ANA House of Delegates adopted a new set of by-laws that would restructure the professional association. ANA by-laws implemented COAR recommendations on the structure, function, and inter-organizational relationships of the professional association.[23] The amendment that stirred the greatest debate concerned membership for "second level practitioners of the future." The new by-laws stipulated that members of state nurses associations be registered nurses. Due to a 1987 by-laws amendment granting membership to registered nurses and associate nurses at a future time, a proviso was adopted. If state nurses associations at a future period were to enact legislation for a professional/associate nurse licensing system to include second-level practitioners as members, the ANA House of Delegates would determine the responsibilities, rights, and privileges of this group.[24]

TWO NEW ANA CONGRESSES FORMED

At the ANA House of Delegates meeting in June 1990, a Congress of Nursing Practice and a Congress on Nursing Economics were formed. The focus of each Congress was on "long range policy development, standard setting, program development and evaluation in their area of expertise."[25] Another notable by-laws change suggested ways to involve specialty organizations in the ANA House of Delegates and the Congress of Nursing Practice. Organizational affiliates (other national nursing organizations) and ANA Councils have the opportunity to participate in the House of Delegates without voting. In summarizing the vision embodied in the COAR Report, Styles concluded by stating

> As I see it, we must choose to lift off, to free ourselves from the gravity of immutable positions and the decay of structured senescence, free ourselves to create a new world for the association and for nursing. . . . As I see it, we cannot turn back.[26]

Aydelotte reminded the nursing community that "an association may be powerful, but its power stems from the power and influence of its leadership, the individual members, and the collective [and] the power image the profession conveys to the public is a reflection of the self-concept held by these two groups."[27] Or as Beletz points out, "In the continuum of professionalization, qualitatively nursing and many individual nurses excel far beyond contemporary recognized professions in many areas . . . quantitatively, the road ahead is very long."[28]

THE CHALLENGE OF PROFESSIONALIZATION OF NURSING

From the previous discussions on characteristics of a profession and nursing's position on the occupation-profession continuum, it is readily apparent that nursing as an occupation has several areas of weakness that should be remedied before full professional status is achieved. For many nurses, these problem areas are recognized as a challenge that they have accepted as a stimulus to advance the process of professionalization.

Nursing's Specialized Knowledge Base

Because professional knowledge is held by only a few—the professionals—it conveys an aura of mystery distinguishing it from more common knowledge. The neophyte professional is initiated into certain "mysteries," that is, contact with essentials usually thought of as sacred to the values of society (access to confidential information or information of all intimate nature). It is interesting to note that the three oldest professions—medicine, law, and the ministry—have strongly embraced these essentials. Thus, clients observe in the tasks performed by professionals an air of mystery the ordinary man or woman does not possess.[29] In other words, the theoretical aspects of professional knowledge, knowledge gained through practice and long periods of training, are what create the air of mystery surrounding the established professions. An occupation aspiring to full professionalism has to be able to control a more substantial body of knowledge than that controlled by other occupations.[30] Without a solid knowledge base recognized by the relevant public, occupations cannot justify their claim to autonomy.[31]

It is evident that many occupations aspiring to professionalism function in organizations that present a threat to the ideals of autonomy and service.[32] Examples are occupations or "quasi-professions," such as pharmacy, hospital administration, and nursing, whose work environment places them in the "stultifying shadow of medicine."[33] Medicine, by legal and informal means, offers resistance to anyone encroaching on its authority.[34] Stated another way, "the caste-like system" places a wall that is impossible to scale between the physician and semiprofessionals in the hospital.[35]

Most nurses would agree that society lacks understanding of nursing's significant contributions to health care and its specific body of knowledge. The public's image of the nurse is still that of the physician's handmaiden. Nurses' work is primarily viewed as ancillary to medicine.[36] Nursing is striving diligently to remake this image for the public. Although nursing alone should be the judge of measuring the validity of its knowledge base, such validation must be accepted by other professional groups and by the public. The professionalization process is greatly influenced by whether or not society supports and values the services provided by nurses and accepts their claim of special knowledge and expertise in health care.

Autonomy in Nursing

Some nurses are convinced that the problem of male dominance, as observed in the controlling attitudes of physicians, hospital administrators, and boards of trustees toward nursing, prevents it from exercising professional autonomy. This issue is very important. Semi-professions enjoy less freedom from being supervised than do the more prestigious professions.[37] In other words, they lack autonomy. They are frequently told exactly what to do and how it is to be done. Nurses' lack of autonomy is attributed in part to the fact that most nurses work in hospitals or in other types of organizations in which precise definitions of the client are not made. Thus, the bureaucracy weakens the nurses' autonomy and colleague authority.[38,39]

The advantages of achieving full professional status are numerous. Since professional work consists of necessary services that cannot be performed or controlled by other groups, professionals enjoy great power and autonomy. Other advantages are control of entry into the profession, determination of the qualifications needed by those seeking entry and organization of their training, and thus deciding who will be one's colleagues.[40] In addition, "one gets to control the piece of one's services by the control of competition and influence on state and federal lawmakers, through professional associations and other pressure groups, [and by control of] the behavior of the members of the occupation and hence is able to enforce standards and maintain whatever values the occupation thinks are desirable."[41]

These advantages and their accompanying autonomy are granted to the profession by society only if its members can exert self-control over their education and practice. Many registered nurses are convinced that they are professionals because of their license to practice. But license alone has little relationship to what is required of professionals. In fact, effective professional autonomy ensured by licensing boards will be granted by society only when the profession demonstrates that it alone has mastery of its craft, and that no other professions have the right to review its decisions.[42]

Monopoly Over Services

Professionalization, therefore, can be viewed as an attempt to exchange special knowledge for social and economic rewards. By keeping essential services in scant supply, professions acquire a monopoly over the services that society needs. If an occupation validates its right to be called a profession, it achieves a monopoly in the interests of the public. A monopoly over a valued service supports the standing of an occupation as prestigious.[43]

Nursing is currently in the process of redefining its function in order to claim a monopoly over its services. Occupations desiring to use professional authority must locate a technical basis for it, state their exclusive jurisdiction, connect skill and jurisdiction to standards of training, and persuade the public of its uniquely trustworthy services.[44] To date nursing has not succeeded in establishing a monopoly over its special knowledge as acquired through an intense period of training. Unlike medicine, it lacks power and is unable to control the supply of nurses. However, controlling nursing's body of knowledge alone will not provide a monopoly. It is only by controlling its unique services, which society wants and deems necessary, that nursing can acquire a monopoly. According to W. J. Goode, "occupations as varied as pharmacy and nursing . . . have set up formal curricula and have succeeded . . . in attaching themselves to colleges and universities, but they have not thereby moved far toward professionalization."[45] In other words, recognition of an occupation's knowledge base and unique services by the general public will not occur unless related occupations also recognize them and are willing to validate their worth to society.

Level of Commitment to Nursing

One reason for nursing's slow progress in professionalization is attributed to the fact that many nurses do not make a lifetime commitment to their work, viewing it as a temporary job rather than a full-time career. It should be pointed out that this attitude is also true of many women in other fields and may be attributed to the other roles that many women fulfill, such as housewife and mother. The doctor assumes responsibility twenty-four hours a day, seven days a week, having made a lifetime commitment. When compared with members of other established professions representing lifetime careers—lawyers, engineers, university professors— nurses tend to leave their occupation at a much higher rate. The fact that a lifetime commitment is stronger in medicine and other related professions is due in part to the higher rewards and long period of professional socialization, which makes members less likely to leave their respective professions. Where nurses' specialized knowledge base is limited, their intrinsic commitment to the work tends to be quite low. Thus, it is not surprising that the ideology of profession and strong colleague orientations observed among professionals is less developed in nursing, since specialized knowledge and lifetime commitment are not greatly in evidence.

Furthermore, semiprofessionals usually obtain rewards from their position in the organization, not from performance of work. As members lack strong intrinsic motivation, they frequently require more supervision and encouragement than professionals do. As a result, they tend to be less resistant to bureaucratic control, more accepting of orders from administrators or supervisors, and less inclined to seek autonomy in their work situation. Nevertheless, nurses desiring to increase their professional status do look for more independence, prestige, greater autonomy, and higher extrinsic rewards. As stated earlier, professional autonomy is based on both specialized knowledge and strong commitment to the service ideal.

The Service Ideal

A service orientation means that professional decisions should be based not on the professional's self-interest but on the client's needs.[46] Professions were established to address specific needs of society. Society, in turn, confers prerogatives of self-regulation on a profession as long as its services are competent and rated highly by the public. Unless society believes a given profession is regulated by a collective organization, it will not grant autonomy or freedom from external control. In other words, the service ideal becomes the pivot on which any moral justification for having professional status revolves.[47]

Limiting the Number of Professionals

One of several suggestions offered by the economist Eli Ginzberg over thirty years ago to nurses concerned about the professional status of their occupation was for nursing to begin "developing a more delimited group of graduates of good college and university programs" that could be properly called professional nurses.[48] To be sure that nurses would understand his meaning of profession, he defined it as a group that (1) possesses extensive training; (2) provides "intellectual leadership" recognized in its field; (3) conducts research of worth; and (4) has independence in defining its specific area of work.[49] Ginzberg stated that nursing should recruit and educate only the number of professional nurses that nursing believes are needed. He was convinced that there were too many RNs for the economy to support at the salary level of a professional. By limiting the group to a maximum of 70,000 the occupation could hope to receive professional pay.[50]

To date, Ginzberg's suggestion of developing an "elite corps" of professional nurses has not been well received. Nurses shy away from such a possibility, although it has been suggested by numerous nursing groups. However, unless nursing can achieve an economic status that will attract highly qualified people, it will be unable to upgrade substantially the level of skill required for professional nursing.

It is interesting to note that Mary Mundinger, a well-recognized leader and author, expressed a similar concern twenty years later by asking, "Are enough health care dollars available in this country to pay for professional nursing?"[51] The answer would be a definite "no" if the current practice continues of considering as professionals all RNs licensed to practice nursing. If nursing concentrated on developing a group of *professional* nurses, according to Ginzberg, it could still encourage licensed practical nurses and associate degree and diploma graduates to move upward toward the top, if they so desired.

One way for an occupation to prove its high status is by being able to choose the very best of young people ready to enter the labor market and then to prolong their schooling before allowing entrance to the prestigious circle.[52] This idea presupposes a pool of prospective applicants with adequate social and educational background and finances. Autonomy for the profession can be realized more readily if the occupation consists of individuals coming from this type of background. Ultimately, this situation would assist nursing in progressing toward the fulfillment of its professional goals.[53] That a declining percentage of nurses is being recruited from the upper classes is apparently no longer true. New recruits are coming from families of higher socioeconomic backgrounds than in the past and they appear to be more autonomous, self-directed, and less willing to conform to authority.[54] Some members of this group represent older students and students with academic degrees in other disciplines.

In order to restrict the labor supply of professional nurses, the occupation of nursing needs *power.* Nursing's power base continues to stay at a very low level. Because of the disunity that exists over professional preparation of its practitioners, nursing is unable to control the number of admissions to all types of nursing programs. As a result, Ginzberg's suggestion of limiting numbers continues to be filed away in the archives of nursing's embattled past.

Most nurses would agree, that the occupation of nursing continues to improve its position and certain significant changes in its character are observable, (upgraded educational requirements, advances in research, successful efforts in legislation, and improved distribution of manpower). Increasing nursing's knowledge base implies an increase in the number of those people performing specialized intellectual work as compared with those doing manual labor or unspecialized routine activities.[55] As nursing's body of knowledge advances, an increase in the number of professional nurses having baccalaureate, master's, and doctoral degrees in nursing should occur, giving nursing the intellectual leadership and professional knowledge required in professional practice.

Nursing's Progress Toward Professionalism

An objective appraisal of nursing, as measured by the characteristics of professionalism, supports the conclusion that nursing has made great strides toward professionalism over the past decade. Two examples of nursing's progress in improving its status are (1) the collective bargaining activities of the ANA in obtaining adequate salaries and improved working conditions for its members and (2) changes in licensure, as seen in modification of nurse practice acts that provide legal sanction and greater flexibility for nurses in assuming expanded roles. Some nurses feel that state nurses' associations (SNAs) have been "saddled" with the task of collective bargaining under the new federation model of the ANA. They believe that other programs have suffered due to the funding for collective bargaining. However, many other nurses are very much in favor of supporting the SNAs' collective bargaining program.

The following points are presented to indicate why nursing is prevented from rising within the professional hierarchy. For instance, although nursing's service orientation continues at a very high level, more effort is needed to continue developing a theoretical base of knowledge, which would enable nurses to implement their functions more effectively. It becomes apparent that nursing's upward movement toward authentic professionalism is still inhibited by a lack of autonomy and a scientific knowledge base. Many nurses do not fully realize or understand the importance of overcoming a subservient role. Nor do they comprehend the need for a scientific knowledge base in order to perform their professional responsibilities. In fact, some nurses have not yet grasped the idea that clients are served best only when nurses fulfill their role in a professional manner.

Nursing's knowledge base has tended to be drawn from experience. It has been built up over a long period of time and relying on intuition in applying such knowledge. Although there has been a substantial increase in the number of college and university nursing programs granting the baccalaureate degree, the sizable number of diploma programs and the increase in community college programs continues to make a standardized form of professional nursing education virtually impossible, at least for the present. Moreover, it is difficult for nursing to prove its right to "exclusive competence" resulting from *highly specialized knowledge and skills,* which no other group can claim, when the bulk of practicing nurses has not acquired such preparation (33.9% of RNs employed in nursing hold a diploma; 53.5% have acquired an associate degree; and 12.6% have a baccalaureate in nursing degree.)[56]

The importance of a knowledge base for nursing should not only be developed but also accepted by outsiders as well as by those within the occupation. This acceptance would have to come from "physicians and hospital administrators and would probably require drastic rearrangement of social roles in the hospital."[57] Over twenty years have elapsed since this observation was made, which raises the question of how many significant changes have or are occurring in "rearrangement of social roles in the hospital." In many hospitals these changes are occurring at a fairly rapid rate. It is important for nursing's future professional status that such changes in social roles take place. Nursing cannot continue to aspire toward full professionalism while remaining under the control of either the medical profession or hospital administration.

Recognizing that no profession remains static but is constantly changing to improve its services, a look at law, the ministry, and medicine reveals how professions can and do change their status. The field of law, for example, has shown a decline in the number of cases that involve direct contact with an individual client. Cases pertaining to personal problems have been replaced by those involving property settlements and corporate business problems. In the ministry, the clergy are not playing an vital a role in directing people's lives in life and death matters as they have done in past centuries.

Medicine has acquired numerous specialty groups in recent years with some splintering from the main professional association in favor of smaller specialty associations. However, the professional status of medicine remains firm since "in the world of health, the doctor so far has been in a privileged position [but] . . . needs to move toward cooperation and shared power."[58] Medicine has more recently made greater efforts to improve its overall image with the public, particularly in the area of interpersonal relationships with clients. Redefining professional roles, breaking down professional barriers, and opening up new channels of communication should be on the agenda for most professions.[59] Whether medicine will become more accepting of nursing's independent role in health care delivery remains to be seen.

Each of these examples points to the fact that change is occurring in even the established professions. Nursing, too, can move forward and achieve all of the characteristics on the professional side of the continuum. The time is ripe for nursing to move rapidly into its own as a profession and exert influence over health care delivery in this country.

Transformation Needed
to Advance Professionalism

To accomplish the professionalization of nursing requires a transformation of nurses in their nursing role. Many nurses seek only socioeconomic advantages while ignoring the fact that professionalization implies having to assume greater responsibilities in their professional role. Transformation implies an improvement over what was. Occupations that desire an improvement in professional status are endeavoring to better themselves. Nurses are realizing the need to *act* as professionals, attend professional meetings, assist in policy formulations, and take responsibility for their professional lives. The important question is whether or not most nurses are willing to pay the cost of such transformation. They will have to decide how much of themselves, their time, energy, and resources they will be willing to invest in this undertaking of professionalism. If they decline to act, nursing will be delayed in achieving its goal of full professional status.

Much of the tension in nursing revolves around the issue of profession, which group is rightfully qualified to use the title of professional and which group is not. Pressures created by splintering groups into those that are "in" and those that are "out" must be resolved so that nursing can forge ahead in its determined effort to claim the right of being a full profession. Thus far, no immediate solutions have been available to relieve such pressures, other than the possible use of a "grandfather" clause to assist many nurses who will not be able to meet requirements for professional nursing in the future.

THE IMPACT OF SIGNIFICANT STUDIES ON NURSING'S PROFESSIONALISM

The history of nursing in this country provides evidence of numerous and repeated efforts to achieve professionalism. A review of nursing studies over a sixty-five year period attests to nursing's concern to upgrade the occupation. The legacy of Florence Nightingale, which nurses are rediscovering as a rich cultural heritage, conveys the importance of nursing as a profession comparable to other professions. Miss Nightingale believed that schools of nursing should have their own identity as educational institutions and be financed independently.[60] At the turn of the century, professionalism was receiving high priority among various occupational groups.

In the second decade of the twentieth century, Abraham Flexner discovered a deplorable lack of standards and facilities in medical education in the United States. Lack of standards was particularly noticeable in relation to admission and curriculum requirements. As a result of the Flexner Report published in 1910 by the Carnegie Foundation for the Advancement of Teaching, sixty-five medical schools were closed by 1915.[61, 62] Consequently, the number of graduating physicians declined markedly. Through the combined efforts of the American Medical Association and the American Public Health Association, a veritable revolution in medical education took place. Within a ten-year period the majority of the reforms outlined in this report, including educational requirements and licensure of physicians, were completed due to the strong leadership of the medical association and the cooperation of medical educators and practitioners who welcomed the need for change.

Flexner's reforms for the medical profession reflected his philosophy of the importance of university-based education for medical practitioners. By raising the standards of medical schools as well as limiting their numbers and thereby reducing the number of graduating physicians, it was possible to obtain a monopoly over medical services. Physicians would always be in demand and thus could charge higher fees for their services. By means of a "restrictionist" policy, women and other minorities were severely limited in obtaining a medical education. As a result of all of these reforms, the prestige, status, income, and power of the medical profession were enhanced far beyond what the reformers had ever anticipated. In the decade from 1910 to 1920, expenditure of power and money was required to raise educational standards in medicine, but such an investment increased the physician's prestige, the profession's power in legislation, and the average doctor's income.[63]

Undoubtedly, the Flexner Report served to put medical training out in front of other traditional forms of professional education, if by no other means than making it unequivocally postbaccalaureate.[64] Flexner's famous report, which produced epochal changes in medical education, was the first instance of a survey of higher education that was national in scope. Although it had no direct bearing on nursing at the time, it continues to challenge nursing, demonstrates the impact of strong leadership and shows how acceptance of its recommendations quickly standardized university preparation as the educational requirement for medical practitioners.

Efforts to upgrade nursing education were facilitated by the Rockefeller Foundation in 1919. By organizing a Committee for the Study of Nursing Education, it was the intent of the Foundation to have a comprehensive study of this field conducted. This committee, recognizing the inadequacies of the majority of nursing schools that were controlled and financed by hospitals, published the Goldmark Report in 1923. The report recommended that more schools of nursing offering five-year programs be established as independent units in universities and that all nursing schools should be supported independently of hospitals.[65] In addition, it listed standards of university education with strong recommendations for the inclusion of the fundamental sciences, liberal arts, and professional training. For nursing practice to improve, the committee was convinced that the system of nursing education would have to be drastically altered.

Unlike the Flexner Report, the Goldmark Report provided little impetus for change until the 1950s, when associate degree nursing programs began and diploma programs started to decline. To date, almost seventy years have elapsed and its main recommendation for sound educational policy and standardization of nursing education has still not been heeded. Why the contrast between these two reports, with the first (1910) literally changing the face of medicine in the United States and worldwide, and the latter (1923) having no impact for so many years on influencing the direction of nursing? Apparently, the 1,760 hospital schools of nursing in existence were unable or unwilling to take specific action on these recommendations, thus preventing nursing from acquiring full professional status at that period. Examining this issue from another viewpoint reveals that in this period nurses and nursing were dominated by hospital administrators and physicians. Nursing units were staffed primarily by student nurses, and the expectation that hospital-based diploma programs must continue was great.

The Goldmark Report, however, stimulated other studies. The Committee on the Grading of Nursing Schools, directed by May Ayres Burgess, published several significant reports between 1927 and 1934 on the status of nursing schools and nursing service. For example, the Burgess

Report, published in 1928, focused on the economics of hospital-based nursing schools, the supply and demand for graduate nurses, working conditions, salaries, and the geographic distribution of nurses throughout the country.[66]

In 1934, the Committee published the results of a study by Blanche Pfefferkorn and Ethel Johns, entitled *An Activity Analysis of Nursing*, describing the activities engaged in by nurses in various health care institutions.[67] This report helped nurse educators correlate theory and practice in a more realistic manner. However, in that period theory was concerned only with disease, pathology, and illness care. Development of nursing theory as it is currently known was not even conceived of by most nurse educators or nursing administrators in the 1920s.

Recognizing the increasing responsibilities that were required of nursing and the lack of a collegiate level of education in the hospital-based nursing schools, the Committee in its final report, *Nursing Schools: Today and Tomorrow*, recommended that nursing education be placed on a true professional level.[68] In 1943, Isabel Stewart, an astute nurse leader, expressed her concern that nurses had not yet accepted the idea of professional education:

> The question of whether at least two grades of nurses should be recognized and prepared has been debated pro and con for a long time. Nurses have been much divided on this issue and have been inclined to side-step it, but cannot delay much longer in reaching a decision.[69]

With the continued growing concern over the poor quality of nursing education programs, another study conducted by social anthropologist Esther Lucille Brown, entitled *Nursing for the Future*, was funded and published by the Russell Sage Foundation in 1948.[70] Focusing on nursing service and nursing education, Brown stressed the importance of collegiate preparation for nursing. "Almost without a dissenting voice those who are conversant with the trend of professional education in the United States agree that preparation of the professional nurse belongs squarely within the institution of higher learning."[71] Brown continued,

> [W]ithin a democratic society there is no person, group of persons, or organized voluntary body that has power to order sudden and drastic change. Such changes as are effected will result from long and careful planning at the conference table of national, state, and local nursing associations and other bodies.[72]

Brown, if alive today, might well consider over forty-five years of "long and careful planning" since the publication of her report more than sufficient time to opt for needed change.

Around the middle of the century, several other nursing reports were published: (1) in 1948, a report by the Committee on the Function of Nursing chaired by Eli Ginzberg entitled *A Program for the Nursing Profession;* (2) a study by Mildred Montag in 1951 describing an educational program to prepare nursing technicians; and (3) Margaret Bridgman's critique of collegiate education for nurses in 1953.[73-75] Each of these studies echoed similar calls for drastic changes in the prevailing system of nursing education. In 1958, Hughes and colleagues published *Twenty Thousand Nurses Tell Their Story,* in which they confirmed the existence of considerable discontent among the nation's nurses.[76] In 1963, the Surgeon General's Consultant Group on Nursing published a report emphasizing the need for a national study of nursing that would focus on the profession's needs and resources. It recommended upgrading the nursing profession by increasing the number of schools of nursing in universities and colleges, by emphasizing research, and by increasing enrollments for minority students, males, and older adults.[77]

An historic landmark for nursing was reached in 1965 when the ANA Committee on Education issued its first position paper on educational preparation for professional nursing and for those assisting them. This paper recommended that education for nursing take place in institutions of higher learning within the general system of education. It further recommended that a baccalaureate degree in nursing should be considered minimum preparation for beginning professional nursing practice and an associate degree in nursing should be the minimum preparation for beginning technical practice.[78]

In 1970, the Secretary of Health, Education, and Welfare appointed a committee to study extended roles for nurses. Recognizing that many nurses lacked the educational preparation for such roles, this report had considerable impact on nursing education and nursing practice.[79] To implement the earlier recommendation of the Surgeon General's Group on Nursing for a national study of nursing, funds were obtained from the Avalon and W. K. Kellogg Foundations in 1966 for a three-year investigation. A final report of the National Commission for the Study of Nursing and Nursing Education (NCSNNE) entitled *An Abstract for Action* was published in 1970 under the directorship of Jerome P. Lysaught.[80] It was anticipated that by analyzing and improving nursing, the delivery of health care would be improved.

Recommendations for the reshaping of nursing education, nursing roles and functions, and nursing careers, were presented in this report. Again, emphasis was placed on redirecting nursing education into the mainstream of general education. A follow-up study by the NCSNNE from 1970 to 1973 resulted in a full report in 1973, *From Abstract into Action,* detailing the outcome of activities carried out to strengthen the recommendations of the 1970 report.[81]

With funds from the W. K. Kellogg Foundation, a longitudinal study to determine progress made on twenty-one of the NCSNNE's 1970 recommendations to improve nursing was undertaken by Jerome Lysaught and his staff from 1977 to 1979. Findings and conclusions from this study were published in 1981 in *Action in Affirmation: Toward an Unambiguous Profession of Nursing.*[82] The report indicated that considerable progress had been achieved by nursing in most of the recommendations for nursing roles and nursing education: "On the 21 specific proposals, the evidence is that some have been realized in full, most have been accomplished in large part, and a small number have suffered from insufficient implementation."[83]

In 1978, the ANA House of Delegates passed resolutions on "entry into practice" supporting two levels of nursing practice by 1985—the professional nurse requiring a baccalaureate education and an unnamed category requiring associate degree education. Additional resolutions emphasized that competencies for both levels were to be developed by 1980 and opportunities for career mobility to facilitate movement from the "yet-to-be-named" level to the professional level be increased.[84] Competencies for both levels have been identified and reviewed by nurse educators and practitioners since 1980.

The Study of Credentialing in Nursing: A New Approach, published in 1979 and sponsored by the ANA, included a history of the credentialing movement, an account of the adequacy of credentialing mechanisms in nursing for accreditation, certification, and licensure, and the need for a National Credentialing Center. The Committee for the Study of Credentialing in Nursing, composed of ten nurses and five other individuals and chaired by Margretta Styles, former Dean of the School of Nursing at the University of California, San Francisco, made several recommendations, which were forwarded to the national nursing organizations for their review and approval. Due to a lack of consensus on the part of these various organizations, no further action on the committee's recommendations had occurred.[85]

BARRIERS TO THE EMERGENCE
OF FULL PROFESSIONAL STATUS

Evidence presented in the numerous and frequent studies conducted over many decades reflects the persistence of barriers to nursing's professionalism. However, barriers to professionalization should not be considered insurmountable but rather as challenges to be overcome. The primary obstacles preventing nursing from achieving full professional status are outlined below.

The first major barrier to nursing's drive toward professionalism is that of *disunity* and *divisiveness* within nursing. R. Bowman and R. Culpepper, for example, have deplored the divisiveness in nursing and have called for unity among its members.[86] Nursing continues to experience dissension within its own ranks, which has tended to compromise its distinction as a profession. And yet without consensus within nursing about its competencies and purpose there can be no identity.[87]

Styles, observing that divisiveness and disunity are a significant problem, cites a few examples of this disunity:

- Conflicting positions and solitary actions regarding basic education and licensing issues
- Competition over accreditation rights
- Division and the resulting flattening of the power base, under the guise of decentralization, in nursing service organizations
- Controversies over collective bargaining as a means of self-determination and access to the economic rewards system
- Dissension about dimensions and standards of practice
- The artificial bifurcation of nursing service and nursing education[88]

Styles concludes that the volume of numbers and services is nursing's greatest power to shape its destiny in society at large. She asserts that this concealed energy can be realized as power only through nursing's capability to engage in unified action.[89]

A second barrier to professionalism is the lack of prepared leaders for the profession. Undoubtedly, there is a severe shortage of nursing scholars and professionals, but the failure is also due in part to the number of nursing scholars and professionals who have not assumed responsibility for leadership within nursing.[90]

Several other barriers to the full professionalization of nursing were discussed earlier in this chapter: a lack of an identifiable scientific knowledge base; the need for a standardized educational system; a lack of autonomy and control over nursing practice; no monopoly over nursing services; and a lack of strength in overcoming the preexisting power structure controlling nursing activities.

TRADITIONALIZERS, PROFESSIONALIZERS, AND UTILIZERS

Over thirty-five years have elapsed since Habenstein and Christ formulated three descriptors to point up differences in motivation among nurses carrying out their various nursing responsibilities: traditionalizers, professionalizers, and utilizers.[91] It is interesting to note how relevant these same terms are in describing the current situation in nursing. As an example of the divisiveness and disunity that exist within the occupation of nursing, frequent reference is made to the "factions" or separate "camps" that continue to create confusion and division among nurses. The "traditionalizers" are those who see nursing as low-status, self-sacrificing, personal service of clients based on past generations of experience, rather than on complex knowledge and skills. Traditionalizers have been described as individuals for whom "expediting the physician's orders is viewed as a primary responsibility and a part of their *raison d' etre*," while the *professionalizers* are concerned with "*achieving occupational advancement.*"[92]

Unfortunately, the number of nurses desiring professionalization who are occupied in implementing significant advances within nursing is very small. These professionalizers represent those who are advancing their professional status by means of the political process and "who are dedicated to inquiry and scholarship; to designing and offering new approaches to preparing nurse practitioners, administrators, educators, and investigators and to planning and evaluating innovative means for delivering high quality nursing care."[93]

Many physicians and health care administrators voice opposition to those nurses who supposedly speak for all nurses in this country. "There are some nurses who seem to be equally committed to enlisting all the help they can muster in order to guarantee that nursing will forever be essentially a vocation or technology whose practitioners are other-directed, minimally educated, and subservient, and ill-prepared to fulfill nursing's unique professional role in society."[94] In addition, they lack awareness of societal forces that will, of necessity, produce changes having an impact on how they will function in the foreseeable future.[95] Furthermore, they remain uncommitted to furthering professional goals and are unwilling to accept the fact that nonprofessional nursing practice is slowly disappearing. The problem results from the slow pace in which this type of nursing *is* disappearing.

Many nurses do not envision themselves as practicing in an autonomous, professional manner. However, "how can a few nurses develop and identify one kind of practice if the majority continues to practice in another way [and] how can clients tell the difference and choose between them?"[96] These pertinent questions are posing serious concerns for nursing in its efforts to upgrade the nursing practice. The issue of providing a grandfather clause enabling many nurses who lack a baccalaureate degree to practice as professionals will continue to delay progress in upgrading clinical practice.

During the past twenty years, a growing tension has existed between those nurses practicing technical nursing and those providing a high level of professional nursing. It has been alluded to that a "cleavage" exists between small numbers of professional nurses and the vast group of registered nurses who provide the greatest amount of skilled technical service to clients.[97] I am of the opinion that conflict between these two groups results from different perceptions about the ideology of professionalism. Many nurses in the latter group believe that nursing has always been a profession, and so they manifest little interest in its professional advancement. However, "the most important and powerful idea in the belief system of nursing is the idea of professionalism [and] ideology is strongest when all segments of the occupation share in the goals and aspirations expressed by the leadership—hence the strength of the early campaigns for organization, licensure, and education."[98] Why this contradiction between what many nurses believe is professionalism and what is actually true professionalism?

Performance of clinical tasks as assistants to the physician provides intrinsic rewards that substitute for the value of the true professional. Concern over salary and other working conditions providing extrinsic rewards leaves little energy for involvement in professional organizations to assist the body of nursing in improving its self-identity. There are some who feel that most nurses remain at the "security" level of Maslow's hierarchy of needs because they exert so much energy over these issues and are thereby hindered from moving toward higher needs. Some nurses question whether nursing care provided by the majority of practicing nurses is valued enough by them to be worth improvement and further development. And yet "nurses in the 1990s must become a far more sophisticated group [since] improvement in nursing and health care will require many intelligent, highly educated, and skilled practitioners of nursing."[99] In fact, "the complexity of health care problems cannot be resolved without the acquisition of a broader base of knowledge and the use of research to address specific problems."[100]

Finally, the so-called "utilizers" in nursing are unrepresentative of either of the two categories previously described. Lacking motivation in their work, they are uninvolved in activities to improve nursing's status. They view nursing solely as a job. They often use their nursing position to further their own personal gains. These nurses expect to be evaluated on their work by the limits of individual tasks or procedures and not on how their performance affects the larger scene. Nursing, in considering its future, should endeavor to increase the number of its professionalizers to ensure that the goal of professionalism will be achieved. Traditionalizers can change their attitudes without negating the richness of nursing's past. Change will occur because the challenge involved in improving nursing and health care for society cannot continue to be ignored. Perhaps nursing will always have utilizers, but if even a few of them begin to change their attitude toward nursing it can only strengthen nursing's position.

SUMMARY

In this chapter, perspectives on the status of nursing's professionalism were presented. In attempting to describe the current progress achieved by nursing in its drive toward full professional status, it was important to consider nursing's early efforts to improve its position among the various occupational groups. The steps involved in the professionalization process were discussed to emphasize nursing's need to evaluate its present position as it moves forward in this process. Because two specific weaknesses in nursing were noted—the lack of an agreed upon scientific knowledge base and lack of autonomy in determining the future of nursing education and practice—these areas provide the central theme for the remaining chapters of this book. By way of comparison, it was interesting to observe the dates when several occupations became full-time, established their first training school, university school, national professional association, state licensing laws, and code of ethics. Although nursing has yet to achieve *full* professional status, it has made great strides over the past ten or fifteen years. Several noticeable improvements have occurred in schools of nursing, in state board examinations, in national and state accreditation of nursing education programs, in efforts to improve nursing's image, and in the self-confidence exhibited by nurses in fulfilling their nursing functions.

A review of nursing's position in the Pavalko occupation-profession model revealed that nursing services are relevant to social values and motivated by a strong service ideal, and that nursing has a professional association and a code of ethics. However, in my opinion, as indicated in this model, nursing's theory is not sufficiently advanced. Its education is not standardized with university preparation as a minimum requirement. Its autonomy and power are limited, and a united membership has yet to be realized. It was pointed out further that the importance of nursing's knowledge and contributions to health care will have to be recognized and esteemed to a greater extent by the public if autonomy and control over nursing practice are to be achieved.

Emphasis was placed on the importance of nurses being transformed in their nursing roles, with commitment and accountability being stressed. In addition, the impact of several significant national studies on nursing were reviewed. Recurring themes on the necessity of improving the professional status of nursing and its educational and practice systems were frequently stressed in these studies. The question was raised as to why the Flexner Report of 1910 was so effective in revolutionizing the medical profession, as compared with the Goldmark Report of 1923, whose recommendations only recently have begun to be heeded. The fact that nursing is composed primarily of women, who have been and continue to be dominated by physicians and hospital administrators in many health care institutions, is an important factor that should not be overlooked.

The chapter concluded with a reminder that nursing in the 1990s will require a high degree of intellectual knowledge and skills to meet the growing demand for an improved health care system. There are external factors working against this goal, which delays nursing in its efforts to achieve *full* professional status. However, as nursing further develops its knowledge base and gains autonomy over its education and practice, these external factors may be greatly diminished. With strong determination on the part of thousands of nurses throughout the country, the goal of professionalism can be reached but not before vast improvements are made in these two specific areas.

REFERENCES

1. Maraldo, P. "The League's 1986 Legislative Agenda," NLN, *Executive Director Wire* (January–February 1986), 1–2.
2. "Health Costs Still Escalating: Findings & Forecasts," *American Journal of Nursing* 90:4 (April, 1990), 132.
3. Maraldo, P. NLN *Executive Director Wire* (Winter, 1989), 5.
4. Wilensky, H. "The Dynamics of Professionalism: The Case of Hospital Administration," *Hospital Administration* 7 (Spring, 1962), 15.
5. Wilensky, H. "The Professionalization of Everyone?" *American Journal of Sociology* 70:2 (September, 1964), 143–144.
6. *Ibid.*, 157.
7. *Ibid.*
8. *Ibid.*, 144.
9. *Ibid.*
10. *Ibid.*, 137–157.
11. Greenwood, E. "Attributes of a Profession," *Social Work* 2:3 (July, 1957), 44–55.
12. Etzioni, A. (ed.), *The Semi-Professions and Their Organization: Teachers, Nurses, Social Workers.* New York: The Free Press, 1969, 328.
13. Pavalko, R. *Sociology of Occupations and Professions.* Itasca, Ill.: F. E. Peacock Publishers, 1971, 234.
14. *Ibid.*, 17–25.
15. Conway, M. "Prescription for Professionalization," in N. Chaska (ed.), *The Nursing Profession: A Time to Speak.* New York, McGraw-Hill Co., 1983, 30.
16. Styles, M. *On Nursing: Toward a New Endowment.* St. Louis: C. V. Mosby, 1982, 54.
17. Lewis, E. "The Professionally Uncommitted," (editorial), *Nursing Outlook* 27:5 (May, 1979), 323.
18. Phone conversation with ANA Research Dept., Kansas City, Mo., on February 1, 1990.
19. American Nurses' Association. "Forty-nine Groups Attend Nursing Organization Liaison Forum," *American Nurse* 16:2 (February, 1984), 5.
20. American Nurses' Association. *Facts About Nursing 84–85.* 1985, 6.

21. Lewis, E. "The Professionally Uncommitted," 323.
22. Grimaldi, C. "COAR Study Enters Fifth and Final Stage," *American Nurse* 21:3 (March, 1989) 22.
23. Selby, T. "House Adopts New Structure for ANA," *American Nurse* 21:7 (July–August, 1989), 1.
24. McCarthy, P. "Bylaws Revisions Based on COAR Report," *American Nurse* 21:6 (June, 1989), 3.
25. Selby, T. "House Adopts New Structure for ANA," 16.
26. Styles, M. "We Cannot Turn Back," *American Nurse* 21:4 (April, 1989), 16.
27. Aydelotte, M. "The Evolving Profession: The Role of the Professional Organizations," in N. Chaska (ed.), *The Nursing Profession: Turning Points*. St. Louis: C. V. Mosby, 1990, 14.
28. Beletz, E. "Professionalization—A License is Not Enough," in N. Chaska (ed.), *The Nursing Profession: Turning Points*. St. Louis: C. V. Mosby, 1990, 21.
29. Wilensky, H. "The Professionalization of Everyone?" 149.
30. Goode, W. "The Theoretical Limits of Professionalization," in A. E. Etzioni (ed.), *The Semi-Professions and Their Organization: Teachers, Nurses, Social Workers*. New York: The Free Press, 1969, 281.
31. Goode, W. "Librarianship," in H. J. Vollmer and D. L. Mills (eds.), *Professionalization*. Englewood Cliffs, N. J.: Prentice-Hall, 1966, 40.
32. Wilensky, H. "The Professionalization of Everyone?" 156.
33. *Ibid.*
34. *Ibid.*
35. Katz, F. "Nurses," in A. E. Etzioni (ed.), *The Semi-Professions and Their Organization: Teachers, Nurses, Social Workers*. New York: The Free Press, 1969, 69.
36. Hughes, L. "The Public Image of the Nurse," *Advances in Nursing Science* 2:3 (April, 1980), 55–72.
37. Simpson, R. and Simpson, I. "Women and Bureaucracy in the Semi-Professions," in A. Etzioni (ed.), *The Semi-Professions and Their Organization: Teachers, Nurses, Social Workers*. 1969, 240.
38. Monnig, G. "Professionalism of Nurses and Physicians," in N. Chaska (ed.), *The Nursing Profession: Views Through the Mist*. New York: McGraw-Hill, 1978, 37.
39. "Academy Fellows Explore Nursing's Role in the 80's," *American Journal of Nursing* 78:11 (November, 1979), 1825.
40. Gross, E. "When Occupations Meet: Professions in Trouble," *Hospital Administration* 7 (Spring, 1962), 45.
41. *Ibid.*
42. Goode, W. "Encroachment Charlatanism and the Emerging Profession: Psychology, Sociology, and Medicine," *American Sociological Review*, 25 (December, 1960), 903.
43. Dibble, V. "Occupations and Ideologies," *American Journal of Sociology*, 67 (September, 1962), 229–241.
44. Wilensky, H. "The Professionalization of Everyone?" 138.
45. Goode, W. "Librarianship," 37.
46. Goode, W. "The Theoretical Limits of Professionalization," 308.
47. Wilensky, H. "The Professionalization of Everyone?" 140.

48. Horgan, P. D. "Is Nursing Really a Profession?" *RN* 23 (January, 1960), 50.
49. *Ibid.*
50. *Ibid.* (February, 1960), 64–65.
51. Mundinger, M. *Autonomy in Nursing.* Germantown, Md: Aspen Systems Corp., 1980, 3.
52. Hughes, E. "Professions," in K. Lynn and the editors of Daedalus, *The Professions in America.* Boston: Houghton Mifflin, 1965, 8.
53. Baldridge, J. (ed.), *Academic Governance.* Berkeley, Calif.: McCutchan Publishing, 1971.
54. Bloom, J., O'Reilly, C. and Parlette, S. "Changing Images of Professionalism: The Case of Public Health Nurses," *American Journal of Public Health* 69:1 (January, 1979), 43–46.
55. Carr-Saunders, A. and Wilson, P. *The Professions.* Oxford: Clarendon Press, 1933, 493.
56. Rosenfeld, P. *Nursing Student Census* 1989 (Pub. No.: 19-2291) New York: National League for Nursing, 1989, 6.
57. Katz, F. "Nurses," 72.
58. Stensland, P. "Old Professionals in a New World," in Barbara Stevens (ed.), *Focus on Professional Issues.* Wakefield, Mass.: Contemporary Publishing, 1975, 101.
59. *Ibid.*
60. Nightingale, F. *Notes on Nursing: What It Is and What It Is Not.* New York: D. Appleton & Company, 1860, 140.
61. Flexner, A. *Medical Education in the United States and Canada,* Carnegie Foundation for the Advancement of Teaching, Bulletin No. 4. Boston: Merrymount Press, 1910, 346.
62. Brubacher, J. and Rudy, W. *Higher Education in Transition.* New York: Harper & Row, 1958, 205–206.
63. Goode, W. "The Theoretical Limits of Professionalization," 268.
64. Brubacher, S. and Rudy, W. *Higher Education in Transition,* 206.
65. Goldmark, J. *Nursing and Nursing Education in the United States.* New York: Macmillan, 1923, 585.
66. Burgess, M. *Nurses, Patients, and Pocketbooks: A Report of a Study on the Economics of Nursing.* New York: The Commonwealth Fund, 1928, 618.
67. Johns, E. and Pfefferkorn, B. *An Activity Analysis of Nursing: A Report of the Second Study Sponsored by the Committee on the Grading of Nursing Schools.* New York: National League of Nursing Education, 1934, 213.
68. Committee on the Grading of Nursing Schools. *Nursing Schools: Today and Tomorrow.* New York: National League of Nursing Education, 1934, 268.
69. Stewart, I. *The Education of Nurses.* New York: Macmillan, 1943, 371.
70. Brown, E. *Nursing for the Future.* New York: Russell Sage Foundation, 1948, 198.
71. *Ibid.,* 138.
72. *Ibid.,* 14.
73. Committee on the Function of Nursing. *A Program for the Nursing Profession.* New York: Macmillan, 1948, 108.
74. Montag, M. *The Education of Nursing Technicians.* New York: G. P. Putnam's Sons, 1951, 146.

75. Bridgman, M. *Collegiate Education for Nursing.* New York: Russell Sage Foundation, 1953, 205.
76. Hughes, E., Hughes, H. and Deutscher, D. *Twenty Thousand Nurses Tell Their Story.* Philadelphia: J. B. Lippincott, 1958, 280.
77. Surgeon General's Consultant Group on Nursing. *Toward Quality in Nursing: Needs and Goals.* U.S. Department of Health, Education, and Welfare, (Pub. No.: 992), Washington, D.C., DHEW, 1963, 43.
78. American Nurses' Association. *A Position Paper: Educational Preparation for Nurse Practitioners and Assistants to Nurses.* Kansas City, Mo.: American Nurses' Association, 1965, 16.
79. U.S. Department of Health, Education, and Welfare. *Extending The Scope of Nursing Practice.* Washington, D.C.: Supt. of Documents, U.S. Government Printing Office, 1971.
80. Lysaught, J. *An Abstract for Action.* New York: McGraw-Hill, 1970, 167.
81. Lysaught, J. *From Abstract into Action.* New York: McGraw-Hill, 1973, 363.
82. Lysaught, J. *Action in Affirmation: Toward an Unambiguous Profession of Nursing.* New York: McGraw-Hill, 1981, 192.
83. *Ibid.,* 190.
84. American Nurses' Association. "Resolutions." *American Nurse* 10:9 (September, 1978), 9–10.
85. Committee for the Study of Credentialing in Nursing. *The Study of Credentialing in Nursing: A New Approach, I, II.* Kansas City, Mo.: American Nurses' Association, 1979.
86. Bowman, R. and Culpepper, R. "Power: Rx for Change," *American Journal of Nursing* 74:6 (June, 1974), 1054–56.
87. Mundinger, M. *Autonomy in Nursing.* Germantown, Md.: Aspen Systems Corp., 1980, 222.
88. Styles, M. "Declaring our Future," Paper presented at the Indiana League for Nursing annual meeting, Indianapolis, Ind., October 9, 1976, 4.
89. *Ibid.*
90. Schlotfeldt, R. *A Brave New Nursing World.* Washington, D.C.: American Association of Colleges of Nursing, 1982, 3.
91. Habenstein, R. and Christ, E. *Professionalizer, Traditionalizer, and Utilizer.* Columbia, Mo.: University of Missouri, 1955, 171.
92. Corless, I. "Nursing Professionalization and Innovations," in B. Flynn and M. Miller (eds.), *Current Perspectives in Nursing,* vol. 2. St. Louis: C. V. Mosby, 1980, 141.
93. Schlotfeldt, R. *A Brave New Nursing World,* 1.
94. *Ibid.*
95. Naisbitt, J. *Megatrends: Ten New Directions Transforming Our Lives.* New York: Warner Books, 1982, 290.
96. Mundinger, M. *Autonomy in Nursing.* 3.
97. Glaser, W. "Nursing Leadership and Policy: Some Cross-National Comparisons," in F. Davis (ed.), *The Nursing Profession: Five Sociological Essays.* New York: John Wiley & Sons, 1966, 1–59.
98. Gamer. M. "The Ideology of Professionalism," *Nursing Outlook* 27:2 (February, 1979), 108.

99. Aydelotte, M. "Governance, Education Are Watchwords for the 80s," *American Nurse* 12:4 (March, 1980), 4.
100. *Ibid.*

SUGGESTED READINGS

Altman, S. "Can We Control Health Care Costs?" *Health Management Quarterly* 10:1, 17.

Flanagan, L., "A.N.A. Monograph Examines 'Professional Collectivism' " *American Nurse* 16:5 (May, 1984), 7.

Barritt, E. "Florence Nightingale's Values and Modern Nursing Education," *Nursing Forum* 12:1 (1973), 12.

Dock, L. *A Short History of Nursing.* New York: G. P. Putnam's Sons, 1920.

Fitzpatrick, M. *Prologue to Professionalism.* New York: Athenaeum Publishers, 1983.

Harrington, C. "The Political Economy of Health: A New Imperative for Nursing," *Nursing and Health Care,* 9:3 (1988), 121.

Kalisch, P. and Kalisch, B. *The Advance of American Nursing.* Boston: Little, Brown & Co., 1978.

Kelly, L. "Swords into Plowshares," *Nursing Outlook* 31:5 (September–October, 1983), 261.

Kimball, M. C. "Nation's Health Bill to Rise 10.4% in 1990, U.S. Says," *Healthweek* 4:1 (April, 1990), 1, 52.

Koff, T. *New Approaches to Health Care for an Aging Population.* San Francisco: Jossey & Bass Co., 1988.

Kuntz, S. "Professionalism and Social Control in the Progressive Era: The Case of the Flexner Report," *Social Problems* 22:16 (October, 1974), 16–27.

Nutting, M. "The Future," *American Journal of Nursing* 29 (1929), 903–910.

Reverby, S. "The Search for the Hospital Yardstick: Nursing and the Rationalization of Hospital Work," in S. Reverby and D. Rosner (eds.) *Health Care in America: Essays in Social History.* Philadelphia: Temple University Press, 1979.

Roberts, K. "Nursing: Profession or Pretender?" *Australian Nursing Journal* 9:10 (October, 1980), 33–35, 51.

Roberts, M. *American Nursing, History and Interpretation.* New York: Macmillan, 1954.

Roemer, R. "The Right to Health Care—Gains and Gaps," *American Journal of Public Health* 78, 241–247.

Stewart, I. "Professional School or Trade School?" *Proceedings of the Thirty-fifth Annual Convention of the National League of Nursing Education* 1929, 130–135.

Velsor-Friedrich, B. "The Emerging Profession of Nursing: Commitments and Constraints," (Unpublished doctoral dissertation) Evanston, Ill.: Northwestern University, 1986.

Wolf, M. "Group Stages: One View of the Development of the Nursing Profession," *Image: the Journal of Nursing Scholarship* 9:5 (October, 1977).

Development of a Scientific Knowledge Base for Nursing Practice

3

INTRODUCTION

In the previous chapter, the need for a scientific body of knowledge was emphasized as a means to acquire autonomy and provide direction for nursing practice. Furthermore, most scholars have agreed that a theoretical body of knowledge is one of the indispensable characteristics of a profession. To control the tasks to be performed, professional practitioners should have at their disposal a well-defined body of knowledge that will enable them to comprehend the basis and consequences of their actions.

> The autonomy of a profession rests more firmly on the uniqueness of its knowledge—knowledge gathered ever so slowly through the questioning of scientific inquiry. Nursing defined by power does not necessarily beget knowledge but knowledge most often results in the ascription of power and is accompanied by power.[1]

Over thirty years ago, nurses were raising vital questions about nursing's unique content. Although some nurses today still believe that an acceptable body of knowledge will not be identified in their lifetime, others believe that it will occur within the span of their careers.[2] In the early 1980s it was noted that "although nursing has an impressive cadre of bright, capable, visionary, and courageous leaders, the profession as a whole remains weak, other-directed, and indeed other-controlled."[3] Nevertheless, the number of nurse scholars who are contributing significantly to the advancement of nursing knowledge is steadily increasing.[4] The 1980s have shown accelerated growth in knowledge development by nurse scholars and in its use by clinicians in nursing practice.

Increased research efforts to build nursing's body of knowledge are essential, yet the essence of research and the ability to interpret the research findings are not highly appreciated by many nurses.[5] As mentioned earlier, society will grant prestige and professional status to nursing only if a theoretical body of knowledge and a strong service ideal are readily observable. Therefore, if nurses are to be granted full professional status, they should identify and continue to increase the theoretical knowledge upon which their clinical practice is based. "If nurses clearly direct their goals toward theory development and testing that are congruent with the domain of nursing, then social relevance will occur."[6]

Full professional status for nursing can occur only if it is not controlled by other means. When nursing's body of knowledge is more fully developed, it will require society's control, and only then will eligibility be granted for full professional status by society.[7] For "if an occupation is not allowed to control itself in a central matter, and need not be controlled in others, it will not be granted high prestige for its moral stature, nor will it ever assert its right to that grant."[8]

The answer to why the emergence of nursing knowledge and theory has been such an extremely slow process may be due to the fact that the discipline of nursing began with Florence Nightingale's emphasis on tasks and procedures. Gradually it changed to have a strong illness and disease orientation. Only more recently has it been concerned with health, health promotion, and wellness. The lack of a scientific knowledge base for nursing is understandable, since "nursing stands today, as a field of practice without a scientific heritage—an occupation created by society long ago to offer a distinctive service, but one still ill-defined in practical terms, a profession without the theoretical base it seems to require."[9]

Nursing is reflecting an orientation indicative of professionalism as compared to technology. Although a high level of technical competence is expected of professional practitioners, they are expected not only to be knowledgeable but also to use that knowledge creatively and with vision in their practice and research.[10] "The task to which nursing as a professional body must devote its greatest efforts over the next several decades is the further development of a knowledge base for its professional practice."[11] In other words, nursing's highest priority is that of theory development and testing of the developed theories.[12] Unfortunately, nursing care is frequently conceived of in terms of task performance and not as using independent thought or decision-making skills to fulfill its responsibilities.[13]

HOW THE PUBLIC VIEWS
NURSING'S KNOWLEDGE

The public's image of nurses and their occupation has been an obstacle to achieving full professional status. The general perception of nursing continues to reflect the belief that nurses are the "handmaidens" of physicians, whose main function is to implement "orders" of the medical profession at their bidding in a subservient manner, without having decision-making responsibilities in their own right.

The public still thinks of the nurse in sex-linked, task-oriented terms: a female who performs unpleasant technical jobs and functions as an assistant to the physician.[14] Undoubtedly the impact of contemporary views on women and women's professions as portrayed by the media are factors influencing the public's image of nursing. As nurses assume more responsibilities for patient care and health promotion, they are becoming dissatisfied with the public image that does not incorporate the realities of modern nursing, including the expanded role of nursing and the independence that is beginning to characterize the profession.

> Although many nurses are now assuming independent and innovative roles in health care, the public continues to view the physician as the sole authority and as the primary provider of health care. Nursing potential has not been fully recognized or utilized by the public, and this has led to wasted nursing talent and inadequate care for society.[15]

Nurses should make their contribution to health care known in order to enhance the public's awareness and demand for nursing's services. Programs to educate consumers about nursing and the real value of its services are increasing. Research conducted by Philip and Beatrice Kalisch has made a significant contribution to awakening nurses and the public about nursing's poor public image and the need to improve it.[16, 17] Nurses now realize that outdated images of nurses must be supplanted with intelligent, accurate descriptions of the vital services that nursing provides to society.[18]

Is this image static? If it is rooted in stereotypes of women in the past, can nursing affect changes to alter such stereotypes? Perhaps if the public understood the meaning of nurses' professionalism, some significant changes in their views about nursing might occur. Yet "images are merely a by-product of the deeper social reality of the occupation."[19] A public relations campaign can alter this image somewhat, but changing the practice of nursing from one that is controlled to one that is autonomous would change nursing's image to an even greater degree. In comparing the services rendered by medicine and nursing, it is readily acknowledged that the public's appreciation for the field of medicine is far greater than for that of nursing.

> Both types of service require a great deal of knowledge and skill on the part of practitioners. Yet, the privileges and rewards expected by physicians and afforded them by society are in sharp contrast to those generally expected by nurses and accorded by those they serve.[20]

Until the public recognizes the value of nursing services to the extent that it recognizes the value of physician services, the image of nursing will not change substantially. If the public lacks understanding of the contributions nurses make to health care or the benefits received from nursing care, it will not grant nursing full professional status. Therefore, the public needs to be made aware of these contributions and to be more accepting of nursing as an important health discipline. The public's image of medicine remains fairly stable, even though its trust in the physician has somewhat deteriorated since physicians are viewed as less caring than nurses and more concerned with monetary remuneration than with their patients' best interests.

The fact that four national nursing organizations, the American Nurses' Association, the National League for Nursing, the Academy of Nursing, and Sigma Theta Tau, have identified the image of nursing as having high priority reflects the concern that nursing and nurses are expressing about their image and their role in improving health care through improved nursing practice. For example, at Sigma Theta Tau's twenty-seventh biennial convention in Boston in 1983, the overall theme "Image Makers: Richness in Diversity" sought to answer such questions as:

- What image does nursing want to portray?
- What is the best way to present nursing's image in today's world?
- How can we as nurses deal with today's issues and today's opportunities?[21]

In order to project a more acceptable professional image to the public, significant changes must occur within the profession. Perhaps the most significant advance would be the identification of a distinct body of knowledge that would justify nursing's claim to full professional status and enhance the public's image of nursing.

DEFINITION AND NATURE OF NURSING

One of the factors that makes this period such an exciting one in nursing's history is the fact that nursing has begun to recapture the essence and spirit of Florence Nightingale's exhortations on nursing and can answer forthrightly the question—"What is nursing?" Although definitions of nursing have been forthcoming by numerous groups of practitioners, physicians, political scientists, legislators, and various authors since Florence Nightingale's era, only recently has nursing articulated a definition that has substance and meaning for the majority of practicing nurses. Lacking a clearly defined body of theoretical knowledge in the past, nursing has had difficulty focusing its research efforts. Now nursing can state with great self-confidence that its mission is the promotion of health for all people, and thus it can begin to define the services that make it unique as a profession. Since the 1940s, nursing has become highly specialized and complex, with greater emphasis on cure than on the caring and comforting functions that characterized nursing in Florence Nightingale's period. As a result, some of the essential concepts have become fuzzy or blurred. Controversy among nurses has continued over the key question, "What is nursing?" There are many nurses who claim that nursing implies giving care and assisting in curing the acutely ill, primarily in hospitals. However, there are numerous nurses who also perform nursing functions regardless of the client's diagnosed condition, economic status, or location.

Dorothy Johnson, an ardent proponent of a theoretical base for nursing practice, addressed the importance of *function:*

> many of the professions have endured for a very long time . . . they are as recognizable today as they were hundreds of years ago. This enduring identity derives from the basic functions these serve for society in general and for the recipient of their services in particular . . . so long as society requires the social consequences a profession was established to achieve, its basic function will not change.[22]

As far back as 1965, Johnson pointed out that nursing's function, which requires a high degree of knowledge and intellectual capacity, is that of pattern maintenance.[23] One of the early nurse leaders concerned about nursing's function, Virginia Henderson, believed that

> it is self-evident that a profession whose services affect human life, must define its function. . . . nursing's attempt to do so has a long and still unfinished history.
> The unique function of the nurse is to assist the individual, sick or well, in the performance of those activities contributing to health or its recovery (or to peaceful death) that he would perform unaided if he had the necessary strength, will or knowledge.[24]

It has been noted that nursing has been overly preoccupied with functions and has not given sufficient attention to its goal and primary focus.[25] Has nursing identified a specific focus, or is it still depending on one to emerge as its knowledge base increases? Some authors believe that nursing has *not* adequately identified its focus. In fact, the lack of unity among nurses on nursing's main focus has become more evident in nursing literature.[26]

It is my belief, however, that dramatic strides have been made during the past ten years toward defining nursing's primary focus. Moreover, a growing concern about nursing's unique role and the contributions that nurses make to health care is evident. However, to what extent this primary focus is understood and accepted by most practitioners of nursing is still questionable.

Over twenty years ago, Martha Rogers unhesitatingly stated that "nursing is concerned with people, all people—well and sick, rich and poor, young and old, wherever they may be at work and at play."[27] Does consensus exist in support of this definition? Is evidence available demonstrating that nursing care has made a difference in the level of health achieved by the society nursing serves? If nurses can understand the nature and focus of the services nursing provides, they may be able to reach agreement on directions for nursing's future in the health care system.

The ANA Congress for Nursing Practice, chaired by Norma Lang, appointed a seven-member task force to develop a statement defining the nature and scope of nursing practice. This task force developed *Nursing: A Social Policy Statement* published by the ANA in December 1980. The statement provided a description of the social context of nursing, a definition of its scope, and an outline of its areas of specialization. It recommended a high degree of competence for nurses to further advance nursing as a profession. A summary of this statement, entitled "Nursing Defined" is presented as follows:

> **Nursing:** Nursing is the diagnosis and treatment of human responses to actual or potential health problems.
>
> **Phenomena of Concern:** The phenomena of concern to nurses are human responses to actual or potential health problems. Any observable manifestation, need, condition, concern, event, dilemma, difficulty, occurrence or fact that can be described or scientifically explained and is within the target area of nursing practice is of interest to nurses.
>
> **Human Responses:** The following provides an illustrative list rather than a comprehensive taxonomy of human responses that are the focus for nursing intervention:
>
> - Self-care limitations
> - Impaired functioning in areas such as rest, sleep, ventilation, circulation, activity, nutrition, elimination, skin, sexuality, and the like
> - Pain and discomfort
> - Emotional problems related to illness and treatment, life-threatening events or daily experiences, such as anxiety, loss, loneliness, and grief
> - Distortion of symbolic functions, reflected in interpersonal and intellectual processes, such as hallucinations
> - Deficiencies in decision making and ability to make personal choices

- Self-image changes required by health status
- Dysfunctional perceptual orientations to health
- Strains related to life processes, such as birth, growth and development, and death
- Problematic affiliative relationships[28]

A succinct summary of the document's content follows:

> The document publicly acknowledges nursing's social context and the concomitant legal authority inherent in nursing's contract with society . . . the definition of nursing is strong, clear, concrete and challenging. It carries us . . . to a clarion demand upon ourselves to be thinking, scientifically grounded, responsible health care providers and leaders . . . and clarifies the focus of our concern and delineates discipline boundaries.[29]

I concur with Luther Christman, nurse leader and former dean, when he observed that it would be inaccurate to conclude that the functions described in the statement can be carried out by all practicing nurses.[30] Strong leadership is needed to implement these care goals to the degree outlined. Nurses must be reoriented to understand the importance of demonstrating and being accountable for their nursing role, as defined in the *Social Policy Statement.*

Society grants certain rights and privileges to professions in their practice, and it assumes that they can and will function as their focus and goals imply. It must be assured, in the case of nursing, that the practitioners are capable of diagnosing and treating the human responses emphasized in this definition. The profession is responsible for identifying and classifying these various human responses and clearly articulating them to all of its members. Until the collectivity of nursing reaches consensus and accepts responsibility for this focus, society cannot be expected to value or demand such service.

The importance of phenomena as a major focus for the profession and what makes nursing unique is summarized in the following passage:

> The four characteristics of nursing which are part of this definition are phenomena, the theory, the action and, finally, the effect of nursing care. The phenomena of the nurse's concern are the event, the dilemma, the occurrence or effect which can be scientifically described. . . . The phenomenon, the major focus of a profession, is the distinction which makes a profession unique . . . [therefore] nursing must get on with the development, testing, refining and evaluating of the phenomena so we can continue our pursuit of nursing's uniqueness.[31]

According to Ellis, a perspective is what leads to a knowledge system. It identifies the phenomena of interest, defines the knowledge to be organized or developed, and serves to identify the key concepts that characterize a field of knowledge.[32]

The importance of communicating the definition and focus of nursing as presented in the *Social Policy Statement* to all practicing nurses, other health professions, legislators, and the public, is both a challenge and responsibility. However, if all nurses are agreed that nursing is the diagnosis and treatment of human responses to actual or potential health problems, then they must convince others that such responses are nursing's unique focus. And then they must produce a body of knowledge to justify this definition.

In a 1983 ANA conference in Denver on "New Knowledge for Nursing Practice," several concerns that nursing is currently addressing were discussed: "chronic pain, acute pain, loneliness, hopelessness, lack of ability to cope caused by aging or caused by multiple losses, hallucinations, social disabilities, concerns related to sleep, safety, grief, and depression."[33] Each of these concerns is relevant to practicing nurses and nurse researchers and will be addressed more frequently during the coming decade.

CURRENT STATUS OF NURSING AS A SCIENTIFIC DISCIPLINE

Nursing is moving rapidly into becoming a scientific discipline because nurse theorists are utilizing scientific methods to explain, predict, and apply new knowledge in the practice of professional nursing. However, many nurses still lack understanding and appreciation of the value of theory for practice and why nursing should be diligently pursuing its development to further advance professionalism. Commitment to science is essential if nursing is to be recognized as a full profession and contribute accountably to society's needs. "Certainly no profession can long exist without making explicit its theoretical bases for practice so that this new knowledge can be communicated, tested, and expanded."[34] Moreover, "[t]he emergence of nursing science as an independent professional discipline valued by society parallels the professional and social demands to assume full responsibility for nursing decisions, actions, and resulting consequences."[35]

Science has been defined as "a body of knowledge consisting of interconnected concepts and conceptual schemes obtained by methods ultimately based on observation and suggestive of further investigation."[36] In regards to nursing, it has also been defined as "the process and the result of ordering and patterning the events and phenomena of concern to nursing."[37]

The history of nursing science in recent decades has undergone several shifts of emphasis. Early theorists explored the interpersonal relations between patient and nurse. More recently, theorists have emphasized the definition and nature of nursing practice and the movement of patients from illness to health. At the present time, health is considered to be a "dynamic process" moving back and forth over the lifetime of individuals. The need to refine factors observed in the relationship between the patient and the environment is a vital one.[38]

Despite the progress made in theory development, nursing cannot be designated as a true science. Nursing practice is still identified as procedural and task oriented, with routines determined by policies, directives, and physicians' orders rather than by actions based on the findings of nursing research. Undoubtedly, nursing will be greatly influenced in its progress toward professionalism over the next decade by the work of nurse theorists who are accepting the challenge of developing nursing as a scientific discipline. These theorists recognize the importance of developing nursing theory to facilitate progress in the emergence of nursing as a profession. Action was taken by the 1981 House of Delegates of Sigma Theta Tau to accept a decision to implement a ten-year plan for increasing the scientific foundation for nursing practice. This history-making event should greatly aid efforts to further nursing as a unique science.

NURSING'S THEORY DEVELOPMENT SHOWS PROGRESS

Theory is often referred to as an explanation or description of a body of specific knowledge. Past efforts in nursing theory development have resulted in controversy over whether nursing science is basic or applied, unique or borrowed from other disciplines. Theories currently stressed are general systems, adaptation, developmental, interactive, self-care, and needs, as the notion of borrowing theories from basic sciences has become moot at present. Most nurse theorists have concluded that nursing should develop its own theories and knowledge base in order to direct its practice. For example, Dorothy Johnson, in 1968, recognized the need for prescriptive knowledge in controlling practice. She stressed the fact that nursing's phenomena of interest differs from the basic sciences. Thus a knowledge base unique to nursing would develop.[39]

From reviewing literature on nursing theory development, it is apparent that nursing should continue to define its focus and unique perspective if theories for practice are to be generated. Specific research questions pertaining to observed phenomena should be addressed to develop nursing's knowledge. Susan Gortner, professor of nursing at the University of California, San Francisco, lists "examples of phenomena that have particular relevance for nursing . . . compliance, chronicity, self-care, social support, parenting, family functioning, and stress."[40] She elaborates on chronicity, parenting, and family functioning by raising the following research questions:

- How does chronic illness modify self-image?
- What coping mechanisms are effective with chronic and acute pain?
- What factors influence maternal role attainment?
- What constitutes health-seeking behavior among adolescents?
- What is the relationship of family functioning to recovery from episodic illness?[41]

The importance of developing key questions about phenomena of interest to nursing provides directions for research activities and ultimately assists research development. Since the 1960s and 1970s considerable energy has been directed toward developing knowledge about theories and concepts as a means of guiding and controlling nursing practice. A body of theory consists of positions or relational statements that describe phenomena relating to a profession's focus of interest.

The issues of whether there should be a single theory of nursing or numerous theories and whether there should be a theory *of nursing* or theory *for* practice have yet to be resolved. To date there seems to be agreement that theories for nursing practice should be developed, but different opinions exist regarding the best scientific methodology to be used to develop them. The hypothetico-deductive or inductive research methods are not preferred as the primary means of developing nursing knowledge. Rather a more generalized approach that includes other scientific methodologies, specifically historical or philosophical research, has received favorable response from nurse researchers.

The preparadigm stage of science is marked by confusion, dispute over theory, and power struggles among various factional groups, making it difficult to develop theory and utilize nursing knowledge.[42] If nursing science is still at the preparadigm stage, it may have to continue struggling until a paradigm acceptable to nurse researchers can be developed.

Nursing has made progress in theory development, but there remains much to accomplish before it can be recognized as a scientific discipline. Recently it has been observed that nursing knowledge is in a preparadigm stage of development, and since a paradigm and community of scholars develop concurrently, nursing has yet to achieve either one of these.[43] If nursing is to guarantee its respectability as a science, then advances in theory development and testing theories through research should be high priorities.[44, 45]

> The discipline of nursing will advance only through continuous and systematic development and testing of nursing knowledge. Several recent

reviews of the status of nursing theory development indicate that nursing has no established tradition of scholarship. Reviewers have pointed out that most work appears unfocused and uncoordinated, as each scholar moves quickly from one topic to another and as few scholars combine their efforts in circumscribed areas.[46]

Only through advancing theory development can the goals of the profession be achieved. Other issues in theory development revolve around the focus of nursing. Should nursing consist of mastery of knowledge and techniques in clinical practice or be more concerned with interpersonal relationships?

NURSING: APPLIED SCIENCE OR NURSING SCIENCE

In the late 1800s and early 1900s, nursing knowledge was concerned solely with advances in medical sciences. It concentrated on development of nursing procedures and techniques needed for the treatment of patients. Little research was conducted to guide nursing practice until the 1950s, when emphasis was placed on integrating concepts from the biological and behavioral sciences. These efforts failed to provide answers to the question of "What is nursing?" Nurses continued to exert energy in studying *nurses* rather than *nursing*, which led to confusion, fuzziness, and many unanswered questions about the practice of nursing.

Some authors believed that nursing knowledge or practice should not be developed by applying basic principles from other disciplines. They recommended that nursing develop its own knowledge base and nursing practice theory.[47] In response to a proposal for nursing practice theory, Dickoff and James produced a four-level model of theory in a practice discipline: (1) factor-isolating, (2) factor-relating, (3) situation-relating, and (4) situation-producing theory.[48] Moreover, they stressed that nursing theories must be situation-producing or prescriptive, because if the aim of nursing is not practice then nursing can no longer be distinguished from some mere academic discipline.[49]

Dickoff and James maintained that if nursing is a practice discipline, then it needs prescriptive theory to determine the goals to be achieved and the activities needed to meet these goals. However, more recent writers such as Diers, Fawcett, and Beckstrand have agreed that descriptive, explanatory, and predictive theory and ethical knowledge are adequate for practice, and prescriptive theory is therefore unnecessary for practicing nurses.[50–52] Unfortunately, efforts to develop situation-producing theory or practice theory did not produce a perspective for advancing nursing practice theory. Nurse theorists such as Dorothy Johnson and

Martha Rogers offered other perspectives within the practice theory movement. For example, Johnson viewed nursing science as an applied science in which findings from several fields are synthesized and provide a perspective for nursing. She defined nursing science as "a synthesis, reorganization, or extension of concepts drawn from the basic or other applied sciences which in their reformulation tend to become 'new' concepts."[53]

Johnson provided an interesting perspective on the nature of the knowledge required for nursing practice. In her view, nursing theory should address knowledge of order, knowledge of disorder, and knowledge of control.[54] Knowledge of order refers to order in nature and describes the normal state and natural scheme of things. On the other hand, knowledge of disorder is classified as that knowledge that provides understanding of undesirable events that could threaten the well-being of individuals or society. Knowledge of control allows the prescribing of a course of action, which, if and when performed, could change the sequence of events in a desired way toward specific outcomes.

Johnson's opinion was that this third type of knowledge represents what others have described as prescriptive theory. Since a "unified theory of human behavior" has yet to emerge from the basic sciences, Johnson believed that nurse theorists would have to develop their own theory and ask questions about events in the universe that are of specific concern to nursing.[55] She stressed the need for knowledge to go beyond description or prediction to that of prescription. Over thirty years have elapsed since Johnson pointed out that it may take a prolonged period of time before consensus will be reached and a sound beginning made in developing theory for nursing practice.[56]

In contrast to Johnson's views, Martha Rogers asserted that nursing is a learned profession. There *is* an organized body of scientific knowledge in nursing characterized by an "identifiable system of concepts, explanatory, descriptive, and predictive principles, and hypothetical generalizations [and] . . . this organized body of theoretical knowledge is the science of nursing."[57] She explained further that "the science of nursing is not a summation of facts and principles drawn from other sources; it is a science of synergistic man—unitary man—characterized by an organized conceptual system from which are derived the hypothetical generalizations and unifying principles essential to guide practice."[58] Rogers emphasized that mankind is at the center of nursing's purpose and that nursing science is concerned with understanding the human life process:

> In the unification and organization of knowledge that constitutes the theoretical basis of nursing practice lies the uniqueness of nursing science. The nature of the knowledge determines the scope and limitations of nursing practice. The vision and creativity, the energy and imagination, that are invested in its on-going elaboration further define the expansion and clarification of nursing's substantive base.[59]

Whether nursing utilizes knowledge from other disciplines is no longer debatable; however, this knowledge should be redefined according to nursing's perspective. It can then be used to foster the development of theories unique to nursing.

NURSING PRACTICE BASED ON THEORY AND RESEARCH

It was pointed out earlier that as an occupation moves toward full professional status it increases its research productivity, concentrating on the occupation or on the phenomena with which it is concerned. Research, as an integral part of nursing's professional development, is needed to increase nursing's professionalism. If nursing practice is to move beyond the ritual stage and improve the quality of nursing care, then research is needed to test and refine nursing's scientific knowledge and ethical and aesthetic bases for such practice.

Nursing is beginning to resolve its identity crisis. Its focus is more clearly defined as the diagnosis and treatment of human responses to health problems that are nursing's phenomena of concern. Questions have shifted from what do nurses do to what does nursing remedy or restore? With impetus from this defined focus, nurse researchers are identifying phenomena of concern to nursing. Some nurse leaders believe that most practicing nurses in the United States have limited knowledge of or interest in nursing research.[60]

> . . . they fail to recognize the link between research and professionalization, and that link is, in fact, essential. Without question, one of the hallmarks of a profession is grounding of practice in scholarly inquiry. . . . To date, nursing has failed to meet this single, mandatory criterion. . . .
>
> Our practice is almost entirely founded on personal wisdom rather than scientific conclusions.[61]

As phenomena are identified and explained by nurse researchers, the body of knowledge required to advance nursing practice to the stage of predicting outcomes should occur. However, unless research is directed by theory, it will not be relevant to nursing practice. Thus, it is important to understand the relation of theory and research to nursing practice, if our aim is to upgrade and improve the quality of nursing care.

Research is the best means to test and validate the usefulness of knowledge for nursing practice. Since the 1970s, nurses have begun to value practice research more than in previous decades, with the major focus now on the nature of the knowledge base underlying nursing practice. By utilizing nursing conceptual models, nurses are able to conduct *nursing* research rather than research in only the basic sciences. Practice research can lead to the production of practice theories, which in turn can contribute to the body of nursing science. Within the last decade research studies have increased significantly, in part because there are more nurses with doctoral and master's degrees available to conduct research programs. However, very few studies are based on theoretical formulations. Nursing has just begun to understand the need for replication studies that proceed from developing a theory to the testing and evaluating stages in clinical settings. When nursing develops its own theory, validates research knowledge in the practice setting, and relies on this knowledge to direct nursing practice, it will become recognized as an independent, autonomous profession. At that point nursing will no longer direct its practice based on knowledge from other sources, but will rely on its own knowledge base to guide nursing practice.

An example of the concern evidenced by the ANA to facilitate nursing research was noted in a conference sponsored by the ANA Council of Nurse Researchers entitled "Nursing Science: Today and Beyond" in Minneapolis, Minnesota, in 1983. This conference was designed to generate interest in conducting and using research findings in nursing practice. Kathryn E. Barnard, Professor of Nursing at the University of Washington, presented the keynote address on the "State of the Art" of nursing research. She defined three distinct phases of nursing science: (1) search/discovery, (2) knowledge building, and (3) dissemination (sharing results with the scientific community). It is the second and third phases that provide authority for nursing practice in the United States. In her opinion, the majority of nurse scientists are at the search and discovery phase. She recommended that greater networking occur among nurse scientists as new technologies (computers, teleconferencing) facilitate improved communication.[62]

Jean Johnson, Professor of Nursing at the University of Rochester, is optimistic that the ANA's definition of nursing will allow nurse researchers to gain relevance as scientists and proceed with the study of responses to human health problems.[63] She believes there is much work needed to study these responses, to focus on theory that brings about the response, and to link interventions with outcomes, that is, knowing the emotional reactions of patients and how to deal with them in the practice of nursing. The roles of researchers in health care agencies are described as developers of new core activities, overseers of clinical trials in nursing, primary gatekeepers of new knowledge and feeding this knowledge back to practitioners and teachers of basic nursing students, and encouraging questioning behavior.[64]

Some authors concur that a commonality among nursing's scientists is not readily noticeable. There is a lack of spirit of colleagueship and collaboration in communicating and sharing one's work with scholars of like interests.[65,66] However, there are encouraging signs that improved communication and collaboration are occurring through activities of the ANA Council of Nurse Researchers and nursing research departments or centers in universities and hospitals.

NURSE PRACTITIONERS AND NURSE RESEARCHERS IN COLLABORATION

As mentioned previously, many practicing nurses have little knowledge of or interest in research. Some even consider efforts in nursing theory development to prove the worth of nursing actions irrelevant and unnecessary. But if the discipline of nursing, based on scientific knowledge, is to be recognized by other professions as well as nursing, then the need to foster collaborative efforts between nurse researchers and practicing nurses is essential.

The fact that nurse researchers have been primarily educators has created a chasm between researchers and their counterparts in nursing practice. If a lag in theory development exists, it may be the result of nurse researchers working isolated from the practice setting and failing to communicate adequately with practicing nurses. This void is beginning to lessen, however, as nursing research becomes an important part of the nursing department. Nursing researchers now collaborate more frequently with practicing nurses in sharing responsibility for developing and testing new nursing knowledge. In order to make this knowledge more relevant, it must be communicated to practitioners and nursing students in an understandable, meaningful way. To emphasize the importance of collaboration between nursing education and nursing service, the following resolution was passed by the delegates at a National League for Nursing (NLN) convention in 1983:

> *RESOLUTION 9:* **For Collaborative Research by Nursing Education and Nursing Service**
> *WHEREAS,* The ultimate goal of nursing is excellence in providing nursing/health care to the consumer; and
> *WHEREAS,* There is a need to improve the delivery and practice of nursing/health care, and
> *WHEREAS,* There is a need to further expand and refine the knowledge base for nursing; and
> *WHEREAS,* There is a need to foster the spirit of inquiry in students and practitioners of nursing; and
> *WHEREAS,* There is a need to foster improved communication and cooperation between nursing educators and nursing practitioners; therefore, be it
> *RESOLVED,* That the National League for Nursing, through its appropriate councils and divisions, work to promote collaborative research between nursing education and nursing service.[67]

Until recently, nursing practice theory has evolved through a trial-and-error method or common sense approach. Practitioners have relied on wisdom acquired from practical, day-to-day experiences. Nurses are now beginning to understand the need for knowledge derived from scientific description, explanation, and prediction. The practice setting is necessary for the validation and application of theory, not only to prove its usefulness but also to refine and revise the theories as needed. Nurse researchers and practitioners should recognize the mutual contributions each can make toward improving nursing care and developing better means of collaborating with each other.

One effort to reduce the divergent views that separate nurse practitioners from nurse researchers was the Fourth National Conference on Nursing Diagnoses. A theoretical model for nursing was presented to motivate the testing of nursing diagnoses acceptable to nursing and as a means to classify nursing phenomena of concern to nursing. Practitioners at the conference engaged in active discussion with nurse scholars about the relevance of this model in establishing nursing diagnoses for practice. The conference concluded in support of using a nursing model in practice and as a generally recognized means to develop links between nursing diagnoses and theories for nursing practice.

A four-day conference in San Francisco cosponsored by four ANA councils (Continuing Education, Nursing Administration, Intercultural Nursing, and Nurse Researchers) centered on nurses working together. Lucie Kelly, a professor of nursing and present editor of *Nursing Outlook*, used her keynote address to describe a study that demonstrated the effectiveness of nurses collaborating together. The study, involving about 100 nurses at nine New York City hospitals, revealed that collaboration among administrators, researchers, and continuing educators facilitated improved communication among nurses and led to better nursing care:

> It was the networking, the sponsorship, the support system and the colleagueship that made the difference in the long run. It was the system of nurses working with nurses for better quality care that was the heart of this study.[68]

Nursing theory has been slow to develop in part because of a lack of shared understanding of nursing practice between nurse researchers and practitioners. Now that nurse scholars have ceased studying nurses and are concentrating their research endeavors on the practice of nursing, evidence is mounting that exciting developments for improved nursing practice are beginning to surface. Florence Downs, Associate Dean and Director of Graduate Studies, University of Pennsylvania School of Nursing, was optimistic when she observed:

given the resources available to us, I think we have done a very good job in a deliberate and responsible fashion—in an extremely short time period. Of course, we have a long way to go, but I believe we are on the edge of a breakthrough to a more cogent and coherent explanation of nursing phenomena than we have been able to set forth until now.[69]

There appears to be substantial agreement among nurses on definitions of the key concepts of personhood, health, nursing, and environment. Moreover, consensus is growing on acceptance of the ANA definition of nursing, which emphasizes the phenomena of concern resulting from human responses to acute or potential health problems. The contribution made by the classification of nursing diagnoses is another means of involving practicing nurses and furthering progress in nursing theory and acquiring a unique knowledge base. The astute observations and clinical interventions that nurses in practice are implementing can further such knowledge considerably. Furthermore, as nurse theorists generate theories or view phenomena of interest to nursing, they frequently rely on practicing nurses to test their validity and relevance for nursing practice. As clinical investigations occur they must be supported and given widespread publicity among practicing nurses. Nurses in practice are recognizing the importance of contributing to theory development and are realizing that a body of nursing knowledge can greatly enhance their practice.

As more nurses are prepared at the doctoral level in nursing, additional researchers will be added, improving the quality of studies and increasing the possibilities for further progress in theory development. However, until scientific activity or commitment to science in nursing are valued more highly by practicing nurses, development of a knowledge base for practice will be greatly impeded.

CLINICAL NURSES ASSIST NURSE THEORISTS IN ACQUIRING A KNOWLEDGE BASE

Although the number of nurses who can add substantially to nursing's body of knowledge is and will continue to be relatively small, the potential for developing a scientific outlook among the over 2,000,000 registered nurses in the U.S. is substantial. If each nurse would agree on the ANA definition of nursing, the possibility of adding new knowledge about phenomena would be significantly increased. Yet, Martha Rogers, in her keenly penetrating manner, asserts that "only professionally educated nurses are competent to guide nursing practice and to make the complex judgments that require substantial knowledge and a high degree of intellectual skill."[70] Still, many practicing nurses can participate in research projects under investigation in the practice setting and add their valuable insights and observations about patients and their care. Today, comparatively few nurses are practicing in a truly scientific manner, but their number is steadily increasing as more nurses accept professional practice as a goal to be achieved. "If nursing is, in fact, a profession to which society grants a monopoly of judgment in the management of problems of considerable social significance, then emphasis must be placed in any description of professional practice on the responsibility and accountability of the practitioner, on her skill and vision in making decisions, and on her command of the knowledge needed to make wise decisions."[71]

Nurses should be encouraged to review their historic roots, the essence of their practice, and their role in assisting clients (sick or well) to improve their health status if they are to contribute a unique, humane service to society. Undoubtedly there is a need for increased knowledge and skill in clinical nursing practice based on research and theories for nursing practice. As the knowledge base for professional nursing is more firmly established, nursing will be recognized as a professional discipline whose services are comparable to that of other health disciplines.

The definition of nursing articulated by the ANA has motivated nurse theorists to ask significant questions about observable phenomena unique to nursing and to direct their investigations toward theory development for nursing practice. Esther Lucille Brown's advice to nurses over four decades ago is relevant even today:

> What is needed at this moment is a decisive reversal of attitudes. By every means at its disposal the nursing profession, collectively and individually, must take a positive position concerning itself and the significance of its function. It must be as unquestioning in that position as are the medical and legal profession. . . . Only when abiding conviction of social worth replaces lack of self-confidence, negativism, and carping comment, will that climate of opinion be created whereby nursing can move forward to greater selectivity of personnel and to a level of nursing care that bespeaks growth and development for the nurse herself and more and better health services for society.[72]

Traditionally, the model uniting research and practice is a collaborative one, whereby researchers work with clinicians as they study phenomena in the clinical setting. Researchers are continuing to involve clinicians in research projects by reporting at inservice programs on the implications found in patient care research and by informing nursing staffs of research being conducted in their practice area.[73]

Do the public and third party payors recognize nursing's capability for "improving the quality of health care and controlling health care costs?"[74] To improve nursing's image and inform the public of the benefits provided by nurses in patient care, major nursing organizations have placed high priority on these agenda items. National nursing leaders holding key positions as nurse administrators, researchers, and educators gathered in Washington, D.C. in May 1990 for a conference to explicate nursing's role in effective health care delivery. The conference "marked a milestone" in efforts of the ANA to exert leadership in developing "standards, guidelines and national clinical data bases." This conference, cosponsored by the American Nurses Association, the Agency for Health Care Policy, the National Center for Nursing Research, and the Division of Nursing of the Department of Health and Human Services, was entitled: "Effectiveness and Outcomes of Health Care Services: Implications for Nursing." It represented "a significant step toward gaining visibility before public and private policymakers for nursing's distinct contribution to patient outcomes," according to ANA President Lucille Joel, Ed.D., RN, F.A.A.N. (Fellow in American Academy of Nursing).[75] In a recent analysis of nursing practice research, all of the studies examined focused on nursing practice, which should rule out a long standing opinion that nursing practice phenomena are rarely studied by nurse researchers.[76,77] There appears to be a growing consensus about the "nature and focus of nursing as a practice discipline."[78]

According to Jane Norbeck, Dean of the School of Nursing at the University of California, San Francisco, the school has enhanced its support for faculty researchers in a variety of ways. For example, a pilot peer review project has been established for grant proposals to assure their accuracy and competitiveness. Linking research expertise available in the School of Nursing with clinical expertise located in the UCSF Medical Center should facilitate an increase in funding to support further research efforts.[79]

National Center for Nursing Research

With the establishment of the National Center for Nursing Research (NCNR) within the National Institute of Health (NIH) on April 18, 1986, nursing research ushered in a new era in the development of nursing science.[80,81] The center represents society's expectations that nursing is accountable for developing new knowledge for its practice. Research findings at the center are intended to promote high standards of nursing research and assist nurses in adding to the scientific base of their practice.

Under the direction of Ada Sue Hinshaw, Ph.D., RN, F.A.A.N., Director of NCNR, a conference was sponsored in 1988 entitled "Nursing

Resources and the Delivery of Patient Care." Nurse scientists addressed four primary research issues relevant to nursing resources (1) assuring the delivery of quality patient care, (2) developing strategies for allocating nursing resources, (3) identifying factors influencing retention of nursing staff, and (4) determining the influence of organizational structure and management on nursing resources.[82] Among other areas of research, they recommended further studies on outcomes of patient care and development of research models to enhance quality care.[83]

International Center for Nursing Scholarship

Another significant development in nursing's quest for scholarship was evidenced by Sigma Theta Tau International, the international nursing honorary society. On November 15, 1989 the International Center for Nursing Scholarship and Nursing Library was dedicated in Indianapolis as a part of its thirtieth Biennial Convention.[84] As a result of the vision and hard work of nurses, non-nurses, faculty and clinicians, individuals and organizations, the center stands as a testimony to all those who made contributions to this effort. The significance of nursing, nursing scholarship, and Sigma Theta Tau International is evident throughout the entire structure. Incoming president Billie J. Brown spoke about the society's future, pointing out that it will "continue to provide a broad slate of scholarly services to its 185,000 plus active members and ever growing roster of chapters (301)."[85] Later in her presidential address, Dr. Brown stated that "the Center for Nursing Scholarship is no longer a dream, it is a physical reality, and as we add additional facets, Sigma Theta Tau's International image will continue to change."[86]

Nurses should not lose sight of the ultimate significance of their collaborative efforts—*to ensure that the recipient of nursing care will receive the highest quality of care possible.* Acceptance of this challenge by professional nurses can be very demanding, but ultimately it can provide the greatest reward. The future of theory development for nursing appears bright, which indeed makes this an exciting time for nursing.

SUMMARY

The need for nursing to develop a scientific knowledge base has increased throughout the 1980s and into the 1990s. Several authors have been optimistic in believing that such a knowledge base will be forthcoming within the next decade or two. The public's image of nursing is, however, still that of the physician's handmaiden. That the public places less value on nursing's services compared to those of other health professions is delaying nursing's advance toward professionalism.

The need for nursing to make its contributions to health care known to the public so that its image may be improved is recognized by each of the professional organizations. Until such time as nursing can identify a distinct body of knowledge that will enhance its professional status and public image, nursing and nurses will have to increase their efforts to achieve this all-important goal.

The ANA document *Nursing: A Social Policy Statement* provides a clear definition of nursing's scope, including a description of the various phenomena of concern to nursing. Communicating this definition and focus of nursing should be the responsibility of all practicing nurses. The importance of research in the development of nursing knowledge and the need for improved communication, collaboration, and networking among nurse scholars are requisites for acquiring a sound knowledge base. Contributions of practicing nurses to the development of theory for practice, especially their active participation in research projects, are of significant value to nursing. Because the development of a scientific knowledge base is one means to move nursing rapidly ahead toward full professional status, practicing nurses should make every effort to cooperate with nurse researchers and theory builders, whose pioneering efforts will assist nursing to achieve this goal.

REFERENCES

1. Fuller, S. "Holistic Man and the Science and Practice of Nursing," *Nursing Outlook* 26:11 (November, 1978), 700–740.
2. Norris, C. "Toward a Science of Nursing," *Nursing Forum* 3:3 (1964), 10–11.
3. Schlotfeldt, R. "Nursing in the Future," *Nursing Outlook* 29:3 (May, 1981), 296.
4. *Ibid.*
5. Feldman, T. "Nursing Research in the 1980s: Issues and Implications," *Advances in Nursing Science* 3:1 (October, 1980), 85.
6. Kemp, V. "Themes in Theory Development," in N. Chaska (ed.), *The Nursing Profession: Turning Points.* St. Louis, C. V. Mosby, 1990, 613.
7. Corless, I. "Nursing Professionalization and Innovation," in M. Miller and B. Flynn (eds.), *Current Perspectives in Nursing.* St. Louis: C. V. Mosby, 1980, 143.
8. Goode, W. "The Librarian: From Occupation to Profession?" *The Library Quarterly* 21 (1961), 20.
9. Johnson, D. "Development of Theory: A Requisite for Nursing as a Primary Health Profession," *Nursing Research* 23:5 (September–October, 1974), 373.
10. Schlotfeldt, R. "On the Professional Status of Nursing," *Nursing Forum* 13:1 (1974), 25.

11. Conway, M. "Prescription for Professionalization," in N. Chaska (ed.), *The Nursing Profession: A Time to Speak.* New York: McGraw-Hill, 1983, 33.
12. Roy, S. "Theory Development in Nursing: Proposal For Direction," in N. Chaska (ed.), *The Nursing Profession: A Time to Speak.* New York: McGraw-Hill, 1983, 455.
13. Hughes, L. "The Public Image of the Nurse," *Advances in Nursing Science* 2:3 (April, 1980), 69.
14. Beletz, E. "Is Nursing's Public Image Up-to-Date?" *Nursing Outlook* 22:7 (July, 1974), 432.
15. Hughes, L. "Public Image," 55.
16. Kalisch, P., and Kalisch, B. "Perspective on Improving Nursing's Public Image," *Nursing and Health Care* 1 (1980), 138–164.
17. Kalisch, P., and Kalisch, B. "Reflections on a Television Image: The Nurses 1962–1965," *Nursing and Health Care* 2:5 (1981), 248–255.
18. Schlotfeldt, R. "On the Professional Status of Nursing," 27.
19. Goode, W. "The Librarian," 21.
20. Schlotfeldt, R. "Opportunity in the Decanal Role," in *The Decanal Role in Baccalaureate and Higher Degree Colleges of Nursing.* Bethesda, Md.: Dept. of Health, Education, and Welfare, Division of Nursing, 1975, 26.
21. "Image Makers: Richness in Diversity," Program for Twenty-seventh Biennial Convention of Sigma Theta Tau held in Boston, Mass., October 12–14, 1983.
22. Johnson, D. "Today's Action Will Determine Tomorrow's Nursing," *Nursing Outlook* 13:9 (September, 1965), 38.
23. *Ibid.,* 39.
24. Henderson, V. "The Nature of Nursing," *American Journal of Nursing* 64:8 (August, 1964), 62.
25. Schlotfeldt, R. "Planning for Progress," *Nursing Outlook* 21:2 (December, 1973), 766–768.
26. Schlotfeldt, R. "On the Professional Status of Nursing," 21.
27. Rogers, M. "Nursing: To Be or Not To Be," *Nursing Outlook* 20:1 (January, 1972), 43.
28. "Five Nurse Leaders Discuss Social Policy Statement," *American Nurse* 15:2 (February, 1983), 4.
29. Kritek, P., "Five Nurse Leaders Discuss Social Policy Statement," 4.
30. Christman, L., in "Five Nurse Leaders Discuss Social Policy Statement," 4.
31. Steel, J. "Statement Moves Us to Focus on What Nurses Fix," *American Nurse* 16:1 (January, 1984), 4, 21.
32. Ellis, R. "Conceptual Issues in Nursing," *Nursing Outlook* 30:7 (July–August, 1982), 406.
33. McCarty, P. "Meeting Explores New Focus, New Knowledge for Practice," *American Nurse* 16:1 (January, 1984), 1, 23.
34. Johnson, D. "The Nature of a Science of Nursing," *Nursing Outlook* 7:5 (May, 1959), 291.
35. Bilitski, J. "Nursing Science and the Laws of Health: The Test of Substance as a Step in the Process of Theory Development," *Advances in Nursing Science* 4:1 (October, 1981), 15.

36. Greene, J. "Science, Nursing, and Nursing Science: A Conceptual Analysis," *Advances in Nursing Science* 2:1 (October, 1979), 60.
37. Jacobs, M. and Huether, S. "Nursing Science: The Theory-Practice Linkage," *Advances in Nursing Science* 1:1 (October, 1978), 66.
38. Newman, M. "The Continuing Revolution: A History of Nursing Science," in N. Chaska (ed.), *The Nursing Profession: A Time to Speak.* New York: McGraw-Hill, 1983, 390.
39. Johnson, D. "Theory in Nursing: Borrowed and Unique," *Nursing Research* 17:3 (May–June, 1968), 206–209.
40. Gortner, S. "The History and Philosophy of Nursing Science and Research," *Advances in Nursing Science* 5:7 (January, 1983), 6.
41. *Ibid.,* 7.
42. Hardy, M. E. "Perspectives on Nursing Theory," *Advances in Nursing Science* 1:1 (October, 1978), 37–48.
43. Hardy, M. E. "Metaparadigms and Theory Development," in N. Chaska (ed.), *The Nursing Profession: A Time to Speak.* New York: McGraw-Hill, 1983.
44. Fawcett J. "The Relationship Between Theory and Research: A Double Helix," *Advances in Nursing Science* 1:1 (1978), 49–62.
45. Fawcett, J. *Analysis and Evaluation of Conceptual Models of Nursing.* Philadelphia: F. A. Davis Co., 1984.
46. Fawcett, J. "The Metaparadigm of Nursing: Present Status and Future Refinements." *Image: The Journal of Nursing Scholarship* 16:3 (Summer, 1984), 84.
47. Wald, F. and Leonard, N. "Toward Development of Nursing Practice Theory," *Nursing Research* 13 (Fall, 1964), 309–313.
48. Dickoff, J. and James, P. "Theory in a Practice Discipline," Part I, *Nursing Research* 17:6 (November–December, 1968), 421.
49. Dickoff, J. and James, P. "A Theory of Theories: A Position Paper," *Nursing Research* 17:3 (May–June, 1968), 31–37.
50. Diers, D. *Research in Nursing Practice.* Philadelphia: J. B. Lippincott, 1979.
51. Fawcett, J. "Contemporary Nursing Research: Its Relevance to Nursing Practice," in N. Chaska (ed.), *The Nursing Profession: A Time to Speak.* New York: McGraw-Hill, 1983.
52. Beckstrand, J. "The Notion of a Practice Theory and the Relationship of Scientific and Ethical Knowledge to Practice," *Research in Nursing and Health* 1:3 (1978), 131–136.
53. Johnson, D. *Nature of a Science,* 292.
54. *Ibid.*
55. *Ibid.,* 290.
56. *Ibid.*
57. Rogers, M. "Doctoral Education in Nursing," *Nursing Forum* 5:2 (1966), 76.
58. Rogers, M. "Nursing: To Be or Not To Be," 43.
59. Rogers, M. *Reveille in Nursing.* Philadelphia: F. A. Davis, 1964, 39.
60. McClure, M. "Promoting Practice-Based Research: A Critical Need," *Nursing Administration* 7:6 (November–December, 1981), 66.
61. *Ibid.*
62. Barnard, K. "'State of the Art' of Nursing Research," Keynote address at a

conference of the ANA Council of Nurse Researchers, entitled "Nursing Science: Today and Beyond," held in Minneapolis, September 22–24, 1983.

63. Johnson, J. "Nursing Research for the Future," Paper presented at a conference of the ANA Council of Nurse Researchers, entitled "Nursing Science: Today and Beyond," held in Minneapolis, September 22–24, 1983.

64. *Ibid.*

65. Fawcett, J. "On Development of a Scientific Community in Nursing," *Image: The Journal of Nursing Scholarship* 12:3 (October, 1980), 51–52.

66. Gortner, S. "Nursing Science in Transition," *Nursing Research* 29:3 (May–June, 1980), 180–183.

67. Lewis, E. "Report on the 1983 NLN Convention," *Nursing Outlook* 31:5 (September–October, 1983), 247.

68. "Conference Illustrates Nurses Working Together," *American Nurse* 15:1 (January, 1983), 3.

69. Downs, F. "Doctoral Education in Nursing: Future Directions," *Nursing Outlook* 26:1 (January, 1978), 60.

70. Rogers, M. "Nursing: To Be or Not To Be," 43.

71. Johnson, D. "Professional Practice in Nursing," in *The Shifting Scene—Directions for Practice.* Paper presented at the Twenty-third Conference of the Council of Member Agencies of the Department of Baccalaureate and Higher Degree Programs held in New York, May 6, 1967. New York: Dept. of B.H.D.P., National League for Nursing, 1967, 9.

72. Brown, E. *Nursing for the Future.* New York: Russell Sage Foundation, 1948, 198.

73. Nelson, L. and Cronin-Stubbs, D. "Mildred Kemp, Ph.D., R.N.: Researcher and Clinician," *CHART* 86:10 (November–December, 1989), 7, 17.

74. Maraldo, P. NLN *Executive Director Wire* (Spring, 1989), 4.

75. Meehan, J. "Leaders to Study Effective Care," *American Nurse* 22:5 (May, 1990), 9.

76. Moody, L., Wilson, M., Smyth, K., Schwartz, R., Tittle, M. and Van Cott, M. "Analysis of a Decade of Nursing Practice Research: 1977–1986," *Nursing Research* 37:6 (November–December, 1988), 374–379.

77. Fawcett, J. and Carino, C. "Hallmarks of Success in Nursing Practice," *Advances in Nursing Science* 11:4 (1989), 6.

78. Stevenson, J. "Research Programming: Past Successes and Future Needs," *Reflections* 15:3 (Fall, 1989), 6.

79. Holzemer, W. "Collaborative Directions," *Research Brochure, School of Nursing, UCSF, 1989–90.* San Francisco: University of California, 1989, 5.

80. Stevenson, J. "The Development of Nursing Knowledge" in N. Chaska (ed.), *The Nursing Profession: Turning Points.* St. Louis: C. V. Mosby, 1990, 605.

81. Jacox, A. "The Coming of Age of Nursing Research," *Nursing Outlook* 34:6 (November–December, 1986), 276–281.

82. "Report on Nursing Research Conference is Now Available," *American Nurse* 21:4 (April, 1989), 34.

83. *Ibid.*

84. "The Dedication," *Reflections* (Winter, 1989), 1.

85. *Ibid.*

86. Brown, B. "Sigma Theta Tau International Presidential Charge," *Reflections* 1 (Winter, 1989), 9.

SUGGESTED READINGS

Alexander, J. "How the Public Perceives Nurses and Their Education." *Nursing Outlook* 27:10 (October, 1979), 654–656.

Berkstrand, J. and McBride, A. "How to Form a Research Interest Group." *Nursing Outlook* 38:4 (July–August, 1990), 168–171.

Benner, P. "Uncovering the Knowledge Embedded in Clinical Practice." *Image: The Journal of Nursing Scholarship* 15:2 (Spring, 1983), 36–38.

Betz, C., Paster, E., Randell, B. and Omery, A. "Nursing Research Productivity in Clinical Settings." *Nursing Outlook* 38:4 (July–August, 1990), 180–182.

Chinn, P. and Jacobs, N. *Theory and Nursing.* St. Louis: C. V. Mosby, 1983.

Davis, M. "Promoting Nursing Research in the Clinical Setting." *Journal of Nursing Administration* 11:3 (March, 1981), 22–27.

Donnelly, G. "How to Break the Handmaiden Image," *Nursing Life* 1:3 (November–December, 1981), 50–53.

Downs, F. *A Source Book of Nursing Research,* 3d ed. Philadelphia: F. A. Davis, 1984.

Fawcett, J. "A Declaration of Nursing Independence: The Relation of Theory and Research to Nursing Practice," *Journal of Nursing Administration* 10:6 (June, 1980), 36–39.

Fawcett, J. "Hallmarks of Success in Nursing Theory Development," in P. Chinn (ed.), *Advances in Nursing Theory Development.* Rockville, Md.: Aspen Systems Corp., 1983.

Fawcett, J. "Another Look at Utilization of Nursing Research," *Image: The Journal of Nursing Scholarship* 16:2 (Spring, 1984), 59–62.

Fawcett, J. *Analysis and Evaluation of Conceptual Models of Nursing* 2d ed. Philadelphia: F. A. Davis Co., 1989.

Fitzpatrick, J. and Whall, A. (eds.), *Conceptual Models of Nursing: Analysis and Application.* Bowie, Md.: R. J. Brady, 1983.

Jennings, B. and Meleis, A. "Nursing Theory and Administrative Practice: Agenda for the 1990's," *Advances in Nursing Science* 10:3, 1988, 56–69.

Kalisch, B. and Kalisch, P. "Improving the Image of Nursing," *American Journal of Nursing* 83:1 (January, 1983), 48–52.

Kim, H. *The Nature of Theoretical Thinking in Nursing.* Norwalk, Conn.: Appleton-Century-Crofts, 1983.

King, I. *A Theory for Nursing: Systems, Concepts, Process.* New York: John Wiley and Sons, 1981.

Lindeman, C. "Role of Nursing Theory and Research in Advancing Practice," in R. Piemonte and I. Hirsch (eds.), *Issues in Professional Nursing Practice.* Kansas City, Mo.: The American Nurses' Association, 1984.

Mariano, C. "Qualitative Research." *Nursing and Health Care* 11:7 (September, 1990), 354–359.

Meleis, Afaf I. *Theoretical Nursing.* Philadelphia: J. B. Lippincott, 1985, 2d ed., 1991.

Meleis, A. "Revisions in Knowledge Development: A Passion for Substance," *Scholarly Inquiry for Nursing Practice: An International Journal* 1:1, 5–19.

Moccia, P. *New Approaches to Theory Development.* (Pub. no.: 15-1992), New York: National League for Nursing, 1986.

Research in Nursing: Toward a Science of Nursing. Kansas City, Mo.: American Nurses' Association, 1987.

Schorr, T. "It's Time to Make the Invisible Nurse Visible," *American Nurse* 16:9 (October, 1984), 4.

Walker, L. and Avant, K. *Strategies for Theory Construction in Nursing.* Norwalk, Conn.: Appleton-Century-Crofts, 1983.

Wilson, H. *Research in Nursing.* Menlo Park, Ca.: Addison-Wesley, 1985.

THE NURSING SHORTAGE

What Can Be Learned from the Nursing Shortage?

4

INTRODUCTION

The national nursing shortage of this past decade has made visible to the public and other professionals how important nurses are to the health and well-being of this nation. "The shortage is unlike any other in history—the country is demanding more nurses to provide increasingly technical, complex and cost-effective patient care, yet, fewer people are choosing nursing as an attractive career alternative."[1] According to Fagin and Moraldo,

> Major changes in health care delivery—high-technology treatment, cost controls, and an aging society—have made the need for knowledgeable, sophisticated, caring nurses more critical now than at any time in the profession's history. If the downturn in student interest continues, in ten years we will have a nursing shortage of dangerous proportions.[2]

If the vast array of health care providers and consumers were to submit their opinions about the nursing shortage, undoubtedly numerous responses and solutions would be readily forthcoming. Everyone agrees that quick-fix remedies will not suffice for the long-term. Nursing's history provides ample evidence of recurring shortages when emphasis is placed solely on short-term solutions to the problem. Will the nursing shortage issue ever be fully resolved? To answer this question, several related questions of continued concern need to be explored. For example, how did this acute shortage arise? What factors have contributed to it? What strategies are being used to overcome this dilemma? And how successful are the results?

The present nursing shortage, which is affecting health care both within and outside health care institutions, reached a severe level in 1983 and again in 1988. It continues to plague government officials, all sectors of the health field, and especially nursing—the chief provider of nursing services in hospitals, Health Maintenance Organizations (HMOs), nursing homes, and home health care agencies. In reviewing recent statistics on nursing personnel, it seems incredible that a shortage exists. Employed registered nurses numbered 1,627,035 in 1988 compared to 1,123,200 in 1978. These figures represent an 80 percent increase in contrast to 70 percent in 1977 and should dispel the myth that the nursing shortage is the result of nurses leaving the profession.[3] Interestingly enough, 50 percent of nurses were employed in hospital staff-level positions—more than two-thirds (69.7 percent) of employed registered nurses.[4,5]

The nursing shortage issue reflects society's demand for adequate health care. For example, "demand for registered nurses will rise by 38.9 percent by the end of the century, predicts the federal Labor Department [and this] agency forecasts that RN jobs will increase from 1,577,000 in 1988 to 2,190,000 in the year 2000."[6]

FACTORS AFFECTING SUPPLY AND DEMAND FOR NURSES

Several factors not prevalent in the 1960s and 1970s are influencing the rising demand for nurses in the marketplace and creating a need for nursing personnel for the chronically ill and elderly. Increased longevity of Americans and early discharge of patients from hospitals have increased the need for nursing personnel in nursing homes and rehabilitation centers and created an additional need for nurses in home health care services.

The acuity level of illness in hospitals as a result of complex medical technology has heightened the use of intensive care units, with patients frequently experiencing severe health crises and requiring sophisticated scientific knowledge and expert clinical skills. Moreover, as a result of the HIV virus epidemic and problems associated with drugs and alcohol abuse, an added strain has been placed on the health care personnel, particularly on nursing's over-worked labor force. Thus, the skill level and quantity of nursing care required has been substantially increased. One consequence has been an increase in the nursing intensity and workload, raising the demand for nursing personnel and the expression of concern about nursing shortages.[7]

HIV VIRUS EPIDEMIC—ITS IMPACT ON THE NURSING SHORTAGE

One factor among those just listed, Acquired Immunodeficiency Syndrome, more frequently referred to as AIDS, has reached a crisis stage. The causative agent of AIDS, human immunodeficiency virus (HIV) has infected one to two million Americans who are at risk for developing this devastating disease. The Centers for Disease Control note that "while the first 100,000 cases of AIDS took eight years to develop, the second 100,000 will come within the next twelve months."[8] They predict that 348,000 cases will occur over the next few years.[9, 10] Nursing continues to play a crucial role in providing support services for individuals with AIDS.

> Persons with AIDS, often young and facing death, confront the health care system with extraordinary physical, psychological and spiritual needs. Perhaps more than any other discipline, nursing has been challenged to meet these needs.[11]

Traditionally, nurses always have accepted the responsibility of providing care to persons needing their services. Individuals with the HIV virus are indeed a challenge to nursing since they motivate nurses to provide humane care and support to a population sorely in need of health care. According to a New York City professional nurse, nursing care is crucial for persons with HIV infection since "the intervention in AIDS is primarily nursing . . . AIDS care is nursing care."[12]

DEMAND VERSUS SUPPLY OF NURSE PERSONNEL

Unlike previous shortages caused by a shrinking supply of nurses, this shortage is the result of a steady increase in demand, which is projected to continue into the late 1990s. As a result of an imbalance between supply and demand, nurses tend to focus on increasing supply as a remedy for this severe problem. However, "continually increasing the supply of RNs is not the primary answer to the current shortage."[13] In fact, the established professions have tended to restrict supply in order to increase both income and status. However, "the shortage can be an opportunity for R.N.s to use the increased demand to advance the profession's standing to its appropriate place in the health care industry."[14] Eli Ginzberg, a noted economist at Columbia University reflects this same view.

> . . . any occupational group or profession frequently faces a simple dilemma: if it wants to improve the economic circumstances of its members, the sensible thing is to control its members. The medical profession, surely through the 1930s and later, followed such a policy.
> On the other hand, an inherent obligation of a profession is to respond to

the public's need for services. That frequently means increasing its numbers.

Therein lies [the] dilemma: the worst way to try to improve the economic returns to a group is to continue to increase the supply.[15]

In planning for the future of nursing personnel, a wide gap exists between supply and the requirements for active registered nurses. It is important to know not only the numbers of nurses but also their educational preparation as they fulfill their professional nursing responsibilities. Therefore, a criteria-based model was used by the Department of Health and Human Services in distinguishing the various types of educational programs for nurses.[16] Table 4-1 is a summary of the full-time equivalent supply and requirement projections for nurses. It indicates that by the year 2000, there will be approximately one-half as many nurses as needed with BSN, master's and doctoral degrees. Although the estimated supply of associate degree/diploma nurses is substantially higher than the requirements for the year 2000, these same supply and requirement figures are almost equal by the year 2020.

The greatest imbalance between supply and requirements occurs for registered nurses with baccalaureate and higher degrees. Baccalaureate graduates required are 43 percent higher than the estimated supply in the year 2000. Estimated requirements were almost three times higher than the supply by 2020. For nurses with master's and doctoral degrees, the estimated requirements were about three times higher than the estimated supply for all three years.[17]

Estimated requirements of nurse supply for the 21st century indicate that the numbers remain almost the same through the first decade. However, during the next ten year period the numbers are in reverse. As a

Table 4-1. Summary of full-time equivalent supply and requirement projections for licensed nursing personnel

	2000	2010	2020
Associate degree/diploma			
Supply	1,027,500	983,500	856,100
Requirements	586,000	794,000	855,300
Baccalaureate (BSN)			
Supply	596,600	656,500	635,500
Requirements	853,800	1,385,300	1,754,300
Master's and doctorate			
Supply	174,900	250,400	314,900
Requirements	377,100	531,800	822,200

Source: Sixth Report to the President and Congress on the Status of Health Personnel in the United States. U.S. Dept. of Health and Human Services. Division of Nursing Public Health Services, Health Resources & Services of Administration, Bureau of Health Professions, Pub. No. HRS-P-OD-88-1. Washington, DC, June, 1988 10-73.

result of fewer graduations and a substantial increase in the age of registered nurses, an estimated decrease in the over-all supply will occur.[18, 19] These long-range projections assist in determining what further steps should be taken to provide nursing personnel in adequate numbers and with qualifications to care for the health needs of the nation's population in a variety of health care settings.

THE DECLINE IN NURSING SCHOOL ENROLLMENTS IN THE 1980s

Although there were many factors contributing to a diminished supply of registered nurses, the drastic decline in overall nursing school enrollment in all basic RN programs (1984–1989) continues to have a serious impact on the overall nurse supply.[20] Over a five year period nursing student enrollments decreased to 182,947 in 1989 compared to 250,553 in 1983.[21] This steep decline of 67,606 nursing students cannot be overlooked. Moreover, a loss between 1983 and 1987 of 5,320 baccalaureate nursing students, from whom graduate nursing students are primarily drawn, can only contribute to a substantial decline in graduate enrollment. Thus, fewer master's degree graduates are available to fill the numerous positions created by demand for their services.[22]

A factor contributing to declining enrollments stems from a lack of interest in traditional women's professions, such as nursing and teaching. Some authors observe that the downward slope results from the women's movement, with its emphasis on seeking challenge in a variety of new fields not predominantly female.[23] The vast opening of career opportunities for women, particularly in law, medicine, dentistry, engineering, computer science programming, and government has created competition for qualified applicants. Furthermore the number of applicants is greatly decreased due to the so-called birth dearth occurring after 1964. Recent statistics on women enrolled in health field professions reveal that "in 1988–1989, the percentage of women enrolled in medical schools reached an all-time high of 35.1 percent . . . [and] . . . one-third of enrollees in dental schools are women, and schools of pharmacy and veterinary medicine have more female than male students."[24]

> Since 1972, the percentage of women physicians has doubled. The percentage of women lawyers and architects has nearly quadrupled. Nearly one third of computer scientists are women. Women make up 49.6 percent of accountants [and] about one-quarter of Wall Street's financial professionals are women.[25]

And yet, the fact that older age groups and more young people are college-bound has resulted in a less dramatic decline than would have otherwise occurred.

SURVEYS REVEAL REASONS
FOR NURSES' DISCONTENT

In the past three years, at least two surveys were conducted to determine what factors most influenced the work experience of practicing nurses. The most frequent responses revealed the following negative factors: inadequate compensation, wage compression, a lack of respect and public recognition from physicians and consumers for nurses' professional contributions, a lack of influence in decision making and policy formation, inflexible work hours, and undesirable schedules.[26] The latter two responses have been a great source of dissatisfaction among nurses in the practical setting. Inadequate compensation also rated high on the list, as nurses described the low pay rates and lack of adequate differential between registered nurses and ancillary personnel. Lesser benefits and higher insurance premiums are other definite trends affecting many staff nurses in hospitals.

Wage compression has been described as perhaps the most serious economic impediment to a career in nursing.[27] Minnick and others point out that wage compression ". . . the difference between average entry wage and average top wage was less than 27 percent" in two metropolitan cities.[28] Hay Management Consultants conducted a survey in 1989 by polling 370 hospitals employing 90,000 nurses. They found that the typical RN earned less than $2,000 more than a beginning nurse graduate.[29] The fact that nurses with ten and twenty years of experience could earn no more than $5,000 or $7,000 beyond a new graduate's salary has prevented many qualified nurses from remaining in the workplace. However, by the fall of 1989, some hospitals in the eastern part of the country had raised their differentials as high as $20,000 for nurses with thirty years of experience.

Mandatory overtime and floating to fill vacancies is a frequent occurrence in several hospitals throughout the country. Nurses dislike floating policies as continuity with their patients is disrupted and orientation to unfamiliar units is required. Mandatory overtime affects their personal life. Moreover, inadequate nurse-to-patient ratios were cited as contributing to nurse dissatisfaction.[30]

STRATEGIES TO REMEDY
THE NURSING SHORTAGE

Despite the severity of the nursing shortage as the 1990s progress, nursing is profiting from certain aspects that are an outgrowth of this problem. With demand for RNs continuing to outstrip the supply, various strategies and proposals have been implemented by government foundations, nursing, and medicine to remedy the imbalance.

Financial Support from Foundations

For example, several key foundations have provided generous grants to assist in alleviating this shortage. The Commonwealth Fund sponsored an interdisciplinary study that focused on hospital nurses and hospitals' decisions in order to provide insight and suggestions to hospital administrators and others on the shortage dilemma.[31] Responses from questionnaires mailed to hospitals (61 percent) and from random samples of registered nurses (51 percent or 15,000 RNs) provided ample information on reasons for and remedies to improve the shortage. An interesting finding in this study was the fact that professional practice issues were not given top priority, but rather salary and benefits, flexible schedules, and stress seemed to be of greater concern to practicing nurses.[32] In Chapter Twelve Maslow expounds on the fact that all humans are concerned primarily with basic physiological needs (housing, nutrition, etc.) that security (salary, benefits) can provide. When these needs are met, problems of achieving self-actualization, esteem, and autonomy can then be addressed. Interestingly enough in this study, significant differences were noted "between master's prepared staff nurses and nurses at all other levels of education; 35 percent of the master's prepared RN staff placed professional rewards first."[33] Is it possible that since nurses with graduate educational preparation are reimbursed at a higher economic level than nurses with less preparation, their security needs have already been met?

In December 1988, the Exxon Corporation awarded the American Nurses Association a $20,000 grant through the American Nurses Foundation to study the extent of the nurse shortage and recommend solutions to resolve the problem. Again in 1989, Exxon provided an additional $25,000 grant through the American Nurses Foundation to assist the ANA in completing a comprehensive study of the nursing shortage. The results of this study were made available in July 1990. According to Barbara Redmond, ANA Executive Director, "this study represents the most up-to-date and comprehensive source of information on the nursing shortage in addition to offering new solutions to resolve a national problem."[34]

The Independence Foundation of Philadelphia, established in 1961, donated $10.8 million in 1989 (the largest single foundation grant ever provided for nursing education) to nine of the top private nursing programs in the following universities: Cleveland's Case Western Reserve, Emory in Atlanta, Johns Hopkins in Baltimore, New York's NYU, Chicago's Rush, University of Pennsylvania in Philadelphia, University of Rochester in New York, Nashville's Vanderbilt, and Yale in New Haven.[35] The grant will endow an Independence Foundation Chair in nursing at each of these universities. Furthermore, an additional $200,000 complemented an existing scholarship program created by this foundation in 1988.

The Pew Charitable Trusts and the Robert Wood Johnson Foundation have funded a $27.8 million dollar project in 1989 for the purpose of restructuring the workplace for nursing services in eighty hospitals around the country. Each hospital was awarded $50,000 and a year later, twenty of the hospitals with the most promising plans received five year grants up to $1 million each to implement their designs.[36] Although 1,110 hospitals had applied for this grant, only twenty were awarded $1,000,000 nationwide over a five year period to restructure nursing roles. Mercy Hospital & Medical Center in Chicago was the only hospital in Illinois in 1990 to receive this coveted grant.

According to Marianne Araujo, vice president for Nursing and General Administration at Mercy, patient care will be improved by a bedside computer system that stores patient information, making it readily available to caregivers to enable them to make decisions and thus reduce professional time and assure more effective communications. "Computerization will be an essential communication linkage in the continuum of care that interfaces with physicians' offices and satellite settings, such as the home, community, or workplace."[37] Support from the Josiah Macy Foundation in 1989 enabled nursing to develop a program that guarantees the quality of nursing care. In addition, the Macy Foundation funded a proposal to create a National Board of Nursing Specialties.

Kellogg Funding for NCNIP

In 1984 the Tri-Council, which includes the National League for Nursing, the American Nurses' Association, the American Association of Colleges of Nursing, and the American Organization of Nurse Executives, received funds from the Kellogg Foundation to conduct the National Commission on Nursing Implementation Project (NCNIP). The main purpose of NCNIP—to help shape nursing's future by identifying trends and action to bring about this future—has engaged the members over a five-year period. Among these trends, identifying a coherent system of education models has been developed for restructuring nursing services more cost-efficiently and for developing nursing data systems.[38] The NCNIP raised over $500,000 for its National Nursing Image Campaign and expected nearly $20 million in contributed television, radio time, and newspaper space through efforts of the Advertising Council. This three year public service campaign conducted jointly by the NCNIP and the Advertising Council, was designed to make the nation aware of nursing's contribution, to improve the *image* of nursing as a rewarding career, and to highlight career opportunities for individuals opting for nursing as a profession.[39]

Additional Foundation Support

In 1989 the NLN received another generous $1.2 million grant from the Kellogg Foundation to "develop consumer-oriented outcome measures."[40] The purpose was "to incorporate these outcome measures into the NLN's Community Health Association Program (CHAP) and thereby enhance accreditation standards for home care providers [and ultimately to] improve the quality of care provided to patients in their homes."[41]

Nurses of America

A high priority on the agendas of nursing professional organizations is that of improving nursing's image. An additional $800,000 grant from the Pew Charitable Trusts to the Tri-Council funded a two-year nationwide multimedia public relations program designed to provide an accurate, up-dated image of professional nursing practice. The project entitled "Nurses of America" (NOA) was administered by the NLN. It emphasized four key nursing roles: health information specialists, case managers, expert bedside caregivers and specialists, and cost effective providers of choice.[42]

NOA is a national multi-media program aimed at both the broadcast and print media, and designed to keep the public informed about nursing's role in delivering high-quality, cost-effective health care services. According to NLN's Chief Executive Officer, Pamela J. Moraldo, "We have to make visible the many changes that have shaped contemporary nursing roles, place the issue of nursing's image on the public's agenda, and provide visibility for models that exemplify these contemporary roles and images."[43]

New Marketing Strategies to Improve Recruitment

In addition to efforts made to change nursing's public image, nursing schools are making serious changes in their methods of recruiting nursing students. Recruitment and retention programs of the 1960s and 1970s are no longer viable in the changing environment confronting nursing in the 1990s. As a result, flexibility in marketing techniques is no longer an *option* but is now a necessary requirement in all recruitment efforts.

Many nursing schools have developed more sophisticated marketing strategies to achieve success in their recruitment programs. In order to attract prospective nursing students, each school has used a variety of creative techniques and materials in communicating the excitement, rewards, and attractiveness of a nursing career choice. Pressure to lower admission requirements continues, but lowering admission standards can only be detrimental to consumers of health care and to nursing.

Decline in the traditional eighteen-year-old applicant pool has necessitated targeting mid-career and older applicants desirous of second careers, along with minority and low income groups and recent college graduates. Many nursing schools have increased efforts to provide remedial assistance for students experiencing academic difficulty in order to retain them in their programs. Launching work/study programs have enabled hospitals and nursing schools to meet their need for additional personnel. Several creative options for educational advancement are observed in nursing programs offering career ladder opportunities. Nursing students are allowed to demonstrate their knowledge, ability and skills without spending unnecessary time in fulfilling requirements of the more traditional programs. Financial assistance (loans, scholarships), proximity of school/home, weekend and evening classes, and flexibility in curriculum offerings and in scheduling clinical experiences, are additional ways to provide for nursing student needs.

REPORT OF THE HHS SECRETARY'S COMMISSION ON NURSING SHORTAGE

The HHS Secretary's Commission on Nursing, appointed in 1987 by the former Secretary of Health and Human Services, Otis Bowen, M.D., was formed to advise the Secretary on the extent of the nursing shortage and provide recommendations for appropriate responses to this problem. The Commission included representatives of ANA and other nursing organizations, medical and hospital associations, the insurance industry, and consumer groups—all experts in the field.[44] The ninety-nine-page report included sixteen major recommendations and eighty-one strategies for their achievement.[45] Table 4-2 lists the Commission's sixteen remedies for the shortage. "Presented in six major groups, the recommendations address utilization of nursing resources, nurse compensation, health care financing, nurse decision-making and the development and maintenance of nursing resources."[46] In reviewing these recommendations, it becomes readily apparent that economic and professional benefits in the work environment comprise more than eighty percent of the recommended items. The fact that the Commission was federally sponsored provided additional clout to these recommendations. The Commission finally concluded that without these necessary changes taking place, the nation's health will be at risk. The twenty-five-member Commission, chaired by Carolyne Davis, Ph.D., would have ceased functioning with the completion of its final report in December 1988. An extension allowed the Commission to remain viable until June 1989. Meanwhile, Congress budgeted $275,000 to retain the Federal Commission for an additional year, shifting its operative base to the National Center for Nursing Research in Washington, D.C.[47]

The Department of Health and Human Services established a new advisory Commission on the National Nursing Shortage on February 12, 1990, to "advise the U.S. Assistant Secretary for Health and the adminis-

Table 4-2. The commission's 16 remedies for the shortage

1. Providers should strengthen staff support to save the RN's time for patient care.
2. Staffing patterns should take account of RNs' different levels of education and experience.
3. Computers and other labor-saving technologies should be applied to support nursing.
4. To better manage nursing resources, providers, professional groups, and the government should track staffing, costs, and utilization.
5. Nurses' "relative wages" should be increased by a "targeted, one-time increase."
6. Government and private payers should reimburse at levels allowing for recruitment and retention of nurses.
7. Nursing should play a more active role in policy making in government, regulatory bodies, and employment settings.
8. Employers should ensure active nurse representation in governance.
9. Employers should foster collaboration among all health care providers.
10. Financial aid to students should increase.
11. Non-financial barriers to nursing education should be eliminated for nontraditional students and nurses seeking advanced degrees.
12. Schools should work with employers and state boards to ensure that curricula and clinical learning experiences are kept "relevant."
13. Nursing must actively promote "positive" images of the profession.
14. The Secretary's Commission on Nursing should be extended by at least five years.
15. Public and private groups should increase research in the factors influencing nursing supply and demand.
16. The federal government should develop the data neded to assess nursepower problems.

Source: Copyright 1989, American Journal of Nursing Company. Reproduced with permission from the *American Journal of Nursing,* February, Vol. 89, No. 2, 278.

trator of Health Resources and Services Administration on specific projects underway to meet the recommendations of the Secretary's Commission on Nursing."[48] Among several areas targeted were recruitment, retention, restructuring nursing services, data collection and analyses, and information systems. Caroline Burnett, Ph.D., RN, was chosen as the Executive Director for the new Commission.[49]

A conclusion drawn by Kramer in a second visit to Magnet Hospitals and another by Roundtree, consultant of the Hays Management Group, a top management consulting firm, was simply that shortages least affect those hospitals that emphasize nurses' professionalism.[50, 51] Roundtree predicted that the imbalance between supply and demand will continue for the next three to five year period. Kramer further observed that hospitals recognizing the professional autonomy and expert clinical practice of their nursing staffs were not experiencing a nursing shortage.[52, 53]

VAST IMPROVEMENTS
IN HOSPITAL WORKPLACE

Significant changes in the work environment for nurses have been occurring in the last two to three years. Development of more attractive working conditions for professional practice in hospitals is slowly occurring. Components are improved nurse to patient ratios, more opportunity for decision making in patient care, increased flexibility in scheduling, improved salaries and benefits with differentials included in salary structures, and other incentives. Everyone agrees that the best publicity campaign cannot overcome deficiencies in the workplace. Among other concerns, hospitals and nurse administrators must improve their management style in order to make hospitals and other health agencies more attractive places to work. "Burnout" is still occurring and will continue until drastic reforms in the workplace are implemented.

An example of improved salary structures occurred in New York City in 1990 with the new contracts negotiated with its unions. Substantive pay increases from $30,000 to $35,000 and continuing on to $42,000 are the starting salaries at Beth Israel Hospital.[54] Mandatory overtime for nurses with five years experience has been prohibited. A peer review based on staffing has also been implemented at Beth Israel. Salary structures have "simply not reflected the great and growing shortage of nurses . . . and the growing technical knowledge and responsibility that are required of nurses in acute-care hospitals today."[55] Beginning salaries of $40,000 will also be operative at Lenox Hill Hospital by 1992.[56] Table 4-3 indicates salary ranges in 14 metropolitan areas. Fortunately higher rates are beginning to reflect remarkable improvement.

AMA'S CREATION OF A
NEW HEALTH WORKER

Concern over the nursing shortage led the American Medical Association (AMA) to introduce a proposal to create the registered care technologist (RCT). People in this new category of "bedside caregiver" would be trained in hospitals in demonstration programs ranging from two to eight months to "carry out medical protocols."[57]

A basic RCT would be prepared to give 'low-tech care' in a 9-month program and would be licensed by state medical boards. Another nine months of training would certify an 'advanced' RCT to function in all types of critical-care units.[58]

Table 4-3. What staff RNs earn in 14 metropolitan areas

City	Range of starting rates reported	Range of top rates reported	Increase in CPI
Boston	$11.05–15.93 $22,984–33,134	$15.15–$26.93 $31,512–56,014	5.3%
New York	$13.70–15.87 $28,500–33,000	$16.10–21.39 $33,500–44,500	5.4%
Miami	$9.16–13.52 $19,053–28,122	$13.75–20.30 $28,579–42,224	4.1%
Atlanta	$10.34–12.00 $21,507–24,960	$15.00–18.50 $31,200–38,480	—
Houston	$9.05–15.02 $18,824–31,242	$12.05–19.90 $25,056–41,388	3.7%
St. Louis	$10.00–10.52 $20,800–21,882	$13.26–15.34 $27,581–31,904	6.1%
Chicago	$10.66–13.56 $22,173–28,205	$14.50–20.48 $30,160–42,598	5.2%
Milwaukee	$9.67–11.54 $20,114–24,003	$12.47–18.13 $25,938–27,710	—
Minneapolis/ St. Paul	$12.09–12.48 $25,147–25,958	$16.84–17.89 $35,023–37,003	—
Detroit	$10.34–13.82 $21,507–28,746	$11.37–18.38 $23,650–38,230	3.9%
Denver	$11.00–12.61 $22,880–26,289	$13.24–19.95 $27,539–41,496	—
Portland	$12.10–12.97 $25,168–26,978	$15.32–16.52 $31,866–34,362	—
San Francisco	$13.96–18.85 $29,037–39,208	$16.76–22.06 $34,861–45,885	5.0%
Los Angeles	$11.25–16.60 $23,400–34,524	$16.12–24.60 $33,528–51,168	5.1%

Note: The salaries found in AJN's October survey, based on a forty-hour week represent the range of base rates for new graduates and top rates for experienced RNs. (Differentials are excluded.) The Consumer Price Index changes are BLS estimates of price increases since mid-year 1988.

Source: Copyright 1989, American Journal of Nursing Company. Reproduced with permission from the *American Journal of Nursing,* December, Vol. 89, No. 2, 1675.

In an updated version, a third category of RCT was proposed: an assistant with two months preparation who could move up to the 'basic' level with seven months added training."[59]

The nursing shortage continues, but attempts to create a new type of health worker that could possibly imperil the welfare of patients was undesirable and unacceptable to organized nursing. In opposing this issue, nurses demonstrated a remarkable degree of unity and were unanimous in their opposition to the RCT proposal. The Association of Academic Health Centers and the American Hospital Association were among those who saw no justification for the AMA's plan. Interestingly enough, with numerous nursing and other groups fighting to prevent this move, the AMA, at its June 1990 delegates meeting in Chicago, agreed to cease its activities to pursue further the recruitment of possible RCT locations.[60]

NURSING SCHOOL ENROLLMENTS IMPROVE

Schools of nursing throughout the country experienced a turn-around in nursing enrollments after four years of decline. This improvement was due in part to the innovative recruitment programs and tremendous effort exerted in projecting nursing as an attractive, rewarding, career choice. Nursing schools have doubled their efforts to recruit minorities, men, and non-traditional students.

According to a survey conducted by the American Association of Colleges of Nursing (AACN) in the fall of 1989, enrollment in university and four-year college nursing programs rose by 5.8 percent in 1989–1990 (60,522 in 1990 compared to 57,154 in 1985).[61] There were increased numbers of RNs with hospital diplomas or two-year associate degrees seeking baccalaureate degrees (6,010 in 1989 compared to 4,151 in 1985) and increased numbers seeking master's degree nursing programs (8.2 percent above 1988—an overall increase of 16.5 percent over the past five years). Such statistics are very encouraging. Doctoral enrollment in 1989 was 9.2 percent above 1988, reflecting a five-year increase of 40.1 percent. Other findings of this survey indicate that nine new baccalaureate nursing programs, forty new master's and nineteen new doctoral nursing programs were in the planning stage.[62]

Shortage of Nurses Slowly Receding

Despite the improvement in nursing school enrollments, the shortage will not go away overnight. In fact, nurse administrators believe that the nursing shortage may very likely continue for another five to ten year period, nor is the end in sight. Their concern is that improvement in wages and in nursing student enrollments may provide a false security and thus encourage less effort to improve reward systems for practicing nurses and to actively recruit prospective nursing students for the future.

In retrospect, the nursing shortage has indeed been a gift to the nursing community.

Nursing has gained much in terms of public support, new infusions of funds, new opportunities to educate policy makers and the public about the value of quality nursing care to the health care delivery system and to society.[63]

SUMMARY

The national nursing shortage that surfaced in the 1980s and continues on into the 1990s has captured the attention of physicians, other health professionals, and the general public. Many agree that this particular shortage differs from previous ones. New factors, including the increase in the number of elderly and chronically ill, acuity of illness (particularly in hospitals), advanced technology, the HIV virus epidemic, and early patient discharge from hospitals, necessitating nursing home and client home care, among others, have placed undue pressure on nurses in their professional practice.

Decreased enrollments in schools of nursing have resulted from a declining interest in the traditional fields of nursing and teaching and from greater opportunities for women to enter professions such as medicine, law, dentistry, engineering. and government. The problem of retention of nurses in the workplace has been increased due to dissatisfaction with inflexible scheduling, wage depression, low salaries, and lack of autonomy and decision making. Generous funding from several foundations has enabled nursing to develop new programs to change the public's poor image of nursing and to attract prospective students to a nursing career.

Tremendous improvements in nursing school enrollments and in financial assistance are beginning to reverse the nursing shortage, although many in the health field believe this problem will not be solved in the foreseeable future. Ultimately, the nursing shortage has made the public realize the importance of quality health care. Legislators are also cooperating as they have a better knowledge of nursing's contribution to the health care of all citizens in this country.

REFERENCES

1. Selby, T. "Nurse-Supply, Demand Reach All-Time High," *American Nurse* 21:3 (March, 1989), 1.
2. Fagin, C. and Moraldo, P. "Feminism and the Nursing Shortage: Do Women Have a Chance?" *Nursing and Health Care* 9:7 (September, 1988), 367.
3. *Selected Findings from the 1988 National Sample of Registered Nurses.* Washington, D.C.: U.S. Department of Health and Human Services, Division of Nursing, Bureau of Health Professions, Health Resources and Services Administration. 1989, 1.
4. *Ibid.*, 2.

5. *Facts About Nursing, 1987.* Kansas City, Mo.: American Nurses' Association, 1987, 3.
6. "613,000 New RN Jobs Projected," Newscaps (ed.) *American Journal of Nursing* 90:7 (July, 1990), 74.
7. Seventh Report to the President and Congress on the Status of Health Personnel in the United States. U.S. Dept. of Health and Human Services, Division of Nursing, Public Health Services, Health Resources and Services Administration, Bureau of Health Professions, Washington, D.C.: (March, 1990), IV--C1.
8. "AIDS Cases Top 100,000 Will Double Next Year," *American Nurse* 21:8 (September, 1989), 2.
9. *Ibid.*
10. Smith, J. "Acquired Immunodeficiency Syndrome (AIDS): A Message for Nurses," (editorial) *Journal of Abnormal Nursing* 15:5 (May, 1990), 235–247.
11. Fauci, A. "Nurses Play Critical Role in Care of AIDS Patients," *American Nurse* 19:7 (July–August, 1987), 17.
12. Selby, T. "Nurses Rise to Challenge of AIDS Epidemic," *American Nurse* 21:6 (June, 1989), 1.
13. Rosenfeld, P. "Myth, Reality and the Nursing Shortage," *Nursing and Health Care* 9:7 (September, 1988), 1347.
14. *Ibid.*, 348.
15. Ginzberg, E. "Facing the Facts and Figures," Keynote Address for a conference entitled "Nurses For the Future: an Invitational Conference to Develop Strategies for Attracting the Best and the Brightest" in Philadelphia (sponsored by University of Pennsylvania School of Nursing and Pew Charitable Trust.) *American Journal of Nursing* 87:12 (December, 1987), 1597.
16. *Sixth Report to the President and Congress on the Status of Health Personnel in the United States.* U.S. Dept. of Health and Human Services, Division of Nursing, Public Health Services, Health Resources and Services Administration, Bureau of Health Professions, (Pub. No.: HRS-P-OD-88-1.) Washington, D.C.: (June, 1988), 10–75.
17. *Ibid.*
18. *Ibid.*
19. *Ibid.*
20. Division of Research. *Nursing Data Review, 1988.* New York: National League for Nursing, 1989, 31.
21. *Ibid.*
22. *Ibid.*
23. Donley, S. Rosemary and Flaherty, S.M.J. "Analysis of the Market-Driven Nursing Shortage," *Nursing and Health Care* 10:4 (April, 1989), 185.
24. *Seventh Report to the President and Congress on the Status of Health Personnel*, Washington, D.C.: U.S. Dept. of Health and Human Services, (March, 1990), 4.
25. Naisbett, J. and Aburdene, P. *Megatrends 2000: Ten New Directions for the 1990s.* New York: Morrow and Company, Inc., 1990, 224–225.
26. Minnick, A., Roberts, M., Curran, C. and Ginsberg, E. "What Do Nurses Want? Priorities for Action," *Nursing Outlook* 37:5 (September–October, 1989), 217.
27. Donley and Flaherty, "Analysis of the Market-Driven Nursing Shortage," 185.
28. "Study Sees RNs Still Gripped by Pay Compressions," *American Journal of Nursing* 90:3 (March, 1990), 93.

29. Minnick, A. *et al.* "What Do Nurses Want?" 217.
30. Kingsbury, A. "RNs Strive to Improve," *American Nurse* 22:3 (March, 1990), 17.
31. Minnick, A. *et al.* "What do Nurses Want?" 217.
32. *Ibid.*
33. *Ibid.*
34. Lichtman, D. "$25,000 Grant from Exxon Funds Study on the Shortage," *American Nurse* 22:3 (March, 1990), 32.
35. "Nine Schools to Share $10 Million," Newscaps (ed.), *American Journal of Nursing* 90:1 (January, 1990), 122.
36. "Million-Dollar Remodeling," Headline News (ed.), *American Journal of Nursing* 89:11 (November, 1989), 1429.
37. Copp, J. "With Grant, Mercy Hospital Hopes to Revolutionize Role of Its Nurses," *The New World* 98:46 (November 16, 1990), 3.
38. Cizmek, C. "Improve Nursing's Image Is ANA Priority," *American Nurse* 21:9 (October, 1989), 14.
39. *Ibid.*
40. Moraldo, P. "The Kellogg Grant to Develop Consumer-Oriented Measures," NLN *Executive Director's Wire* (Winter, 1989), 3.
41. *Ibid.*
42. Cizmek, C. "Improve Nursing's Image Is ANA Priority," 14.
43. Moraldo, P. "NLN To Administer $800,000 Project to Recast the Public's Image of Nursing," *Nursing and Health Care* 10:1 (January, 1989), 37.
44. Not Just Another Nursing Report. NLN Trends and Issues (ed.) *Nursing and Health Care* 10:1 (January, 1989), 11.
45. *Secretary's Commission on Nursing. Final Report, Vol. I.* Washington, D.C.: Dept. of Health and Human Services, Office of the Secretary, 1988.
46. Not Just Another Nursing Report, 11.
47. "RN Commission, Its Term Expired, Gets Reprieve," *American Journal of Nursing* 90:2 (February, 1990), 11.
48. Koeppen, C. "ANA Urges Move on Health Care," *American Nurse* 22:4 (April, 1990), 2.
49. *Ibid.*
50. *Magnet Hospitals: Attraction and Retention of Professional Nurses.* Kansas City, Mo.: American Nurses' Association, 1983.
51. Kramer, M. and Schmalenberg, C. "Magnet Hospitals Part I," *Journal of Nursing Administration* 8:1 (January, 1988), 13–24.
52. *Ibid.*
53. "Misuse of RNs Spurs Shortage, Says New Study; Only 26% of Time Is Spent in Professional Care," *American Journal of Nursing* 89:9 (September, 1989), 1223.
54. "New York City Nurses Win Record-Breaking Raises," *American Journal of Nursing* 90:3 (March, 1990), 93, 106.
55. *Ibid.*
56. *Ibid.*
57. "AMA Votes To Break a New 'Bedside Caregiver': 'Outraged' RN Groups Unite to Block the Plan," Newscaps (ed.), *American Journal of Nursing* 88:8 (August, 1988), 1131.
58. *Ibid.*

59. *Ibid.*
60. "Claiming 'Success,' AMA Members Vote to Abandon the RCT Idea," Newscaps (ed.) *American Journal of Nursing* 90:8 (August, 1990), 75.
61. "Enrollments Up Again in 1989–90," *American Nurse* 22:2 (February, 1990), 27.
62. *Ibid.*
63. Moraldo, P. NLN *Executive Director Wire* (April, 1988), 3.

SUGGESTED READINGS

Barrick, B. "Light at the End of a Decade," *American Journal of Nursing* 90:11 (November, 1990), 37–40.

Buerhaus, P. "Not Just Another Nursing Shortage." *Nursing Economics,* 5:6 (November–December, 1987), 267–279.

Current Statistics on AIDS (Statistics, Tables/Charts.) *Caring* 9:2 (February, 1990), 42.

Curtin, L. "A Shortage of Nurses: Traditional Approaches Won't Work This Time." *Nursing Management* 18:9 (September, 1987), 7–8.

Huey, J. and Hartley, S. "What Keeps Nurses in Nursing: 3,500 Nurses Tell Their Stories," *American Journal of Nursing* 88:2 (February, 1989), 181–188.

"Image Campaign Meets the Public." *American Nurse* 22:4 (April, 1990), 12.

Neros, "NLN's Exclusive Data Projects Nursing Shortage in 1990s," *Nursing and Health Care* 11:4 (April, 1990), 213.

Porter, R., Porter, M., and Lower, M. "Enhancing the Image of Nursing," Journal of Nursing Administration 19:2 (February, 1989), 36–40.

"RN Vacancies Hit 12.66% in '89, says AHA," *American Journal of Nursing* 90:11 (November, 1990), 11.

Selby, T. "RN Supply Still Below Demand," *American Nurse* 22:3 (March, 1990), 1.

Selby, T. "RN Shortage Threatens Quality of Care," *American Nurse* 19:3 (March, 1987), 1, 11.

The Nursing Shortage: Dilemmas and Solutions. Monograph Series, Kansas City, Mo.: American Nurses Association and American Organization of Nurse Executives, 1990.

The Nursing Shortage and the 1990s: Realities and Remedies. Kansas City, Mo.: American Nurses Association, 1990.

Thompson, D. "A Losing Battle with AIDS," *Time* 136:1 (July 2, 1990), 42–43.

Wilensky, G. "Economists Viewpoint: Nursing Shortage More Complex than It Seems," *Hospitals* 62:17 (September 5, 1988), 24.

Weinstein, S. *Restructuring the Work Load: Methods and Models to Address the Nursing Shortage.* Chicago: Center for Nursing, American Hospital Association, 1989.

CONTROL OF PROFESSIONAL NURSING EDUCATION

IV

Status of Nursing Education in the 1990s

5

INTRODUCTION

The present system of diversified nursing education continues to present a powerful challenge to the professionalization of nursing. Achieving consensus on a nationwide system of nursing education that would standardize preparation for each level of practice has yet to be accomplished. In fact, "nursing's lack of consensus on educational requirements makes it vulnerable to the encroachments of other professions."[1] Despite numerous reports and studies recommending baccalaureate preparation for professional nursing, conflict and tension continue to exist over this primary issue. Grass roots resistance to baccalaureate preparation for professional nurses divides nursing groups and postpones united action to move nursing forward as a full profession.

Nursing has been slow to move preparation for nursing practice into higher education. Lacking a unified system of education and a unique body of knowledge, nursing has experienced difficulty in joining with other health professions to influence health care. In comparing education for nursing with educational standards of the recognized professions, it is noted that nursing is one of few evolving professions that does not require a minimum of baccalaureate preparation for entry into practice. Actually, no other profession prepares its practitioners in the confused mixture of programs that presently describes nursing's educational system. Other professions, such as dentistry, law, theology, medicine, and clinical psychology, consider a doctoral degree essential for socializing their practitioners. A true colleague relationship cannot exist between physicians and nurses when nurses' academic preparation is at a much lower level. The discrepancy weakens nursing's influence as a collaborator with other health professionals. Unless educational preparation for nursing practice is at the same level as that of the medical profession, and equal to or better than the other major health professions, nursing will continue to remain dependent.[2]

Nursing has gained entry into institutions of higher learning and thus, is beginning to achieve recognition as a full profession. However, forward movement toward full professionalism will be delayed until the collectivity of nursing can reach agreement on future directions for preparation of its practitioners. Professional nurses should be socialized as learned individuals in institutions of higher education. The rich resources of the liberal arts foster the spirit of inquiry and the knowledge that is essential to professional practice. In viewing the dilemma that continues to exist over this issue, several pertinent questions are raised.

> Is nursing considered to be merely the execution of uncomplicated tasks, carried out at the direction of others and, therefore, looked upon as a vocation for which short-term technical training will suffice? Or is it that highly educated, knowledgeable, competent nurses pose threats to the stability of an entrenched health care system—a system judged to be inadequate? Perhaps the key factor is control; educated nurses cannot be controlled.[3]

Present efforts to upgrade nursing's educational system are viewed by "such forces as organized medicine and hospital administration . . . as potentially upsetting to the sensitive, economic and power bases in the health field and [they] have been blinded to the potential cost-effective health care benefits."[4]

Rozella Schlotfeldt asserts that to institute an appropriate system of nursing education, "only highly qualified professionals have the requisite competence to (1) explicate the subject matter of a discipline; (2) determine its scientific, humanistic, and ethical content; (3) identify its legitimate practice strategy; (4) direct its research; (5) identify its strengths and shortcomings; (6) decide the focus and scope of its services; and (7) determine the nature and preparation needed for professionals and their assisting personnel."[5] Since only highly qualified nurses have the competence to accomplish each of these responsibilities for nursing, it is hard to believe that other professions would consider themselves knowledgeable enough about nursing to dictate the contents of its educational programs.

Can you imagine members of any other professional field permitting others outside their profession to define the nature and scope of their practice? Or to accept decisions made by other than their own peers relative to the content, length, rigor, and pattern of education necessary to prepare generalist and specialist practitioners in their field of work?[6]

Sharing similar concerns, Martha Rogers pointed out as far back as 1964 that "integrity of professional education demands professional autonomy: in the determination of its theoretical content and the purposes for which its knowledge will be used; in the selection of its students and in the setting of standards by which the excellence of the educational program will be measured; in the definition of professional qualifications of its faculty and in the exercise of responsible, self-direction in meeting its obligations to society."[7] Rozella Schlotfeldt and Martha Rogers have emphasized the need for professional autonomy for qualified professionals entrusted with establishing nursing's educational system. The professional practitioner uses a specialized body of knowledge in practice and is capable of judging when to use it. If the body of knowledge and not just the practical skills the professionally educated nurse possesses is what makes nursing unique, then the nurse responsible for making decisions must be educated far differently than the nurse who simply follows orders.[8] Only in colleges and universities can this unique body of knowledge be acquired and the ability to develop it further increased.

NEED FOR TRANSFORMATION OF NURSING EDUCATION CURRICULA

Nursing students are seeking faculty who will transform nursing education. As a result, the challenge for nurse educators in this last decade of the twentieth century is to transform the nursing curriculum by seeking alternatives that emphasize the human aspects of nursing. The so-called curriculum revolution is the result of recognizing that present nursing programs are sorely in need of revision. Nursing should now consider new perspectives for dealing with problems of existing curriculum models and place caring as a core value in the new model. "Nurse educators are among those leading the call for change as we strive to maintain and enhance the quality of our programs; to explore ways to promote educational mobility while guaranteeing the integrity of our programs; . . . (and) to construct curricula that reflect new visions."[9]

At the NLN biennial convention in June 1989, a resolution on nursing education was passed unanimously, whereby innovative curricula were acknowledged that reflect, among other goals, "enhancement of caring practices through faculty-student relationships and faculty to faculty relationships that are . . . humane and characterized by cooperativeness."[10] This resolution is a "move away from content-driven curriculum to one that is a transaction among students, faculty, and the people who are participants in health care."[11]

According to Benner and Wrubel, "Caring as defined from a phenomenological perspective, is the most basic mode of being and is central to all helping professions. . . . Caring means that people, interpersonal concerns, and things matter."[12] In commenting on how the present health care system affects nursing curriculum, Watson points out that it:

> . . . operates within a structure which has to now be openly acknowledged as patriarchal. It is a system that 'treats' normal life processes as illness, and has no formal place for the basic health and human caring concerns of our nation's people.[13]

She continues on to state that:

> In the midst of all the debate about the future of nursing education, it is clear that (it) has historically failed in two significant ways. First, we educators have failed to address the issue of how to educate a person and have continued to prepare a first-level 'product' for institutions. Secondly, we have failed to address the issue of how to prepare educated nurses as full health care giving professionals and have focused instead on how to prepare students to be institutional employees.[14]

Watson believes that nursing schools will have "to reconsider many of the things they have traditionally done, (and among them, for example) fixating on entry into practice and a degree, rather than on how to educate thinking professional people in such a way as to prepare them for a full health and human caring role that is consistent with nursing's social, moral, and scientific mission to society."[15]

In order to consider this issue from another vantage point, it is interesting to note the views of another prominent educator. According to Margaret Newman:

> Nursing practice is riddled with the problem of mixed paradigms. The predominant paradigm, health as absence of disease, is enhanced by the medical model. The nursing model embraces a paradigm of dynamic patterning of relationships. It incorporates the feminine principles of caring, cooperation, collaboration, and mutuality. We have allowed our 'energy' to be dissipated in support of and in opposition to the medical paradigm. It is time to recognize the values and directions of the nursing paradigm and move into the reality of our professional responsibility.[16]

Again, as DeBack points out, "the changing health care environment will require nurses who are educated differently than nurses in the past . . . [and] increased use of technology and the changes already seen in the age and health status of clients will require curricula that teach broad life skills as well as sophisticated technical skills."[17]

Nurse educators are being challenged to assure nursing education's future by being on the alert for health care and market trends that encourage the designing of nursing curricula to meet the needs of students and the public. A question that nursing faculty should be asking is, "What are the trends that are reshaping nursing education at present?" Noticeable among them are the changing population from which nursing students are drawn and the way in which students learn. Many of today's students are adults having family responsibilities. They no longer solely represent eighteen-year-old high school graduates. Frequently they are in their thirties and forties. More minority students and males are also choosing nursing careers. Many people in these age groups enter nursing with advanced degrees in other disciplines. They have chosen nursing as a second or third career. As a result, they exert considerable influence in determining course locations and scheduling. Courses offered only on weekends, evenings, or in summers have been developing to meet student needs. These students usually opt for part-time study in order to maintain their current position, income, and lifestyles.

Success in educating nurses for the next century is occurring in nursing programs that provide multiple entrances and alternate tracks in achieving student goals. "Students of all ages will learn as much from employers, TV, and V.C.R.'s as they will on campus . . . [and] schools of nursing will be expected to prepare a new breed of nurses who are independent experts and capable professionals."[18]

PROFESSIONAL IDENTITY: THE GOAL OF SOCIALIZATION IN NURSING

According to Robert Merton, socialization is "the process by which people selectively acquire the values and attitudes, the interests, skills, and knowledge—in short, the culture current in the groups to which they are, or seek to become, a member. . . . "[19] *Professional* socialization is frequently defined as the practice whereby the values and roles of a profession are internalized through reinforcement by factors in the social environment. Being socialized into a professional role that frequently demands technical or interpersonal expertise can be very stressful. This is true whether the individual enters nursing directly from high school or after completion of another academic degree. Acquiring a professional identity by assuming the role of a professional tends to present conflicts for the neophyte nurse.

The ideal professional is one who becomes socialized and adjusted to the professional culture, which includes the values, norms, rituals, symbols, codes, and behaviors that guide the professional's activities. Through the process of socialization, students develop a self-concept associated with their profession. They acquire a new set of role expectations and behaviors, which indicate professional competence to those observing them. These new expectations reflect the rights and obligations of a profession aimed to assist students in acquiring a professional identity.

Some of the behavior that accompanies the "hierarchical, caste-like structure" of the medical profession is implicitly taught by isolation during the training period.[20] It is interesting to note that "three professions—the clergy, the military and medicine—almost isolate their recruits from important lay contact for several years, furnish new ego ideals and reference groups, impress upon the recruit his absolute social dependence upon the profession for his further advancement, and punish him for inappropriate attitudes or behavior."[21]

Unlike lawyers, ministers, or physicians who realize that their choice of such a career will allow them to become members of an *elite* profession, most nurses do not share this view of their career choice. In fact, many of them consider their nursing role only as a vocation or occupation, which in time can be replaced by marriage, family responsibilities, or another more challenging or satisfying career. It would be helpful for nursing students to be taught at an early period that professional nursing is changing rapidly and that preparation for full professional growth must not stop with the baccalaureate degree. Rather it can continue on to completion of the doctoral nursing degree. Moreover, nursing students should be aware that learning is a lifelong process extending over their entire career. By enlarging the socialization process for nursing students, so that they realize the opportunities and challenges the future holds for nurses with advanced preparation, many of them can develop a long-range outlook and plan for a career embodying such preparation. The faculty has the responsibility of socializing nursing students early in their education to view nursing as a lifetime commitment and inculcating a strong professional identity in students as they commence their educational program.

There is a tendency for students in professional schools to adopt attitudes and values similar to those of the faculty in their institution.[22] The role of faculty in student-faculty contacts is extremely important.

> Our students watch us very closely . . . anything a student learns about us . . . stands a chance of being incorporated into the student's value system.
> This . . . is the challenge for faculty and professional socialization. Pro-

grams, curricula and clinical experience are obviously important but the individual teacher is the critical element.[23]

Success in assisting students "to develop a professional identity" partially depends on the extent to which faculty has internalized the profession's values.[24] Many faculty members exert considerable energy through role modeling and exhortations to students about the values and professional system of nursing. Inducing new members with such ideology stimulates socialization of students and assists them in being assimilated into the occupational group.

In a study by J. Colombotos of the social origins and ideology of physicians, the major theme stressed was the impact made on students' attitudes and behavior by the medical schools.[25] There are profound changes occurring in students during their four years of medical school, but their appearance becomes very similar by the end of that period.[26] Although many of these students are not given opportunities for autonomous practice, they do absorb the elitism of their profession. Upon graduating they assume all of the distinctiveness and autonomy that is the hallmark of every true professional.

In nursing, autonomy is missing from much of professional practice. Until nursing students are allowed to function autonomously, their professional socialization process will be incomplete. Dissatisfaction and withdrawal from nursing will continue to be the pattern that many of them choose to follow.

Marlene Kramer conducted a well-known study of the "reality shock" that new baccalaureate nursing students experienced. A program provided early in the professional socialization process was made available to students to introduce the "professional-bureaucratic conflicts and role strategies to combat such conflicts."[27] Such preparation helped address this difficult problem. In a later publication, she stressed the need for a sound professional socialization process that would assist nurses to adhere to professional values and norms. Nurses would then have the ability to deal successfully with the bureaucracy prevalent in the employment setting.[28]

CRITICAL ISSUES IN NURSING'S SYSTEM OF EDUCATION

In order to meet the needs of society for professional nursing practice, nursing must have an abundant supply of highly qualified nurse specialists, generalists, and technicians. Although there has been a tremendous increase in the number of nurse technicians and practical nurses over the last decade, a severe shortage of university-prepared nurse professionals continues to prevent nursing from adequately fulfilling its obligations to society. This is only one of several issues confronting nursing that must be resolved if full professional status is ultimately to be achieved. To fully understand this and related issues, it is helpful to review statistics on the number and types of educational programs and their admissions and graduations. Some interesting observations can be made by reviewing Table 5-1. It is interesting to note how nursing rapidly increased the number of its schools while medical schools remained relatively stable in number.

For example, over a forty-six year period (1880–1926) the number of nursing schools increased from fifteen to 2,155 and the number of graduates increased from 157 to 17,522. From 1880 to 1900 medical schools increased from 100 to 160. But due to the influence of the Flexner Report, which moved medical education into the university and closed proprietary schools, the number of medical schools decreased to seventy-nine by 1926. "From 1900 to 1930, the number of physicians per 100,000 population declined and then remained essentially unchanged until 1970, when increases in numbers and gender occurred."[29–31]

"Moreover, compared to the controlled number of physicians, the number of registered nurses per 100,000 population in 1970 revealed a three and one half time increase over figures in 1920."[32, 33] Nursing increased its numbers primarily to provide service to the hospitals operating the 2,155 diploma schools. Meanwhile, medicine forth-rightly moved in the opposite direction, which has kept its supply far less than the demand and the economic rewards substantially greater than for most professions. Although monetary compensation for its services is of concern to nursing, it has not blurred the current ideal of service and is a reason for society viewing nursing as contributing a needed service.

A significant moment in nursing education occurred in 1909, when the first collegiate school of nursing in the United States was

Table 5-1. Medical and nursing schools: number of graduates, 1880–1926

Year	Medical schools	Nursing schools	Medical graduates	Nursing graduates
1880	100	15	3,241	157
1890	133	35	4,454	471
1900	160	432	5,214	3,456
1910	131	1,129	4,440	8,140
1920	85	1,775	3,047	14,980
1926	79	2,155	3,962	17,522

Source: Burgess, M.A. *Nurses, Patients, and Pocketbooks*, New York: Committee on the Grading of Nursing Schools, 1928, 35.

established at the University of Minnesota. Another important development was the establishment of the first independent school for professional nursing at Yale University in 1923, which accepted arts and science graduates as enrollees in nursing. Associate degree programs, begun in 1952, increased from eight that year to 174 by 1965, whereas diploma programs decreased from 1,032 to 821 during the same period. Although the growth of collegiate schools of nursing did continue at a slow pace, the number of baccalaureate programs increased from 135 in 1952 to 210 by 1966.[34] In 1960, there were 1,114 programs preparing for RN licensure.

Table 5-2 presents information on the number of basic RN programs from 1969–1988. An examination of its data reveals that from 1969–1979, the number of nursing programs increased from 1,324 to 1,374. By the fall of 1983, the number had increased to 1,466, plus two generic master's and one generic doctoral program.[35] However, by 1988, the total number of nursing programs decreased from 1,466 to 1,442, plus six generic master's and one generic doctoral program.[36] By 1982 there were 1,319 programs preparing for Practical Nurse licensure. By 1984 this number decreased to 1,280.[37]

By type of basic RN program, Table 5-2 reveals that from 1969 to 1979, baccalaureate programs increased from 252 to 363. The number of associate degree programs increased from 384 to 678. The number of diploma programs decreased from 688 to 333. Although nursing education was centered in hospital diploma programs for many years, for the first time in 1972, more nurses graduated from collegiate schools of nursing than from hospital diploma programs. By 1989, the number of baccalaureate and associate degree programs had increased to 479 and 792 respectively, but diploma programs had decreased from 333 to 171. From 1969 to 1988, 517 diploma programs had closed.[38]

From all of this statistical data on basic pre-service nursing programs it appears that associate degree programs are rising at a phenomenal rate, that diploma programs have experienced a severe decline but are showing some increase, and that baccalaureate nursing programs are increasing, but not with the rapidity of the associate degree programs. Although diploma programs have experienced a serious decline in numbers, the increase in associate degree and baccalaureate programs has offset this decline. In the fall of 1982, there were 154 master's programs and twenty-five doctoral programs being conducted in nursing schools as compared to 213 master's degree programs, six generic masters and forty-eight doctoral programs plus one generic doctoral program in 1989.[39]

Table 5-3 presents information on the number of admissions to basic programs preparing for RN licensure from 1968–1969 to 1987–1988. In reviewing Table 5-3, it is readily observed that there has been a tremendous increase in the annual admissions to all basic RN programs (63,408 in 1968–1969 to 94,269 in 1987–1988). Again, it is noteworthy that bacca-

Table 5-2. Basic RN programs and percentage change from previous year, by type of program: 1969 to 1988[a]

Year	Number of schools	All basic RN programs		Baccalaureate programs		Associate degree programs		Diploma programs	
		Number of programs	Percent change	Number of programs	Percent change	Number of programs	Percent change	Number of programs	Percent change
1969	1,313	1,324	+3.6	252	+8.2	384	+18.5	688	-4.6
1970	1,330	1,340	+1.2	267	+6.0	437	+13.8	636	-7.6
1971	1,338	1,349	+0.7	282	+5.6	484	+10.8	583	-8.3
1972	1,350	1,362	+1.0	290	+2.8	532	+9.9	540	-7.4
1973	1,348	1,360	-0.1	302	+4.1	565	+6.2	493	-8.7
1974	1,347	1,358	-0.1	310	+2.6	588	+4.1	460	-6.7
1975	1,349	1,362	+0.3	326	+5.2	608	+3.4	428	-7.0
1976	1,337	1,358	-0.3	336	+3.1	632	+3.9	390	-8.9
1977	1,339	1,356	-0.1	344	+2.4	645	+2.1	367	-5.9
1978	1,340	1,358	+0.1	348	+1.2	666	+3.3	344	-6.3
1979	1,354	1,374	+1.2	363	+4.3	678	+1.8	333	-3.2
1980	1,360	1,385	+0.8	377	+3.9	697	+2.8	311	-6.6
1981	1,377	1,401	+1.2	383	+1.6	715	+2.6	303	-2.6
1982	1,406	1,432	+2.2	402	+5.0	742	+3.8	288	-5.0
1983	1,432	1,466	+2.4	421	+4.7	764	+3.0	281	-2.4
1984	1,445	1,477	+0.8	427	+1.4	777	+1.7	273	-2.8
1985	1,434	1,473	-0.2	441	+3.3	776	-0.1	256	-6.2
1986	1,426	1,469	-0.3	455	+3.2	776	0.0	238	-7.0
1987	1,406	1,465	-0.3	467	+2.6	789	+1.7	209	-12.2
1988	1,391	1,442	-1.6	479	+2.6	792	+0.3	171	-18.7

[a]Excludes American Samoa, Guam, Puerto Rico, and the Virgin Islands.

From *Nursing Student Census 1989*. Division of Research, (Pub. No. 19–2291). New York: National League for Nursing, Copyright 1989, 6. Reproduced with permission of publisher.

Table 5-3. Annual admissions to basic RN programs and percentage of change from previous year, by type of program: 1968–69 to 1987–88[a]

Academic year	All basic RN programs		Baccalaureate programs		Associate degree programs		Diploma programs	
	Number of admissions	Percent change	Number of admissions	Percent change	Number of admissions	Percent change	Number of admissions	Percent change
1968–69	63,408	+4.5	15,901	+7.3	18,536	+27.2	28,571	−7.4
1969–70	74,598	+17.6	18,942	+19.1	25,142	+35.6	30,514	+5.3
1970–71	78,524	+5.3	20,299	+7.2	29,433	+17.1	28,792	−5.6
1971–72	93,344	+18.9	27,228	+34.1	36,454	+23.8	29,662	+3.0
1972–73	103,789	+11.2	30,348	+11.5	43,733	+20.0	29,708	+0.1
1973–74	107,344	+3.4	32,461	+7.0	47,940	+9.6	26,943	−9.3
1974–75	109,020	+1.6	34,956	+7.7	49,368	+3.0	24,696	−8.3
1975–76	112,174	+2.9	36,320	+3.9	52,232	+5.8	23,622	−4.3
1976–77	112,523	+0.3	36,670	+1.0	53,610	+2.6	22,243	−5.8
1977–78	110,950	−1.4	37,348	+1.8	52,991	−1.1	20,611	−7.3
1978–79	107,476	−3.2	35,611	−4.7	53,366	+0.7	18,499	−10.2
1979–80	105,952	−1.4	35,414	−0.5	53,633	+8.5	16,905	−8.6
1980–81	110,201	+4.0	35,808	+1.1	56,899	+6.1	17,494	+3.5
1981–82	115,279	+4.6	35,928	+0.3	60,423	+6.1	18,928	+8.1
1982–83	120,579	+4.6	37,264	+3.7	63,947	+5.8	19,368	+2.3
1983–84	123,824	+2.7	39,400	+5.7	66,576	+4.1	17,848	−7.8
1984–85	118,224	−4.5	39,573	+0.4	63,776	−4.2	14,875	−16.7
1985–86	100,791	−14.7	34,310	−13.3	56,635	−11.2	9,845	−33.0
1986–87	90,693	−10.0	28,026	−18.3	54,330	−4.1	8,337	−15.3
1987–88	94,269	+3.9	28,505	+1.7	57,375	+5.6	8,389	+0.6

[a]Excludes American Samoa, Guam, Puerto Rico, and the Virgin Islands.

From *Nursing Student Census 1989*. Division of Research, (Pub. No. 19–2291). New York: National League for Nursing, Copyright 1989, 26. Reproduced with permission of publisher.

laureate admissions increased while diploma programs decreased. However, the greatest increase in admissions occurred in associate degree programs over a nineteen-year period (18,536 in 1968–1969 to 57,375 in 1987–1988). According to NLN data, in 1989 enrollments in nursing schools increased 8.9 percent, which reflects some optimism for the future. Diploma programs were up 8 percent; associate degree programs increased 11 percent; and baccalaureate programs noted a 6 percent increase. However, poor utilization of nurses continues to be the root cause of the nursing shortage. Increasing the supply cannot be considered a remedy, but rather as an effort to use nurses more effectively in the workplace.[40]

In 1982, a total of 17,085 students were enrolled in master's degree programs and 1,342 in doctoral programs. Of this number, 6,389 (37.4 percent) were full-time master's students, and 655 (48.8 percent) were full-time doctoral students.[41] The fact that the remaining 10,041 (13.8 percent) were part-time students indicated that a time lapse occurred before this vast number of graduate students were available to increase the number of nurse leaders desperately needed. By 1989, 22,157 students were enrolled in master's degree programs and 2,364 doctoral students were enrolled with twenty-seven percent full-time masters students and four percent full-time doctoral students.[42] In viewing the increased numbers of enrollees in nursing programs in 1974, the following observations regarding the control of nursing personnel are of interest:

> Nurse educators have characteristically acted to recruit and to produce increasing numbers of personnel without thoughtful establishment of policy guides concerning the number of nurse professionals, nursing technicians, and nursing assistants actually needed.
>
> The nursing profession urgently needs to address the question of how numbers of nursing personnel can and should be controlled through regulating inputs at the point of admissions into all types of nursing education programs. The well-recognized over-production of assisting and technical personnel and the relative paucity of professionals support this recommendation. The highest quality training and research are being shortchanged in the interest of continued production of large and increasing numbers of personnel trained at lower levels of sophistication.[43]

Almost twenty years have elapsed since this admonition was made, but as in the past, little thought or action has been addressed to the possibility of controlling numbers and proportions of nursing personnel.

During the decade 1969 to 1979 annual nurse graduations from programs preparing for state nursing licensure almost doubled, from 41,801 to 77,132.[44] By 1983, graduations totaled 80,312; and in 1985 totals were 82,075.[45] By 1987, the total number had decreased to 70,561. In 1978–1979 there were 4,621 master's graduations and by 1984–1985, 5,247 master's degrees graduations.[46]

From 1969 to 1973, nurse doctorates increased from 504 to 1,020, but the latter number represented only 0.12% of the 815,000 registered nurses employed in nursing.[47] However, an increase of 826 doctorates from 1973 to 1981 indicated the growing professionalism of nurses and their efforts to achieve professional status. There were 5,193 master's and 137 doctoral graduations in 1981–1982. By 1989, there were 5,558 master's and 320 doctoral graduations, plus forty-eight graduations from generic masters and fifty-two from doctoral programs.[48] Statistics on highest educational preparation of all employed registered nurses from 1980 to 1987 are presented in Table 5-4.

> Among the registered nurse population in March, 1988, who had graduated from initial nursing education programs within the last 5 years, 15 percent were from diploma programs and 53 percent from associate degree programs . . . [and] as of March, 1988, about 821,000 registered nurses have diplomas as their highest nursing education, 512,000, associate degrees, and 557,000, baccalaureate degrees. About 125,000 have nursing or nursing-related master's degrees and 5,400, doctorates [0.26%].[49]

The data on employed, registered nurses reveal the dearth of leadership personnel at the baccalaureate and graduate level and the high percentage of registered nurses with less than a baccalaureate degree.

VARIATIONS IN BASIC NURSING EDUCATION PROGRAMS

On a more encouraging note, Martha Rogers observed in 1964 that "in spite of opposition and harassment on the part of vested interest groups and advocates of the status quo the education of nurses is moving rapidly

Table 5-4. Estimated active supply of registered nurses by educational preparation 1980–1987

Year	Nurses with less than baccalaureate degree		Nurses with baccalaureate in nursing		Nurses with master's and above		Total
	Number	*Percent*	*Number*	*Percent*	*Number*	*Percent*	
1980*	900,562	70.7	297,300	23.4	68,192	5.9	1,272,851
1983†	977,200	69.6	347,100	24.7	79,900	5.7	1,404,200
1985†	1,024,500	66.5	419,900	27.2	93,700	6.3	1,538,100
1987†	1,054,300	64.8	468,860	28.8	103,810	6.4	1,624,000

*Modified from *Facts about Nursing* 1982–1983, 1986–1987, 1988–1989. Kansas City, Mo.: American Nurses' Association 1983, 1987, 1989, 5, 3.
†Division of Nursing, Bureau of Health Professions. Health Resources and Services Administration, Department of Health and Human Services, Washington, D.C., 1989.

and inexorably into the framework of America's educational system."[50] Almost thirty years later, the pace at which education of nurses has moved into colleges and universities is gratifying. But there is much work to be done before a standardized educational system is accomplished.

Among the 1,455 basic nursing schools, the traditional hospital school that offers a three- or two-year diploma program continues, despite the large numbers of programs that have closed in recent years. Approximately 517 diploma programs closed their doors between 1969 and 1988.[51] Massachusetts General Hospital's diploma program in Boston, one of the oldest nursing schools in the United States, graduated its last class in June 1980. However, the increase in diploma program enrollments that occurred in 1989 may continue in the future. With fewer hospital diploma programs offered, associate degree education for nurses has been quite firmly established.

Interestingly enough, some associate degree educators are critical of those in their ranks who prepare students at one extreme merely to move on to senior colleges and who at the other extreme offer mini-B.S.N. programs.[52] This trend concerns many nurse leaders, as the following statement confirms:

> Many A.D.N. [Associate Degree Nursing] programs have tried to be or become all things to all people; they have included leadership, public health nursing content, and other content irrelevant to technical nursing in an effort to become mini-baccalaureate programs. In so doing, they have lost sight of their primary mission and goal—to prepare warm, sensitive, caring nurse technicians who are skilled and competent in the care giver function.[53]

In technical nursing education, the product of the nurse technician's performance is care, and skills are what make the goal of care achievable.[54]

Mildred Montag, the originator of Associate Degree Nursing programs, observes that in viewing present A.D.N. curricula, it appears that the philosophy underlying the concept of this type of program "is now either unknown, unaccepted, or ignored."[55] She refers to two basic premises on which the associate degree program was developed:

1. That the functions of nursing can and should be differentiated,
2. That these functions lie along a continuum with professional at one end and technical at the other.

> If the functions can be differentiated, then it follows that the two kinds of workers should be prepared differently for the two kinds of functions— hence two programs, one professional and one technical.[56]

Presently, resistance continues in associate degree programs about using the term "technician." Some diploma and associate degree educators and graduates of these programs believe that professional status is conferred upon receiving an RN license. Thus, it is not surprising that the public is confused over the variety of basic nursing education programs (one year practical, two year associate degree, three year diploma, four or five year baccalaureate). Even some employers are uncertain as to the expected levels of performance. Many nurses attribute this confusion to the fact that despite four levels of nursing education programs, only two levels of nursing practice for licensure exist—licensed practical nurse and registered nurse. "Quite obviously an examination which is valid for students prepared as professionals cannot also be valid for students prepared as technologists, and the converse is also true."[57]

The question of what constitutes professional education as compared to technical education is an issue still dividing many nurse educators. Professional nursing education is offered only in senior colleges and universities. It provides knowledge from the biological and social sciences, humanities, and nursing and allows for self-enrichment, the creative use of knowledge in decision making, and the implementation of skills in practice. Controversy over what constitutes adequate competencies for professional and technical education still remains a source of heated debate among many nurse educators. A set of characteristics for each level, acceptable to most nurses, has been made available by the national nursing organizations.[58, 59]

In observing how baccalaureate degree graduates function in health care delivery, it has been conjectured that until basic attitudes toward employment reflect major changes, nurses with less than a master's degree will continue to be an unstable work group, noticeable for their high turnover and lack of commitment.[60] However, in future health care delivery, the baccalaureate graduate with additional experience and level of maturity should be able to function as a professional in nursing practice. The reality of preparing baccalaureate students for hospital nursing as generalists is questionable because the demands of health care institutions for technicians outweigh their need for generalists in nursing practice.[61]

Several selected issues related to basic nursing education programs warrant a more in-depth presentation. Evidence continues to mount that there are still many unresolved issues regarding undergraduate nursing education. More and more, nurse educators are concluding that the baccalaureate degree is inadequate due to the increased demands of the health care delivery system. "Nursing has found multiple educational pathways costly, inefficient, out of the mainstream of higher education, and not conducive to career mobility."[62] For some time, nurse educators have recognized that professional nursing education with its generalist preparation no longer belongs at the baccalaureate level. "The economic pressures of the marketplace demand an educational system that prepares nurses for an increasingly complex environment."[63]

To meet the growing demand for nurses prepared beyond the baccalaureate level, a trend is emerging that indicates that post-baccalaureate nursing degrees are increasing and may become the first professional degree in nursing. "Nurse educators are beginning to focus on the increasing need for a sound foundation in the liberal arts before pursuing graduate study."[64-66] Duffy is of the opinion that "all professions involved in caring for people begin their professional preparation at the post-baccalaureate level, except for nursing."[67]

Nontraditional nursing programs, referred to as combined or accelerated, appear to be on the increase.[68-70] Non-nurses have been admitted to master's programs (MSN) that combine generalist and advanced nursing content as preparation for entry into practice at the following schools: Pace University, New York; Yale University in New Haven, Connecticut; University of Tennessee at Knoxville; and Massachusetts General Institute in Boston, Massachusetts. Moreover, several university nursing programs have offered a master's in nursing degree program for graduates of associate degree and diploma programs and for those having bachelor's degrees in other disciplines.[71]

NURSE PRACTITIONER PROGRAMS

Henry Silver and Loretta Ford were pioneers in the nurse practitioner movement. These former faculty members in the schools of medicine and nursing at the University of Colorado initiated a twenty-four-month pediatric nurse practitioner program in 1965. This program had as its goal testing and expanding the scope of practice for professional nurses who held a baccalaureate degree in nursing and who were eligible for admission to the graduate nursing program at the University of Colorado.[72] Since the beginning of this movement, over 20,000 nurse practitioners have been prepared in specialties that include family, geriatric, community, maternity, and pediatric practice. Functioning under protocols acquired by state law, nurse practitioners perform physical examinations, conduct certain laboratory tests, make nursing diagnoses, and prescribe medications. An additional function is that of health promotion, wherein they counsel clients about the importance of staying well.

Since the early 1970s, thirty-eight states have amended laws to allow nurse practitioners to carry out functions previously barred to them by medical practice acts.[73] As a result of such amendments in nurse and physician practice acts, acceptance of nurse practitioners has been accelerated.

Educational requirements for the preparation of nurse practitioners have been very confusing for a number of reasons. For example, the length of these programs has ranged from six weeks to two years. However, eligibility for federal funds now requires practitioner programs to be a minimum of one year in length. After strong recommendations from the ANA, many of these programs are located in universities and award a master's degree upon completion.

According to the third national study of nurse practitioners conducted by the School of Health Related Professions, State University of New York in Buffalo, more than 2,000 nurse practitioners graduated in 1981, which brought the total number of NPs to about 20,000.[74] This report showed a decline in the number of short-term certificate programs, an increase in the number of master's degree programs and an emphasis on adult and family nurse practitioner preparation.[75]

During the ANA convention in New Orleans in 1984, delegates requested ANA to reaffirm its commitment to graduate preparation in nursing for nurse practitioners entering advanced nursing practice. Nurse practitioner programs at the graduate level will undoubtedly continue to have a tremendous impact on the future of nursing practice. Justification for the nurse practitioner movement has been explained by various authors. For example, Jessie Scott, former Executive Director of the Division of Nursing, Bureau of Health Professions in Washington, D. C., made the following observation in reviewing the nurse practitioner movement.

> The fact remains that nursing's purpose and practice is derived from the needs of patients and families. It was clear that health problems were not being addressed and that it was essentially nursing's role to do so. What began as a small circumscribed area of practice has now blossomed into a full-range specialty of primary care practitioners.[76]

Perhaps no one can appreciate the progress made by the nurse practitioner movement as well as Loretta Ford. In reviewing this progress, she noted:

- An estimated 20,000 nurse practitioners have been prepared; 90% are practicing.
- The quality of care and acceptance by patients are unquestioned.
- One-hundred forty master's programs and 133 continuing education programs prepared nurse practitioners.
- Increasingly the master's level clinical specialist programs are including the assessment and management components introduced by the nurse practitioner concept.[77]

SUMMARY

Graduate education is urgently needed to provide leadership and advance professionalism for nursing. The present status and problems associated with master's and doctoral nursing education programs must be addressed if graduate students are to receive programs of excellent quality, whose purpose and goals are clearly defined. Doctoral level entry into nursing practice, including the views of several nurse educators on why nursing needs to expand its knowledge base and work toward a standardized system of nursing education, should be given serious attention during the 1990s.

Directions in doctoral nursing education and issues revolving around the nature, purpose, and scope of existing doctoral programs reveal that further clarification is needed to overcome the confusion noted at this level of nursing education. Emphasis is being placed on certification as a means of validating faculty competence in clinical practice. It was noted that certification may become a requirement for the nursing faculty employed in collegiate settings.

Finally, the responsibility of nurse faculty to include in their curricula preparation for health, wellness, and the caring aspects of nursing, in addition to the present emphasis on illness and disease, is of growing concern to nurse educators. Ultimately, nursing may adopt a health model for all of its educational programs.

Although nursing continues to improve its educational system, the pace of progress will remain slow until consensus can be reached on directions for the future of nursing education. Standardizing a system of nursing education is sorely needed. It should be given high priority on nursing's agenda for the future.

REFERENCES

1. "Education Task Force Offers Recommendations for Transition," *American Nurse* 15:4 (May, 1983), 3.
2. Christman, L. "Accountability and Autonomy are More than Rhetoric," *Nurse Educator* 3 (July–August, 1978), 3–6.
3. Schlotfeldt, R. "Nursing in the Future," *Nursing Outlook* 29:3 (May, 1981), 295–301.
4. Styles, M. *On Nursing, Toward a New Endowment.* St. Louis: C.V. Mosby, 1982, 162.
5. Schlotfeldt, R. "Nursing in the Future," 300.
6. *Ibid.*
7. Rogers, M. *Reveille in Nursing.* Philadelphia: F. A. Davis Company, 1964, 27.
8. de Tornyay, R. *Teaching–Learning Strategies for Baccalaureate Nursing Education* (Pub. No. 15-1622). New York: National League for Nursing, 1976, 7.

9. Moccia, P. "Critiques, Challenges and Common Ground," *Nursing and Health Care* 9:8 (October, 1988), 403.

10. National League for Nursing. Resolution No. 12: Support for Innovative Curricula for Nursing Education. Final session: "The New NLN." *Nursing and Health Care* 10:7 (September, 1989), 386.

11. Tanner, C. "Caring as a Value in Nursing Education," *Nursing Outlook* 38:2 (March–April, 1990), 71.

12. Benner, P. and Wrubel, J. *The Primacy of Caring: Stress and Coping in Health and Illness.* Menlo Park, CA: Addison-Wesley Co., 1989, 7.

13. Watson, J. "The Moral Failure of the Patriarchy," *Nursing Outlook* 38:2 (March–April, 1990), 62.

14. Watson, J. "Human Caring as Moral Context for Nursing Education," *Nursing and Health Care* 9:8 (October, 1988), 423.

15. *Ibid.*

16. Newman, M. "Professionalism," in N. Chaska (ed.), *The Nursing Profession: Turning Points.* St. Louis: C.V. Mosby, 1990, 52.

17. DeBack, V. "Nursing Education," in *Nursing's Vital Signs: Shaping the Profession for the 1990s.* Battle Creek, Mich.: W.K. Kellogg Foundation, 1989, 60.

18. Moraldo, P. "Will National Health Care Become a Reality?" *Nursing and Health Care* 9:6 (June, 1988), 279.

19. Merton, R., Reader, G. and Kendall, P. (eds.), *The Student-Physician: Introductory Studies in the Sociology of Medical Education.* Cambridge, Mass.: Harvard University Press, 1957, 287.

20. Thorne, B. "Professional Education in Law," in E. C. Hughes, B. Thomas, A. DeBoggis, A. Gurin, and D. Williams, *Education for the Professions of Medicine, Law, Theology, and Social Welfare.* New York: McGraw-Hill, 1973, 80.

21. Goode, W. "Community Within a Community: The Professions," *American Sociological Reveiw* 20 (April, 1957), 196.

22. Ondrack, D. "Socialization in Professional Schools: A Comparative Study," *Administration Science Quarterly* 20:3 (March, 1975), 97.

23. Werner, J. "Professional Socialization of Nurses: A Faculty Member's View," *Journal of New York State Nurses Association* 4:4 (November, 1973), 25.

24. Jacox, A. "Professional Socialization of Nurses," in N. Chaska (ed.), *The Nursing Profession: Views Through the Mist.* New York: McGraw-Hill, 1978, 13.

25. Colombotos, J. "Social Origins and Ideology of Physicians: A Study of the Effects of Early Socialization," *Journal of Health and Social Behavior* 10:1 (1969), 16.

26. Eron, L. "The Effect of Medical Education on Attitudes: A Follow-up Study," in H. H. Gee and R. J. Glaser (eds.), *The Ecology of the Medical Student.* Evanston, Ill.: Association of American Medical Colleges, 1957, 25.

27. Kramer, M. "Professional-Bureaucratic Conflict and Integrative Role Behavior," in M. V. Batey (ed.), *Communicating Nursing Research: Is the Gap Being Bridged?* Boulder, Co.: Western Interstate Commission on Higher Education, July, 1971, 56.

28. Kramer, M. *Reality Shock.* St. Louis: C. V. Mosby, 1974.

29. Axelrod, S., Donabedian, A. and Gentry, D. *Medical Care Chart Book,* 6th ed., Ann Arbor, Mich.: University of Michigan, 1976.

30. Cammings, K. and Lazonick, W. "The Development of the Nursing Labor Force in the U.S.: A Basic Analysis." *International Journal of Health Services* 5:2 (1975) 185–216.
31. Aaronson, L. "A Challenge for Nursing: Re-viewing a Historic Competition," *Nursing Outlook* 37:6 (November–December, 1989), 276.
32. Axelrod, S. *et. al. Medical Care Chart Book, 1976.*
33. Aaronson, L. "A Challenge for Nursing," 277.
34. *Facts About Nursing, 1967.* New York: American Nurses' Association, 1967, 113.
35. *Nursing Student Census with Policy Implications, 1984.* Divisions of Public Policy and Research (Pub. No. 19-1960). New York: National League for Nursing, 1984, 3.
36. Rosenfeld, P. *Nursing Student Census,* Division of Research. (Pub. No.: 19–22, 91), New York: National League for Nursing, 1989, 6.
37. *Facts About Nursing, 1983–1984.* Kansas City, Mo.: American Nurses Association, 1984, 92.
38. Rosenfeld, P. *Nursing Student Census,* 6.
39. *Report on 1989–1990 Enrollment and Graduations in Baccalaureate and Graduate Programs in Nursing.* Washington, D.C.: American Association of Colleges of Nursing, 1990, 10.
40. Maraldo, P. "NLN Data Projects Good News for Nursing Shortage," *NLN Executive Director Wire* (Spring, 1990), 4.
41. Vaughn, J. C. "Educational Preparation for Nursing—1982," *Nursing and Health Care* 4:8 (October, 1983), 463.
42. *Report on 1989–1990 Enrollment and Graduation,* 10.
43. Schlotfeldt, R. "On the Professional Status of Nursing," *Nursing Forum* 13:1 (Winter, 1974), 23–24.
44. *Facts About Nursing, 1976–1977.* Kansas City, Mo.: American Nurses Association, 1977, 95.
45. *Facts About Nursing, 1986–1987.* Kansas City, Mo.: American Nurses Association, 1987, 30.
46. *Ibid.,* 55.
47. Pitel, M. and Vian, J. "Analysis of Nurse-Doctorates," *Nursing Research* (September–October, 1975), 340–351.
48. *Report on 1989–1990, Enrollment and Graduation,* 10.
49. "Current Developments in the Registered Nurse Population," in *Seventh Report to the President and Congress on the Status of Health Personnel in the United States.* U.S. Dept. of Health and Human Services, Division of Nursing, Public Health Service, Health Resources and Services Administration. Washington, D.C.: (March, 1990), VIII-10, VIII-11.
50. Rogers, M. *Reveille in Nursing,* 2.
51. Rosenfeld, P. *Nursing Student Census,* 6.
52. Report of NLN Biennial Convention, Philadelphia, in June, 1983, *American Journal of Nursing* 83:7 (July, 1983), 995.
53. Kramer, M. "Philosophical Foundations of Baccalaureate Nursing Education," *Nursing Outlook* 9:2 (April, 1981), 226.
54. *Ibid.*

55. Montag, M. "Looking Back: Associate Degree Education in Perspective," *Nursing Outlook* 28:2 (April, 1980), 248–249.
56. *Ibid.,* 249.
57. Schlotfeldt, R. "The Professional Doctorate: Rationale and Characteristics," *Nursing Outlook* 26:5 (May, 1978), 305.
58. *Essentials of College & University Education for Professional Nursing.* Washington, D.C.: American Association of Colleges of Nursing, 1986.
59. "Characteristics of Professional and Technical Nurses of the Future and Their Educational Programs," in Gretchen Gerds (ed.), *Nursing's Vital Signs: Shaping the Profession for the Future.* Battle Creek, Mich.: W. K. Kellogg Foundation, 1989, 127–134.
60. Aydelotte, M. "The Future Health Delivery System and the Utilization of Nurses Prepared in Formal Educational Programs," in N. Chaska (ed.), *The Nursing Profession: Views Through the Mist.* New York: McGraw-Hill, 1978, 356.
61. Conway, M. "The Place of the Professional School," in M. Conway, and O. Andruskiw *Administrative Theory and Practice.* Norwalk, Conn.: Appleton-Century-Crofts, 1983, 11.
62. DeBack, V. "Nursing Education," 59.
63. *Ibid.*
64. Conway-Welch, C. "School Sets Sights on Bold Innovations," *Nursing and Health Care* 7:1 (January, 1986), 21–25.
65. Sokalys, J. and Watson, J. "Professional Education: Post-baccalaureate Education for Professional Nursing" *Journal of Professional Nursing* 2:2 (February, 1986), 91–97.
66. Carter, M. "The Professional Doctorate as an Entry Level Into Clinical Practice," in *National League for Nursing Perspectives, 1987–1989.* New York: National League for Nursing, 1988, 49–56.
67. Duffy, M. "New Models for Professional Nursing Education," in N. Chaska (ed.), *The Nursing Profession: Turning Points.* St. Louis: C.V. Mosby, 1990, 86.
68. Jaffe-Ruiz, M. "Non-nurse College Graduate," (Letters) *Nursing and Health Care* 11:2 (February, 1990), 61.
69. Feldman, H. and Jordet, C. "On the Fast Track," *Nursing and Health Care* 10:9 (November, 1989), 491–493.
70. Conway-Welch, C. "Emerging Models of Postbaccalaureate Nursing Education," in J. McCloskey and H. Grace (eds.), *Current Issues in Nursing,* 3d ed. St. Louis: C.V. Mosby, 1990, 140.
71. Krauss, J. "Generic Master's Degree in Nursing," Paper presented at the fall semi-annual meeting of the American Association of Colleges of Nursing. Washington, D.C., October 25, 1988.
72. Ford, L. C. "Nurse Practitioners: History of a New Idea and Predictions for the Future," in L. Aiken (ed.), *Nursing in the 1980s: Crises, Opportunities, Challenges.* Philadelphia: J. B. Lippincott, 1982, 233.
73. "For 'New Nurses': Bigger Role in Health Care," *U.S. News and World Report,* 88:1 January 14, 1980, 60.
74. "NP Study Reports 66% of New Grads Find Jobs Quickly," *American Nurse* 16:5 (May, 1984), 12.

75. *Ibid.*, 13.
76. Scott, J. "The Changing Scene: Societal Changes and Their Impact on Nursing Education," Paper presented at Deans' seminar cosponsored by the American Association of Colleges of Nursing and the Council of Baccalaureate and Higher Degree Programs of NLN at Smuggler's Notch, Vermont, (July, 1981), 3.
77. Ford, "Nurse Practitioners," 243–244

SUGGESTED READINGS

Bensman, P. "Focus on Associate Degree Nursing: Have We Lost Sight of AD Philosophy?" *Nursing Outlook* 25 (August, 1977), 511–513.

Bevis, E. and Watson, J. *Toward a Caring Curriculum: A New Pedagogy for Nursing* (Pub. No.: 15-2278) New York: National League for Nursing, 1989.

Brimmer, P., Skoners, M., Pender, N., Williams, C., Fleming, J. and Werley, H. "Nurses with Doctoral Degrees: Education and Employment Characteristics," *Research in Nursing and Health* 6:4 (December, 1983), 157–165.

"Characteristics of Graduate Education in Nursing Leading to the Master's Degree," *Nursing Outlook* 27:3 (March, 1979), 206.

Cole, E. "Support Growing for Nurse Education in College," *American Nurse* 15:5 (May, 1983), 2.

Gorney-Fadiman, M. "A Student's Perspective on the Doctoral Dilemma," *Nursing Outlook* 29 (November, 1981), 650–654.

Holzemer, W. "Quality in Graduate Nursing Education," *Nursing and Health Care* 3:10 (October, 1982), 536–542.

Murphy, J. "Doctoral Education In, Of, and For Nursing: An Historical Analysis," *Nursing Outlook* 29:11 (November, 1981), 645–649.

NLN Competencies of Graduates of Nursing Programs: Report of the NLN Task Force on Competencies of Graduates of Nursing Programs. New York: National League for Nursing, 1982.

Selected Issues
in Nursing Education

6

INTRODUCTION

At the beginning of the 1950s, it was observed that the deeper and broader the scholarship aimed at the more it became evident that general professional competence could not be achieved short of graduate studies.[1] The importance of graduate education for nursing was not fully recognized until the early 1960s, especially at the master's degree level, and prior to the 1970s, graduate content focused on functional preparation for teaching and administration. Availability of federal funds in the 1970s allowed nurses to specialize in the physical and biological sciences. Grants were awarded directly to nursing schools to finance doctoral education (Ph.D.). Shortly thereafter, nurses began to realize a need for specialization in clinical nursing practice. Again, the federal government provided traineeships for graduate nursing students to help defray the cost of these programs.

MASTER'S LEVEL PREPARATION

As it is viewed today, graduate education contains as much confusion and lack of clarity as the issue of entry into practice. In a review of the May 1987 NLN publication "Master's Education in Nursing," numerous descriptions for master's programs have resulted in considerable confusion for prospective graduate students.[2] Differences in the titles of master's degree programs, for instance, raise questions about whether each title purports to accomplish the same objective.

Master's degree programs should provide knowledge in a specialized area of nursing as a means to improve and upgrade nursing practice. However, it is a misnomer to refer to nursing practice as "advanced." The practice of professional nursing can be enhanced by additional knowledge, but it still remains practice. As Janet Williamson, Professor of Nursing at Pennsylvania State University, pointed out, "there is only one level of nursing practice—the professional level—[for] there is really no such creature as an advanced practitioner, there is only a specialized practitioner."[3]

It has been asserted that "there is a need for many more nurses to address the complex problems concerning quality and delivery of care, but the level of preparation of many nurses is not adequate to the scope and complexity of responsibilities expected of nurses today."[4] Observing the present state of nursing and nursing education, Nan Heckenberger, former Dean at the University of Maryland, stated, "while we debate the baccalaureate as entry into nursing practice, other groups such as respiratory therapists are raising their entry to the master's level."[5] She predicts that nursing will follow suit and make advanced educational preparation a requirement for entry into professional nursing. One of the greatest challenges for nursing in the remainder of the 1990s is the development of strong, high-quality graduate programs. Marketing the services of the master's prepared nurse is a responsibility that nurse educators should assume whenever possible.

The lack of doctorally prepared faculty to teach at the master's level is, however, a reason for questioning the strength of present graduate nursing education programs. In 1978 it was considered questionable to prepare master's students for faculty positions. Presently, many colleges and universities require faculty to have an earned doctorate prior to employment.

An innovative Master of Science in Nursing (M.S.N.) program was begun in 1983 at Case Western Reserve University for RN students wishing to pursue additional preparation in nursing at the graduate level. This program is built on a liberal arts and upper division professional education, that is, a first professional degree in nursing or its equivalent. Students who enter without the B.S.N/N.D. enroll for three academic years of full-time study or the part-time equivalent. The M.S.N. curriculum prepares the clinical specialist to be an administrator, clinician, or teacher in a variety of settings. If nursing is concerned with constructing a professional nursing degree program on a liberal arts and science base, this movement represents "a wave of future innovation" in schools offering open nursing education programs for college graduates from other disciplines.[6]

The Yale University master's program for non-nursing college graduates, which began in 1974, prepares students for entry into specialized practice. Like the Case Western program, this one also recognizes the value of graduate nursing education for professional nursing practice. Candidates are required to have earned a baccalaureate degree prior to enrollment. After completing one year of basic sciences and nursing skills, students choose an area of specialization for the two remaining years of the program.

The idea that nursing could profit by encouraging graduates of Ph.D. science programs to consider enrollment in nursing was noted by Luther Christman in 1978:

> There may be another source of richly qualified persons who could enter the nursing profession and enrich it further. Many persons with Ph.D.s in the fundamental sciences are finding their career pathways limited. With a well-conceived post doctoral program, these persons could become first-rate clinicians and pass the state board examinations to function as registered nurses. They would provide a new force within the profession because they entered it in such a nontraditional manner.[7]

Since 1978, there have been numerous non-nurse Ph.D. graduates who have enrolled in nursing programs, especially the Doctor of Nursing Program (N.D.) initiated in 1979 at Case Western Reserve University's School of Nursing. In the fall of 1988, Rush University College of Nursing in Chicago began a Doctor of Nursing (N.D.) degree program also.[8]

A number of nurse educators now believe that the baccalaureate nursing degree as a minimum for professional nursing practice will, in the foreseeable future, be insufficient for meeting the societal demands for health care. For example, Margretta Styles, former Dean of the University of California, San Francisco, asserts that "the baccalaureate must be seen as only a beginning . . . and may very shortly be judged inadequate to fill the increasing demands of professional practice; this would require that the base be raised to graduate level."[9]

Margaret Newman, a well-known nurse leader and theorist, believes that we should consider the four-year baccalaureate nursing program as probably *not* sufficient for preparing a nurse for the depth of independent practice required and insisted on by today's public.[10]

DOCTORAL LEVEL ENTRY FOR PROFESSIONAL NURSING

In 1977, the ANA Commission on Nursing Education placed increased emphasis on the importance of graduate education for nursing. It further recognized the concept of doctoral education as the first professional degree in nursing.[11] Over fifteen years have elapsed, but only two schools now offer the doctorate as the first professional degree for entry into professional nursing. Therefore, this concept will require long and continued debate before becoming a national requirement for entry into practice.

In order that nursing can be given the same recognition as other professions, (who educate for entry into practice by awarding the Doctor of Medicine (M.D.), Doctor of Law (J.D.), Doctor of Dental Science (D.D.S.), and Doctor of Philosophy (Ph.D.)) several nurse educators have concurred that doctoral preparation in nursing should be required for professional nursing practice. Virginia Cleland, author and professor at the University of California, San Francisco, and Margaret Newman, Professor at the University of Minnesota, agree that an academic baccalaureate degree plus three years of professional education leading to the award of a professional doctorate by the school should be the minimum acceptable preparation for professional nursing practice.[12, 13] Cleland is quick to point out that the purpose of the professional doctorate is to prepare a utilizer of research rather than an investigator. Its primary focus is on expert clinical practice.[14]

A firm believer in doctoral preparation for nursing, Rozella Schlotfeldt, is of the opinion that:

> The time is right for instituting education for all health professional students at the doctoral level. Admission to professional schools should require a minimum of 3 to 4 years of liberal education, in addition to prerequisites for professional sciences.[15]

Another nurse leader and educator, Mary Conway, asserts:

> Professional preparation as we now know it at the baccalaureate level will give way to preparation at the master's or doctoral level. That is, entry level education for many professions will require the professional doctoral degree, as distinct from the Ph.D. . . . The trend toward the professional doctorate for entry into the professions is not mere accident or innovation for its own sake; it is impelled by the continuing, rapid expansion of knowledge.[16]

Schlotfeldt asserted again in 1982 that the time had come for nurse faculty nationwide to develop rigorous programs leading to the first professional nursing degree that would be deserving of doctorates.[17]

The professional nursing doctorate (N.D.) degree begun at Case Western Reserve University was opened to college graduates and students having completed three years of liberal education. Upon completion, graduates of the program would be qualified to do the following things:

- Serve as the primary health professional in health maintenance
- Collaborate with physicians in identifying illness and implementing care plans
- Serve as primary health professionals for older persons and those with chronic health problems
- Collaborate with all health professions in helping people through health crises
- Collaborate with all health professionals in planning and providing total health care programs for individuals and their families
- Serve in a variety of settings with referral to other health professionals as the needs for their particular services emerge[18]

From examining the expectations for the N.D. graduate, it becomes apparent that the present baccalaureate programs are unable to provide the level of professional education that is required for the future professional practitioner. With few exceptions, nursing has "developed technical baccalaureate programs and technical practice [but] we have not developed professional programs nor professional practice."[19] A step toward assuring a sound educational base for practitioners would be adopting a professional degree comparable to those of other health professions.[20]

In considering the views of other nurses about the future needs of nursing education, one author made the following statement:

> The most significant shortcoming of the nursing education system has been its slowness to adapt to changes in health care delivery that have warranted greater attention on preparation at baccalaureate and higher degree levels.
>
> Given the increasing amount of scientific knowledge about treatment modalities, and consumer sophistication and desire, the educational base for nursing practice must reflect the increase in scientific and social knowledge.
>
> The need for more nursing education programs in institutions of higher learning necessitates preparation of a greater percentage of nurses at the doctoral level.
>
> [Above all,] there is a need to achieve consensus on a national system of nursing education that clarifies and standardizes the expected competencies and the educational preparation for each category of nursing practice.[21]

Each of these observations points up nursing's need to look to the future in establishing a standardized educational system that will warrant the legitimate title of professional nursing education. While many nurses are convinced that entry into professional nursing practice should be at the doctoral level, other viewpoints on this issue should be considered. Several problems associated with doctoral level entry exist and should be acknowledged: the cost of the program; the length of time required for completion; the size of the qualified applicant pool, the availability of pre-service doctoral nursing programs; the number of faculty qualified to teach doctoral students; the number of faculty qualified to serve as role models in clinical practice and clinical research; and the lack of public awareness of expectations for the performance of N.D. graduates. Each of these problems must be addressed before consensus can be reached on doctoral level entry as the educational requirement for professional nursing.

Some individuals also question why various "entry into practice" levels (two-, three-, and four-year programs) are viewed as a problem by a certain segment of nurses. Doctoral level entry is not seen as an additional problem, but rather it is a goal to be achieved. Preparation for professional nursing, with all that it implies, cannot continue its present course. The health needs of the public already demand a level of preparation that goes well beyond the current provisions of pre-service nursing education programs. Furthermore, the rapid rate at which the knowledge base is expanding demands additional preparation requirements.

Some individuals with doctorates from other disciplines are enrolling in N.D. programs, making these programs innovative. If and when the N.D. program becomes the standard for entry into professional practice, the present confusion over multiple programs preparing graduates for practice may be eliminated. In other words, since there would be only one type of program preparing for entry into practice (the doctoral nursing program), no confusion would exist.

From all of the previous discussion on professionalism, the issue of doctoral level entry will be resolved only when nurses realistically face the question of what is required for preparation for professional nursing practice within a professional discipline. Meanwhile, an interdisciplinary task force on education for nursing practice was appointed by the Cabinet on Nursing Education in 1982. This group was to develop national recommendations and strategies to advance ANAs position on baccalaureate preparation for entry into practice. Their report, published in the spring of 1983, stated that "change in illness patterns, expanded treatment alternatives and a societal commitment to enhance survivability for the newborn and the aged have placed heavy burdens on the nursing profession, burdens which nursing could meet more easily with an expanded educational base, [and] by adopting the baccalaureate degree as the education required for entry into professional practice."[22] Undoubtedly, baccalaureate preparation for professional nursing practice is one of the most important issues that nursing continues to face.

The first doctoral program in nursing began at Teachers College, Columbia University, in 1924, the Doctor of Education (Ed.D.). Ten years later, New York University began an Ed.D. degree (which was phased out in 1960) followed by a Ph.D. degree in that same year. In 1954, the University of Pittsburgh initiated a Ph.D. in nursing. Later, Boston University offered the first professional nursing doctorate (DNS) in 1960, followed by the University of California, San Francisco, in 1964 and the Catholic University of America in 1967.[23]

The variety of doctoral degrees in nursing continues to create a dilemma for nursing as the twenty-first century approaches. There are four major types of doctoral programs that have been developed within the present century. Several issues pertaining to their structure and curricula continue to create serious debate and make it difficult for prospective doctoral students to choose between the different programs. Since other professions are in agreement as to the type of doctoral program that best meets their needs, it is not unreasonable to expect that at some future date one specific type of nursing doctorate may finally be agreed upon.

In the past, nursing has not had large numbers of nurses with research doctorates to provide sorely needed research expertise. Presently this problem has been resolved. Providing schools of nursing with faculty having earned doctorates was one of the goals of nurse educators in recent years. In academia, research doctorates (Ph.D.) are considered more appropriate for faculty because they provide in-depth knowledge of the research process. In the clinical setting, however, a clinical doctorate is considered by many nurses to encompass the kinds of knowledge requisite for excellent clinical practice.

Case Western Reserve University established the first nursing doctorate (N.D.) for non-nurse college graduates in 1979 for entry into practice. Since that time, there has been a dramatic increase in the number of doctoral programs offered in university schools of nursing. In the fall of 1989, forty-eight doctoral nursing programs and one generic doctoral program had begun.[24] It is readily observed that there is a definite trend toward the Ph.D. in nursing degree. Of the forty doctoral programs functioning in 1984, "17 offered the DNS, DNSc, or DSN, one program offered the Ed.D., and 22 offered the Ph.D. degree."[25] This trend was observed in a national survey on the need for doctorally prepared nurses in academic settings and health service agencies. Of the doctoral programs planned for 1990, thirty-six proposed a Ph.D. program while seven planned a DNSc. degree.[26] The two major types of nursing doctorates—the academic and the professional—are producing different products. The thirty-three Ph.D. nursing programs strongly outnumber the twelve professional doctoral programs offered in the 1990s. The result may be fewer graduates having an applied focus relevant to the design and evaluation of improved, cost-effective care.[27]

Nursing currently offers a first professional degree (BSN, MSN or MS, and N.D.), a second professional degree (MSN), and a third professional degree (DSN/DNS/DNSc). In comparing these models to medicine, Forni observes that "in medicine there is only one professional degree, the M.D., and advanced education may be attained in related fields leading to the Ph.D., M.P.H. . . . [and] in dentistry there is also one professional degree (DDS or DMD) with graduate degrees for advanced specialty practice in dentistry leading to the master's degree (awarded post-doctorally)."[28] Meleis believes, "we should focus our energy on developing a first-rate single doctoral degree that includes different options . . . [the discipline of nursing cannot] afford to be divided among different degrees and programs."[29]

DIRECTIONS IN DOCTORAL NURSING EDUCATION

Members of the Council of Baccalaureate and Higher Degree Programs identified several major issues of concern at one of the annual meetings. Issues pertaining to graduate education were discussed, particularly the need for mechanisms for standard setting and quality control in doctoral education in nursing. An evolving trend in doctoral nursing education is evident in the substantial growth in numbers of doctoral programs and doctorally prepared nurses since the early 1960s. The growth from four doctoral programs in 1960, to sixteen in 1976, to twenty-five in 1982, to forty-nine plus one generic program in 1989, along with nineteen additional programs in the planning stage shows a significant increase in professionalism for nursing.

Believing that sound preparation of doctoral students is an important issue confronting nursing in the 1990s, several nurses have expressed concern about the quantity of doctoral programs and their *quality.* In 1978, it was recommended that the nature and goals of doctoral education should be given serious attention in the future.[30] Since that time, evaluation of existing doctoral programs has occurred. But further clarification of their purpose and goals is necessary to ensure sound programs for the future. Some nurse educators predict there will be approximately sixty-eight doctoral programs in nursing by the close of this century. This conclusion was drawn from results of a survey conducted by the American Association of Colleges of Nursing in 1978 on present programs and future plans for doctoral programs in 208 university and college nursing programs. A supporting survey was also conducted in 1989.[31, 32]

In order to avoid problems in the late 1990s over the essential type of doctoral preparation for professional nursing practice, the purposes of these various doctoral nursing degrees should be clarified. Until the distinction between these various programs is clearly defined, nurses may enter doctoral programs without realizing until much later that the programs were not appropriate to their individual needs and goals.

Although these concerns were stressed when the doctoral programs were developing, the present content of these programs indicates that clarification of the issues has not been adequately addressed. For example, should all doctoral nursing programs include a clinical practice dimension? Or should the research doctorate (Ph.D.) include development but not testing of theories? "Doctoral programs are caught up in the cross currents of on the one hand preparing researchers and scholars and on the other hand, maintaining ties to the clinical practice of nursing."[33] However, many nurse educators responsible for doctoral nursing programs agree that doctoral education in nursing should be concerned with the practice components of nursing as well as with the generation and dissemination of high-level nursing knowledge.[34]

Doctoral nursing education can move nursing rapidly into the ranks of major health professions. But nursing should quickly resolve the debatable issues surrounding preparation. Otherwise future professional practitioners may be adversely affected.

CERTIFICATION FOR ADVANCED PRACTICE—A FACULTY REQUIREMENT?

By the year 2000, "faculty in master's programs in nursing should be required to have, in addition to the doctoral degree, specialist certification and each would have a built-in component of clinical work that would end 'ivory tower' teaching and make practice an integral part of the faculty member's role."[35] Interestingly enough, many faculty throughout the country, recognizing the importance of clinical competence, have successfully achieved ANA certification in their clinical specialty area.

Although certification for nurses has progressed, it has not been without serious struggle and even major setbacks. Since 1958, the ANA has continued to seek means by which "formal recognition of personal achievement and superior performance in nursing could be measured."[36] By 1974, criteria for pediatric, ambulatory care, geriatric, community health, psychiatric, and mental health nursing practitioners were established.

A model of certification developed by an ANA interdivisional council on certification during 1976–1978, was presented at the 1978 ANA convention. This model recommended certification for competence in specialized areas of practice at one level and certification for excellence in practice at another. However the model lacked support, so it was agreed that the new certification programs would emphasize only advanced specialty practice.[37] In order for faculty members to be eligible for certification, they must practice clinical nursing at least four hours a week. Since the majority of nurse faculty members have acquired advanced preparation in a specific clinical specialty area, the criteria of clinical practice presents difficulties only for those whose practical skills may not still be current.

NURSE EDUCATORS' RESPONSIBILITY TO TEACH WELLNESS CARE

Another issue of concern for nursing educators is the need to prepare nursing students for wellness. In preparing nurses for professional nursing practice, nurse educators are realizing that society is becoming increasingly concerned with wellness. Health professionals must, therefore, be knowledgeable in assisting patients to attain, maintain, or regain their health.

Maximizing the health potential of individuals can be justified on a purely economic basis. It is economical for society to remain healthy. Not only is illness care far too costly, but cost-containment factors are also posing genuine threats to the health care industry. Health care, health promotion, and prevention of disease have become increasingly appealing in recent times for these economic reasons.

> Health promotion is an idea whose time has come. Where technologic advances were the hallmark in the 1970s, health promotion promises to be the watchword for better health for Americans in the 1980s and beyond.
> But to equate health promotion solely with changing lifestyle behavior would overlook its other important dimensions. Tandem to behavioral change is the fostering of individual self-responsibility for health and the recognition that changes in the environment are also critical to optimum well-being.[38]

Nursing curricula in baccalaureate programs are slowly changing from a medical model to a health model, emphasizing wellness, caring, primary care, and appropriate health behaviors. Because nursing, in the ANA Social Policy Statement, has identified its focus as the diagnosis and treatment of human responses to actual or potential health problems, then wellness and health promotion will be dominant aspects in future professional nursing practice.

Nurse educators have prepared practitioners primarily for the acute care setting, but society's health needs are much broader in scope. Revised curricula should incorporate a health care approach and not simply emphasize illness care.

> The faculty of the professional school and the university have an obligation to prepare practitioners who will be able to meet a broad range of society's needs, not just the needs of one specialized sector. Thus, it is

important that curricula in schools focus on nursing's mission to provide health care rather than sick care only.[39]

Since society delegates autonomy to full professions, it expects that professionals will function independently. Consultation, collaboration, and cooperation between nurses and other workers in the various health disciplines must occur if society's demand for adequate health care is to be met. To function smoothly in the health care industry presupposes that each profession has achieved a high degree of consensus regarding "(1) the role responsibilities, and jurisdiction of its own practitioners; (2) the kinds of assisting personnel that are needed; (3) the ratio of professionals to assisting personnel that is appropriate safe and cost effective; (4) the nature and standards of educational programs through which personnel are prepared for entering into practice."[40]

It would appear that nursing has yet to reach consensus on each of the issues listed above. Many nurses do not believe they should practice independently. Nursing roles and competencies for each level of practice are still unclear. The kind of nursing assistants needed and the ratio of professionals to assistants, have not been generally agreed upon.

The ANA proposal for entry into practice has yet to be resolved nationally. In 1975, ten years after publication of the original position paper, the ANA Commission on Nursing Education released *Standards for Nursing Education* for programs leading to graduate, baccalaureate, and associate degrees and for programs involving diploma and continuing education. These standards provide a means for monitoring quality as well as support for innovation and testing of new nursing goals. Their focus is on education for nursing practice.[41] In developing these standards, the commission described basic assumptions about nursing's approach to education, which reinforced the 1965 proposal.[42] However, some nurses believe these guidelines have not been effective in standardizing the basic nursing education programs that claim to prepare professionals.[43]

To the question "Should health or illness be the dominant concept in nursing's perspective?" it is interesting to observe medicine's concern with diagnosis and cure and how disease becomes their main organizing concept. In nursing, however, disease is not the predominant focus. Rather it is the diagnosis and treatment of actual or potential health problems of clients. "Nursing and medicine may include identical elements in their orienting perspectives or knowledge systems, but focus, emphasis, goals and, therefore, bodies of knowledge, theories, and research will differ, as will many activities of the professional practitioners in the two fields."[44]

Although health promotion, sometimes referred to as prevention of disease, emphasizes health or wellness, prevention concentrates on disease. An important question being asked is, "What meaning should health have in a nursing knowledge system—health and well-being or their opposites, illness or disease?"[45] Believing that health is the absence of disease does not describe nursing's concept of health. Nurses are endeavoring to conceptualize an accurate definition of their view of health and nursing's role in attaining, maintaining, or regaining it. Nursing comprises practitioners who are responsible and accountable for the assessment and promotion of the health status, assets, and potential of the whole community.[46]

For some time, national nursing organizations have strongly recommended changes in patterns of health care services. They have supported autonomy and greater visibility for nursing and have worked to enhance the public's acknowledgment of the value of nursing services. Nurses should recognize the new opportunities generated by shifts in national health policy to advance from an illness care to a wellness care orientation. New health policies are presaging significant changes for health care delivery in the United States.

Nurses, with their emphasis on patient education and on providing a client advocacy role, should be among the leaders in this revolutionary movement. With current public dissatisfaction with the existing health care system, the time is right for nurses to take on a greater advocacy role in the delivery of health care. Thus, the public will better understand and be more receptive to the role of nursing in health care delivery. Actually, nursing's role must be recognized, comprehended, and endorsed by its numerous audiences if health care is to reach the entire American community. Nursing will never achieve full professional status until society bestows such recognition, based on its assessment of nursing's competence and expertise in meeting societal needs. If nurses are to be in the forefront of health promotion and disease prevention, which has become the main concern of health providers and payors of health care, then they should communicate their right to this position and demonstrate their ability, expertise, and professional skill to justify such a claim.

> A nursing practice focusing on health promotion is a professional practice independent of physician guidance and regulation. This supports nursing's autonomy and portends the establishment of health centers administered by nurses for the purpose of health promotion. It also means nurse participation with families in their homes to guide changing patterns in a familiar environment. Nursing then—a science and autonomous profession—enhances human potential by strengthening the integrity of persons, family, and environment.[47]

Nurses should demonstrate that they can produce significant changes in the health status of the public and effect important outcomes through nursing practice. Above all, determining how to reallocate resources in order to bring about changes in health care delivery should be high on nursing's agenda throughout this decade. Nursing should convince the public that it can meet its health needs in collaboration with the other health disciplines. Moreover, now is the time for nursing to persuasively convince the public that it can and will be the best advocate for promoting health and well-being.

SUMMARY

Considerable differences exist among the various types of pre-service and graduate nursing education programs that comprise nursing's present educational system. They indicate a need to work toward greater standardization in nursing education. Nursing needs to achieve autonomy in controlling and maintaining the integrity of its professional education. Professional socialization has been recommended as a means of alleviating the stresses accompanying entrance into a professional role. Unlike physicians or lawyers, many nurses do not believe they are joining an elite profession when they choose nursing careers. Many of them view nursing as an occupation that can be replaced by other responsibilities at a later period. Faculties need to socialize students early in their career to consider nursing as a lifetime commitment. Adherence to professional values and norms also needs to be emphasized.

Statistical data provide information on the number, type, and admissions to basic pre-service nursing programs and on the number and graduations from master's and doctoral programs. These data reveal that associate degree programs are experiencing a tremendous growth pattern to a far greater extent than either the baccalaureate or diploma programs. The dearth of qualified professional nurses prepared at an advanced level is readily observed in the low percentage of employed nurses with master's and doctoral degrees. The large number of currently practicing registered nurses with less than a baccalaureate degree indicates a need to resolve this issue as quickly as possible. Ultimately, the role of nurse practitioners, their remarkable growth, and the ways in which they are influencing nursing autonomy may describe the role of all future professional nurses.

REFERENCES

1. Brubacher, J. S. and Rudy, W. *Higher Education in Transition.* New York: Harper & Row, 1958, 208.
2. *Master's Education in Nursing: Route to Opportunities in Contemporary Nursing.* New York: National League for Nursing, 1987.

3. Williamson, J. A. "Crisis in Academic Nursing," in N. Chaska (ed.), *The Nursing Profession—A Time to Speak.* New York: McGraw-Hill, 1983, 68.
4. Lang, N., McPhail, J., and Spengler, C. "Providing High Quality Care Challenges Profession," *American Nurse* 12:2 (February, 1980), 4.
5. "Report of NLN Biennial Convention," *American Journal of Nursing,* 83:6 (June, 1983), 995.
6. Slavinsky, A. T. and Diers, D. "Nursing Education for College Graduates," *Nursing Outlook* 30:5 (May, 1982), 292.
7. Christman, L. "Alternatives in the Role Expression of Nurses That May Affect the Future of the Nursing Profession," in N. Chaska (ed.), *The Nursing Profession: Views Through the Mist.* New York: McGraw-Hill, 1978, 364.
8. Phone conversation with Barbara Haynes, Associate Dean, Rush University College of Nursing, June 19, 1990.
9. Styles, M. *On Nursing, Toward a New Endowment.* St. Louis: C.V. Mosby, 1982, 164.
10. Newman, M. A. "The Professional Doctorate in Nursing: A Position Paper," *Nursing Outlook* 23:11 (November, 1975), 705.
11. "Assuring Quality in Nursing Education?" (ed.), *American Nurse* 9:7, (July, 1977), 4.
12. Cleland, V. "Developing a Doctoral Program," *Nursing Outlook* 24:10 (October, 1976), 631–635.
13. Newman, M. A. "The Professional Doctorate," 705.
14. Cleland, V. "Developing a Doctoral Program," 632.
15. Schlotfeldt, "The Professional Doctorate Rationale and Characteristics," *Nursing Outlook* 26:5 (May, 1978), 305.
16. Conway, M. "The Place of the Professional School," in M. Conway and O. Andruskiw *Administrative Theory and Practice,* Norwalk, Conn.: Appleton-Century-Crafts, 1983, 17.
17. Schlotfeldt, R. M. *A Brave New Nursing World* (Pub. Ser. 82, No.: 3). Washington, D. C.: American Association of Colleges of Nursing, 1982, 11.
18. "University Offers Doctor of Nursing as Entry Degree," *American Journal of Nursing* 78:8 (August, 1978), 1288.
19. Williamson, J. A. "Crisis in Academic Nursing," 67.
20. Newman, M. A. "The Professional Doctorate," 706.
21. Carroll, M., Fischer, L., and Frericks, M. "Education Must Adapt to Changing Health Care System," *American Nurse* 12:3 (March, 1980), 6.
22. "Education Task Force Offers Recommendations for Transition," *American Nurse* 15:4 (May, 1983), 3.
23. Matarazzo, J. and Abdellah, J. "Doctoral Education for Nurses in the United States" *Nursing Research* 20:5 (September, 1971), 404–414.
24. American Association of Colleges of Nursing. *Report on 1989–1990 Enrollment and Graduations in Baccalaureate and Graduate Programs in Nursing.* Washington, D.C.: The Association, 1990, 10.
25. Marriner-Tomey, A. "Historical Development of Doctoral Programs from the Middle Ages to Nursing Education Today" *Nursing and Health Care* 11:3 (March, 1990), 136.
26. Anderson, E. "A National Survey of the Need for Doctorally Prepared Nurses in Academic Settings and Health Service Agencies," *Journal of Professional Nursing* 1:1 (January, 1985), 23–33.

27. Andreoli, K. "Specialization and Graduate Curricula: Finding the Fit," *Nursing and Health Care* 8:2 (February, 1987), 65–69.

28. Forni, P. "Models for Doctoral Programs: First Professional Degree or Terminal Degree?" in S. Hart (ed.), *Issues in Graduate Nursing Education*. (Pub. No.: 18-2196) New York: National League for Nursing, 1987, 433.

29. Meleis, A. "Doctoral Education in Nursing: Its Present and Its Future," *Journal of Professional Nursing* 4:6 (November–December, 1988), 445.

30. Downs, F. "Doctoral Education," In Nursing: Future Directions, *Nursing Outlook* 26:1 (January, 1978), 61.

31. "Doctoral Programs Increasing," *American Journal of Nursing* 78:8 (August, 1978), 1290.

32. American Association of Colleges of Nursing. *Report on 1989–1990*, 10.

33. Grace, H. K. "Doctoral Education in Nursing: Dilemmas and Directions," in N. Chaska (ed.), *The Nursing Profession: A Time to Speak*. New York: McGraw-Hill, 1983, 147–148.

34. *Ibid.*

35. "Heckenberger Maps Future of Education," *NLN Convention News* Philadelphia, June 4, 1983, 3.

36. *ANA Certification* (Pub. No.: CR. 4-73). Kansas City, Mo.: American Nurses Association, 1973, 7.

37. *Certification—The New Approach*. Proceedings of the 1978 House of Delegates at the Convention of the American Nurses' Association. Kansas City, Mo.: The American Nurses' Association, 1978.

38. Nassif, J. "Health Promotion—An Idea Whose Time Has Come," *American Lung Association Bulletin* 66:5 (September, 1980), 9.

39. Conway, M. "Place of the Professional School," 11.

40. Schlotfeldt, R. M. "Professional Doctorate," 305.

41. *Standards for Nursing Education*. Kansas City, Mo.: American Nurses' Association, 1975, iii.

42. *A Case for Baccalaureate Preparation in Nursing*. Kansas City, Mo.: American Nurses' Association, Commission on Nursing Education, 1979, 2.

43. Schlotfeldt, R. M. *A Brave New Nursing World*, 7.

44. Ellis, R. "Conceptual Issues in Nursing," *Nursing Outlook* 30:7 (July–August, 1982), 407.

45. *Ibid.*, 408.

46. Schlotfeldt, R. M. "Can We Bring Order Out of the Chaos of Nursing Education?," *American Journal of Nursing* 76:1 (January, 1976), 105.

47. Smith, M. J. "Transformation: A Key to Shaping Nursing," *Image: the Journal of Nursing Scholarship* 16:1 (Winter, 1984), 29.

SUGGESTED READINGS

Amos, L. "Issues in Doctoral Preparation in Nursing: Current Perspectives and Future Directions," *Journal of Professional Nursing* 1:3, (May, 1985), 101–108.

"Characteristics of Graduate Education in Nursing Leading to the Master's Degree," *Nursing Outlook* 27:3 (March, 1979), 206.

Cole, E. "Support Growing for Nurse Education in College," *American Nurse* 15:5 (May, 1983), 2.

De Bach, V. and Mentkowski, M."Does the Baccalaureate Make a Difference?: Differentiating Nurse Performance by Education and Experience," *Journal of Nursing Education* 25:7 (September, 1986), 275–285.

"Diploma Schools are Reviving as Enrollments Surge," *American Journal of Nursing* 90:9 (September 1990), 104, 117.

Forni, P. "Models for Doctoral Programs: First Professional Degree or Terminal Degree," *Nursing and Health Care* 10:8 (October, 1989), 428.

Forni, P. and Welch, M. "The Professional Versus the Academic Model: A Dilemma for Nursing Education," *Journal of Professional Nursing* 3:5 (May 1987) 291–297.

Gorney-Faidman, M. J. "A Student's Perspective on the Doctoral Dilemma," *Nursing Outlook* 29 (November, 1981), 650–654.

Hart, S. *Doctoral Education in Nursing*, Pub. No.: 15-2238. New York: National League for Nursing, 1989.

Haussler, S. "Faculty Perceptions of the Organizational Climate in Selective Top-Ranked Schools of Nursing," *Journal of Professional Nursing* 4:4 (July–August, 1988), 271–278.

Holzemer, W. "Quality in Graduate Nursing Education," *Nursing and Health Care* 3:10 (October, 1982), 536–542.

Meshanis, H., "Redefining the Expanded Role," *Nursing Outlook* 36:6, 280–284.

Munro, B. and Krauss, J. "The Success of Non-BSNs in Graduate Nursing Programs," *Journal of Nursing Education* 24:5 (May 1985), 192–196.

Murphy, J., "Doctoral Education In, Of, and For Nursing: An Historical Analysis," *Nursing Outlook* 29:11 (November, 1981), 645–649.

NLN Competencies of Graduates of Nursing Programs: Report of the NLN Task Force on Competencies of Graduates of Nursing Programs. New York: National League for Nursing, 1982.

Rose, M. "ADN vs. BSN: The Search for Differentiation." *Nursing Outlook* 36:6 (November–December, 1988), 275–279.

Schroeder, B. "Entry-Level Graduate Education in Nursing: Master of Science Programs," in *Perspectives in Nursing 1987–1989*. New York: National League for Nursing, 1988.

Snyder-Halpern, R. "Nursing Doctorates: Is There a Difference?" *Nursing Outlook* 34:6 (November–December, 1986), 284–285.

Other Issues
in Nursing Education

7

INTRODUCTION

Perhaps one of the most critical issues facing nursing education in the 1990s is that of entry into practice. Controversy over minimal preparation for professional nursing practice is a recurring theme throughout nursing's history: "It appears that at a critical time, when retrenchment can affect professional nurses and there is competition from other health fields, the profession lacks consensus concerning the appropriate level and type of preparation."[1] In 1976, it was observed that "directors of nursing across the country are now beginning to recognize that the quality of patient care will not begin to improve unless and until the required educational preparation for entry into nursing practice is at the baccalaureate level."[2]

VIEWS ON ENTRY INTO PRACTICE

The entry into practice issue began in 1960 with a report of the Committee on Current and Long-term Goals to the American Nurses' Association House of Delegates. The Committee proposed that within the next twenty to thirty years the ANA should strongly promote the baccalaureate degree nursing program. Eventually it was to become the basic educational foundation for professional nursing. Even now this proposal is continuing to create dissension. Presented as a resolution to the ANA House of Delegates in 1962, it was adopted with recommendations to the ANA Board of Directors to implement after careful review of the various implications involved.

In 1965, the ANA formally issued a position paper on educational preparation for professional and technical nursing practice. Reverberations from this position paper, which called for the baccalaureate nursing degree for professional nursing practice and the associate nursing degree for technical nursing practice, have lessened considerably in the intervening years. However, consensus on the issue of whether or not there should be two categories of nursing personnel—professional and technical—has yet to be achieved by the various nursing groups throughout the country. Presently, graduates of hospital diploma programs, associate degree programs, and baccalaureate degree programs are eligible to take state examinations and be licensed as registered nurses. However, it is difficult to clearly differentiate the skills and competencies of the graduates of these different programs to the public and to other health professionals.

Throughout the period of 1965 to 1974, this issue remained in abeyance, although some state nurses' associations conducted studies of needs and resources for nursing personnel. In 1972, Rogers emphasized that there are two separate levels of nursing responsibilities. These two levels should be taught by two different educational programs.[3] According to Montag, the originator of the associate degree concept, "it is an advantage to have two kinds of nurses and two kinds of programs [since] it simplifies curricular problems and makes it less likely that the associate degree nurse will be misused . . . [and] it makes it easier for teachers to know what to teach and prospective nurses to decide which program they want to enter."[4]

A resolution was introduced and adopted by the New York State Nurses Association (NYSNA) in 1974 regarding entry into professional practice. It would have made it mandatory for all applicants for registered nurse licensure in New York to have a baccalaureate nursing degree by 1985.[5] This resolution also called for legislation to change the educational requirements for the licensed practical nurse to an associate degree. According to the resolution, by means of a "grandfather" or waiving clause, licenses and practice privileges of all current registered and licensed practical nurses would be protected. Any nurse licensed as either an RN or LPN prior to January 1984 would retain that license without having to meet the degree requirements. After that date, only new graduates of baccalaureate programs would be eligible for professional nurse licensure, and only new associate degree graduates would be eligible for associate degree licensure. Introduced as a bill into the New York state legislature in 1976 and again in 1977, it did not progress and has yet to be passed as law. However, this resolution began a national movement that continues to trigger serious debate over the "entry into practice" issue.

In 1976 the ANA Commission on Nursing Education appointed a task force to study the entry issues involved in the New York State Nurses' Association's resolution. At a National Conference on Entry into Nursing Practice in 1978 in Kansas City, Missouri, the task force received recommendations. Based on these recommendations, the Commission on Nursing Education submitted to the 1978 ANA House of Delegates three resolutions on entry into practice. The delegates adopted these resolutions as follows:

1. Resolution 56
   The ANA should ensure that two categories of nursing practice be clearly identified and titled by 1980 and . . . by 1985 minimum preparation for entry into professional nursing practice be the baccalaureate degree in nursing.
2. Resolution 57
   The ANA should establish a mechanism for deriving a comprehensive statement of competencies for two categories of nursing practice by 1980.
3. Resolution 58
   The ANA should actively support increased accessibility to high-quality career mobility programs which utilize flexible approaches for individuals seeking academic degrees in nursing.[6]

A resolution adopted at the March 1979 House of Delegates Convention of the Association of Operating Room Nurses also recommended that all nursing education should be at the baccalaureate or higher degree level in order to reach the ideal of true professional status for nursing.[7] In order to develop strategies for implementing these 1978 resolutions, the Commission on Nursing Education and the Task Force on Entry into Practice, chaired by Lorene Fischer, former Dean of Wayne State University School of Nursing, sponsored regional forums in several cities in 1978. Based on information derived from these meetings, the Commission on Nursing Education presented several resolutions to the 1980 ANA Convention in Houston. The main issues of concern were career mobility for nurses, titling for the two categories, and a mechanism for development of competency statements.[8] A summary of the Commission's work appeared in *Educational Preparation for Nursing: A Source Book* in 1981.[9]

In 1982, the Cabinet on Nursing Education appointed an interdisciplinary National Task Force on Education for Nursing Practice to make recommendations to advance the ANA's position on education for nursing practice. The ANA House of Delegates in 1982 adopted the following resolution: "That the American Nurses Association move forward in the coming biennium to expedite recognition of the baccalaureate in nursing as the minimum educational qualification for the practitioner in professional nursing practice."[10] The National Task Force submitted its report, entitled *Education for Nursing Practice in the Context of the 1980's*, to the ANA Cabinet on Nursing Education early in 1983. After the Cabinet adopted the report, it was approved for publication by the ANA Board of Directors at its March meeting.[11, 12]

The Cabinet on Nursing Education also submitted several proposals to the ANA Board of Directors at the May 18–20, 1983 meeting and the Board took the following actions related to these proposals:

- Directed that the Cabinet's report entitled *Education for Nursing Practice in the Context of the 1980s* be widely disseminated
- Directed that efforts be made to publicize the Cabinet's projection that by 1992, 50% of the states will have adopted educational or legal provision requiring the baccalaureate for professional nursing practice
- Authorized the Cabinet to convene a two-day strategy meeting of representatives of ANA and of state associations that have developed plans to establish the baccalaureate as the requirement
- Allocated funds to the Cabinet to be used to implement the baccalaureate requirement[13]

The Cabinet on Nursing Education's ultimate goal was to achieve "congruence of nurse licensure with the educational base of the baccalaureate."[14]

With the new *Standards for Nursing Education* available, the Cabinet envisioned that with such guidelines, by 1986, five percent of the states would have established the ANA standards of the baccalaureate for professional nursing practice; by 1988, fifteen percent of the states could claim this achievement; and by 1992, fifty percent of the states would have in place those necessary educational or legal elements to enable nursing to meet its social mandate by the twenty-first century.[15] Thus the Cabinet recommended this timetable to the 1984 House of Delegates for implementation of this goal. It won an "unconditional" endorsement with no changes by the House of Delegates. One delegate, noting that nurse leaders have been struggling for over eighty years to upgrade nursing education, stated: " . . . had we done what needed to be done decades ago, we would be admitting and discharging; we wouldn't be a part of the per diem costs; we wouldn't be dealing with DRG's but with nursing care categories . . . we wouldn't be talking about nursing/diagnosis as a basis of payment—we would have it.[16]

For the present, nurse leaders believe that the timetable and approach for getting the requirement of the baccalaureate nursing degree for professional practice enacted into law should rest with each state. One reason given for lack of consensus on acceptance of the baccalaureate requirement for professional practice is nursing's inability to validate competencies for professional and technical nursing practice. The need for a statement of competencies was articulated in 1978 and 1980. But the 1983 report *Education for Nursing Practice* still acknowledged that professional and technical nursing needed to be defined and described and that further work would be required.[17] Since graduations from associate degree, baccalaureate, master's, and doctoral programs have continued to increase, it appears that nursing education has become a vital part of the mainstream of higher education.

As a part of the ANA's efforts to implement the 1965 position paper on entry into practice, representatives of twenty-five state nurses' associations met in Kansas City in 1983 to develop a national plan for achieving the ANA goals on education for nursing practice. Among the issues discussed was that of cooperation among state nurses' associations to accomplish these educational goals.[18] Undoubtedly, the thrust toward demanding higher standards for entry into nursing practice has had a strong impact on professionalization for nursing. More nurses are now pursuing nursing degrees in higher education than ever before. Ultimately, such a development is bound to affect the nurse's expanding role, as more clinical specialists, family nurse practitioners, and critical care specialists become available.

Throughout the period from 1965 to the present, the National League for Nursing (NLN) attempted on numerous occasions to support a resolution that would direct nursing education into colleges and universities. However, tremendous pressure from the American Hospital Association, the American Medical Association, and the National League for Nursing's Council of Diploma Programs prevented the NLN from sustaining such a resolution. After repeated attempts, the Board of Directors of NLN adopted a position statement on February 3, 1982, on "Nursing Roles—Scope and Preparation" calling for the baccalaureate degree in nursing as the academic preparation needed for professional nursing practice, the associate nursing degree for technical nursing practice, and a certificate or diploma for vocational nursing.[19]

Diploma educators were dissatisfied by the term "technical." Appeals to the NLN Board to rescind the statement were unsuccessful, so representatives of diploma programs agreed to present this issue to the total membership at the sixteenth Biennial NLN Convention in Philadelphia, Pennsylvania, June 1–4, 1983. "Culminating a debate that has overshadowed all other issues of the 16th NLN Biennial Convention, membership . . . let stand the controversial NLN position statement . . . by a vote of 1,879 to 1,444."[20] The rejected resolution read as follows:

RESOLUTION 3: **To Rescind the Position Statement "Nursing Roles—Scope and Preparation"**

WHEREAS, The Certificate of Incorporation of the National League For Nursing states: "The object of this organization shall be to foster the development and improvement of hospital, industrial, public health, and other organized nursing service and of nursing education through the coordinated action of nurses, allied professional groups, citizens, agencies, and schools to the end that the nursing needs of the people will be met"; and

WHEREAS, The first function set forth in the N.L.N. Bylaws Article I, is: "To identify the nursing needs of society and to foster programs designed to meet these needs"; and

WHEREAS, The terms *vocational, technical,* and *professional* have not been adequately defined; and

WHEREAS, The verification and validation of competency differences among diploma, associate degree, and baccalaureate graduates have not been established; and

WHEREAS, The N.L.N. Board of Directors adopted and published the 1982 position statement "Nursing Roles—Scope and Preparation"; and

WHEREAS, The said position statement has been interpreted in a variety of ways by the membership; therefore, be it

RESOLVED, That the National League for Nursing Board of Directors rescind the position statement "Nursing Roles—Scope and Preparation."[21]

Table 7-1 summarizes by year the contributions made by the ANA and NLN in facilitating movement toward the accomplishment of the baccalaureate nursing degree as the educational requirement for professional nursing.

The hope of many nurse educators was expressed in the following statement:

> Maybe now we can lay this issue to rest. The need for baccalaureate education for professional nursing is not a new mandate. In one way or another it has been advocated for almost 100 years. Certainly in the last 20 years the majority of nurses have repeatedly voted for both the concept and its implementation in every major nursing organization.[22]

An extensive amount of time, effort, and energy has been given to this one issue. As a possible solution to remedy the existing confusion in nursing education, Janet Williamson suggested that nursing "(1) should allow the continued phase-out of diploma programs; (2) redefine the content of the associate degree to a narrow sphere of technology, and/or workplace, such as intensive care; (3) rename the current baccalaureate degree 'a baccalaureate degree in nursing technology' and maintain current licensure for this degree."[23] This latter degree would not be necessary for

Table 7-1. Significant activities of ANA and NLN on the entry into practice issue (1985–1990)

Year	Activities
October 31, 1985	Adoption of position in support of two levels of nursing practice, professional and associate, by NLN Board of Directors
November 6, 1985	Letter sent from NLN President Jacquelyn S. Kinder, Ed.D., to agency and individual members informing them of the action and rationale of the Board and asking for their support
November 21, 1985	Special meeting of chairs of NLN educational councils held to discuss responses of NLN members to the position on two levels of nursing practice and to discuss needs for further communication regarding the position
December 1985	Coverage of Board action and guest editorial, "Charting Nursing's Future," by President Kinder, appears in *Nursing and Health Care*
January 22, 1986	Meeting of the educational and service council chairs and vice chairs group held to continue the discussion of membership response to the position, to establish the agenda for the meeting with ANA cabinet chairs, and to plan communications to apprise members of activities to date
January 23, 1986	Presidents and executive directors of NLN and ANA and chairs of NLN councils and ANA cabinets meet
February 26, 1986	Meeting of educational and service council chairs and vice chairs held to discuss the NLN/ANA meeting and to draft an interpretive statement designed to clarify the NLN position on two levels of nursing practice
March 1986	Interpretive statement mailed to all NLN members, agencies, and individuals
April 1986	Related activities to be covered in Highlights of February 27–28 Board meeting, and "Questions and Answers on NLN Position in Support of Two Levels of Nursing Practice" to be printed in *Nursing and Health Care*
May 8, 1986	Next meeting of the educational and service council chairs and vice chairs group scheduled to plan the forum on titling and licensure to be held at the ANA convention. Participants in the forum will include NLN, ANA, the National Federation of Licensed Practical Nurses, the National Association for Practical Nurse Education and Service, and the National Council of State Boards of Nursing
February 1987	ANA develops a new scope of practice for nursing
March 18, 1987	NLN President sends letter to membership reporting on letter response to the League's position in support of two levels of nursing practice

Table 7-1. (continued)

Year	Activities
June 18, 1987	NLN members vote at Biennial Convention to put aside ongoing debates on titling and licensure, reflecting a shift in nursing priorities
November 1988	Council of Baccalaureate and Higher Degree Programs supports achieving two distinct levels of collegiate nursing education, which supports two levels of nursing practice and postpones the issue of titling and licensure by majority vote until an indefinite future date
June 1989	NLN's 19th Biennial Convention evidenced signs of new thinking as contentious titling and licensure debates did not surface
June 1990	ANA's House of Delegates adopt a proviso that if SNAs enact legislation that second level practitioners be given membership in the ANA, the House of Delegates must determine responsibilities, rights, and privileges of the group

entrance into a *professional* nursing program, because individuals with a baccalaureate or advanced degree in other disciplines should be permitted to enroll in professional nursing programs.

Moreover, Williamson believed that a decision at that time on baccalaureate nursing education for entry into professional practice would simply see the return of a crisis situation in another decade or two similar to the present confused state.[24] However, a new approach to licensing professionals will be required when preservice professional nursing education becomes regularized.[25] It was proposed that "high priority be given to designing and putting into operation a valid licensing procedure for professionals who should be judged capable and personally and professionally responsible before they are granted the privilege of entering practice."[26] Individuals seeking a license for the practice of professional nursing should be required to meet the following criteria:

1. Present evidence of having an academic credential that attests to their having completed a program of professional study, with that credential recognized by nursing's academic and professional community
2. Present evidence of assurance by faculties from the professional schools from which they were graduated that they have demonstrated mastery of subject matter and practiced competencies and exemplified professional values that have been accepted by

the existing associations of university nursing schools and by nursing's professional society as essential to professional practice

3. Pass the licensing examination designed exclusively to test mastery of professional knowledge[27]

An Issue that Will Not Go Away

"Entry into practice" still remains a crucial issue in the 1990s. However, nurse leaders have agreed to postpone any serious deliberations in order to address more immediate concerns, such as the nursing shortage and the inadequate health care system. Postponement simply means that the issue will have to be addressed later on—it will not go away!

Why then has the entry dilemma remained unresolved, although two levels of practitioners were proposed by the ANA as far back as 1965? Progress on this issue has occurred, but a division still separates those nurses favoring a two-tiered system and those opposing it. Although a vast number of books, articles, and national meetings have provided up-to-date information on the advisability of adopting two levels of practice (professional and technical), some nurses have concluded that nursing and nurses must be satisfied with the present system and are not convinced that nurses' professionalism is really being questioned.

According to Baker, "Professionalism is the basis for collegiality and involves a shared set of values, certain powers, rights, and duties, common goals and equality among colleagues."[28] It is possible that many nurses debating the entry issue are not fully aware of what true professionalism is all about. In fact, nurse leaders question whether many nurses really want to belong to a profession. They may simply be satisfied with remaining at a subprofession or occupational level. Styles urges that the "nursing education system in this country be strengthened and that it be related to license to practice."[29] She considers the entry into practice issue as "a lingering, festering issue that should be looked at again and resolved."[30] Nurses should understand that the "direction and control of basic nursing education come primarily from politics, not professional sources."[31]

> The issue is: Will nursing leaders active in the period just prior to the beginning of the 21st century continue to relegate control of basic education of professionals to governmental appointees who are subject to political pressures or will nursing leaders act to insure that basic nursing education will be guided and controlled by qualified professionals within the field of nursing?
>
> The issue is: Will corporate nursing continue to settle for undifferentiated registration of nursing, or will professionals act to establish a license procedure for its clearly identified professionals?[32]

"In the transition of an occupation to a profession, it is essential that the members hold special and exclusive knowledge essential to its practice."[33]

> The knowledge base for each type of graduate must be sufficiently differentiated so that the practice of each resides upon a different base and the exchange or substitution of one type of practitioner is not possible. The corpus of knowledge for the professional practitioner must be vastly different from the technical and contain far more exclusive knowledge than that which is provided today.[34]

To date, nursing has been unsuccessful in differentiating between professional and technical nursing. Is the problem of differentiation of levels difficult? If so, what efforts are being made to identify the body of knowledge requisite for professional nurses? The American Association of Colleges of Nursing (AACN) final report describing the essentials of collegiate education for professional nursing was prepared to assist nurse professionals in reaching consensus on the subject matter basic to professional nursing.[35] As nursing continues its progress from an occupation to full professional status, the various members must provide evidence that they possess special knowledge and judgment that cannot be substituted by less prepared non-professional personnel.

Unlike other professions that require post-baccalaureate education for their members, nursing continues to educate practitioners in multiple educational preparation levels (associate degree, diploma, baccalaureate degree, entry level master's, and entry-level doctoral) in order for them to obtain a license as a registered nurse. The public, high school and college counselors, and professionals in and outside of nursing, find it impossible to comprehend why nursing has been unable to "put its house in order" and finally offer only one form of basic nursing education for professional nursing.

Minimum Preparation for Entry
Into Professional Practice

Another pertinent issue is whether the baccalaureate degree should be the minimum preparation for entry into professional practice. Since the acuity of illness of hospitalized patients has changed dramatically, due in part to technological advances in medical and surgical treatments, "entry level nursing students are not prepared for the complex medical and nursing requirements . . . found in hospitals today."[36] Moreover, the increasingly complex nature of professional nursing requires educational preparation beyond the baccalaureate nursing degree, even though the BSN has not been approved for entry into practice.

Some nurse educators believe that in the future post-baccalaureate generic graduate degrees (M.S.N. or N.D.) will be required for nurses functioning at a professional level. It is interesting to note that in 1986 physical therapists declared the entry position to be at the master's level. Recognized professions (i.e., medicine, dentistry) require a doctorate as an entry point. Lang optimistically predicted that "if all goes well by the year 2000, nursing will have settled the issue of entry at the professional level so that nursing would be similar to other practice disciplines and practice professions that are moving toward the master's degree as the minimum education for practice."[37]

CLINICAL PRACTICE—A PART OF THE FACULTY ROLE?

An issue that many nurse educators believed to be of little importance in the early 1970s has emerged as vitally important in the 1980s and 1990s. Concerns are being voiced more frequently about the clinical competence of nurse faculty members and the need for appropriate faculty role models as practitioners of nursing. In the past, nursing faculty was not expected to provide direct nursing care to clients. Today, however, clinical practice for faculty is an expectation that is shared by many nurse deans, faculty, and other health professionals in university teaching centers and other nursing education settings. Since there are proponents for and opponents against this issue, viewpoints representative of both groups will be considered in the following paragraphs.

Nurse faculty members continue to exert their energy in a triad of responsibilities for teaching, research, and community service. They have believed for many years that time was unavailable for direct nursing practice and that clinical supervision of students met the faculty's responsibility for clinical nursing practice. Heavy teaching loads, responsibility for clinical supervision, numerous university and school of nursing committee involvements, participation in grant writing, and curricular studies, along with professional responsibilities at the local, state, and national level, have allowed little time for clinical practice. With tenure and promotion criteria so demanding, especially requirements for research and publications, it is understandable why the concept of faculty practice has not been universally accepted by all nurse faculty.

Moreover, the transition from that of practicing nurse to nurse educator is not an easy one. The nurse educator exchanges the role of caregiver for that of a facilitator of learning. In the former role, the nurse may be extremely knowledgeable, but knowing a subject matter does not necessarily make the individual an effective educator of that knowledge. Such role changes necessitate a shift in personal reward systems and in sources of personal satisfaction. A clinical nurse often assumes her teaching responsibilities with a strong emotional tie to the practitioner role. As a result, clinical competence and expertise are altered.[38]

This observation raises some questions. "Should the nurse educator be competent in clinical practice and an expert in her ability to communicate or transmit knowledge to the students?" "Is it reasonable to expect that all nurse educators be clinical experts?" Ideally, if a faculty member is clinically competent, engages in clinical practice, and is expertly qualified to teach, then nursing education will benefit. However, circumstances will affect answers to the latter question because prior nursing experience, age of the faculty member, interest in pursuing clinical practice, and other responsibilities could greatly affect the individual's pursuit of clinical practice.

In the early period of nursing in the United States, the role of teacher and practitioner was combined. Teachers were also head nurses on the various wards. Several of the head nurses were senior students or new graduates with no teaching experience. Interestingly enough, the ability to *do* was equated with the ability to *teach*.[39] It should be mentioned that the latest NLN criteria for accrediting collegiate schools of nursing requests information on the clinical activities of nursing faculty. However, the NLN provides for broad responses, in that clinical consultation and other activities can be used as evidence of maintaining currency in clinical nursing practice.

A review of this issue from the viewpoint of those advocating faculty practice also presents some convincing arguments. For example, some authors have described faculty practice as "those functions performed by faculty within a service setting that have as the principal goal continued advancement of the nursing care of patients/clients, a goal congruent with the role of an academician in a professional discipline."[40] These authors believe that clinical teaching does not meet this criteria because its main focus is on educating the students. Some would exclude clinical practice obtained through "moonlighting"—a part-time position that is concurrent with a part-time faculty position. They would also exclude an occasional rendering of care to patients to maintain one's clinical skills or faculty involvement that is limited to simply discussing and evaluating students' practice.[41]

From the increasing number of articles on unification of nursing service and nursing education and on nursing faculty practice, it appears that the tensions over this issue are increasing. Faculty in nursing are an important variable in measuring the quality of the educational enterprise. Their involvement in clinical practice should be an important requisite of their teaching role. However, due to increasingly heavy teaching loads, faculty members have systematically disengaged themselves from clinical practice. Thus, many of them may begin to doubt their clinical competence. It is only recently that the possibility of nurse faculty contributing to both the quality and improvement of nursing practice has become a topic requiring reflection and study.[42]

Combining practice and teaching was evidenced in a 1979 resolution by the American Academy of Nursing, which stated that "The American Academy of Nursing endorses the idea of cementing the relationship of service and education through such devices as faculty practice."[43] Again in March 1979, thirteen nursing leaders signed a "Statement of Belief Regarding Faculty Practice," which stressed the importance of nursing practice as a legitimate part of the faculty role; the creation of incentives for faculty to integrate practice into research and teaching; and the provision of opportunities for faculty to develop new roles.[44]

Presently there are few institutions that consider expertise in nursing practice as a criteria for reappointment, promotion, or tenure. Nor have many provided release time or other notable rewards for clinical practice.[45, 46] And yet, many universities are beginning to expect faculty to engage in the full professional role of education, research, practice, and service. As more and more faculty are prepared at the doctoral level, movement toward professionalization will be greatly increased, and the "full role" will be accomplished by many university nursing faculty. It is evident that faculty cannot be effective in motivating students to become clinically expert, if the faculty themselves are not expert practitioners who seek improvements in the health field. And yet, how often are students provided the opportunity to observe faculty managing patients in direct care or working to improve standards for quality nursing care? Each component of this "full role" cannot be fulfilled to the same degree at any given period. For example, during the first year of a new teaching responsibility, the main emphasis would be on teaching, whereas in additional years, faculty should be able to negotiate with their administrators as to what percentage of time would be allocated to research, to service, and to clinical practice. Wisdom and prudence should dictate these decisions, so that misunderstandings do not occur and reachable goals are set. Clinical practice as evidence of faculty credibility will be needed by those having major responsibility for clinical supervision of students.[47]

In order to reinforce their 1979 resolution on faculty practice, the American Academy of Nursing sponsored the first annual Nursing Faculty Practice Symposium, entitled "Structure to Outcome—Making It Work," in December 1983, in Orlando, Florida. This symposium was designed to "offer a showcase for advanced concepts and effective models of nursing practice by faculty in a variety of settings, and to provide a forum for discussion and debate among nurse leaders with a view toward clarifying the role, scope, and nature of faculty practitioners."[48] Attended by 235 people, this symposium provided five major presentations and an opportunity for small group discussions on topics suggested by the papers (e.g., faculty organization structures, faculty practice plans, and administrative structures).[49]

As a means of helping faculty maintain and improve their clinical skills, several strategies or options are being made available. Practice modalities, such as joint appointments with appropriate clinical agencies, independent or private practice for some faculty, summer practice in clinical agencies, and reordering or adjustment of faculty teaching loads, are a few strategies currently being used. The latter can be achieved by the use of graduate teaching assistants, reducing committee responsibilities, and encouraging collaboration on research projects of mutual interest. Provision of release time for short or extended periods of time (sabbaticals), educational leaves, planning faculty workloads on a yearly basis, and more flexible scheduling are additional strategies to be used. Also, by changing methods of teaching, reducing class size, using computer-assisted instruction, and using adjunct faculty for course instruction, faculty loads can be considerably lessened. Without administrative support for faculty practice, it will be difficult for faculty to accomplish any of the practice modes just mentioned.

Developing faculty practice plans as a means of supporting faculty and having faculty provide direct care to clients have begun to stimulate interest in clinical practice among faculty in some schools of nursing. Before developing such a plan, agreement on what constitutes clinical practice must be reached. The faculty practice plan developed in the College of Nursing at the University of Oklahoma continues to serve as a model for other university schools of nursing. Characteristics of this professional practice plan are well documented in nursing literature.[50-52]

The primary deterrent to nursing school faculty developing a faculty practice plan, however, is that most nursing faculty do not engage in clinical nursing practice. The real basis for such a plan lies in the value of clinical competence as an important credential in support of faculty credibility, as observed in the day-to-day involvement of faculty as providers of excellent clinical nursing care.[53]

In referring to the personal and professional rewards for the individual as well as for the institution resulting from faculty practice, it has been observed that:

> The respect, credibility, and self-esteem of the faculty member are enhanced considerably by the individual's ability to demonstrate competency in practice and to successfully integrate and synthesize that practice to accomplish the goals of education and research. The institution gains by having experts in clinical nursing who can also provide staff development, give guidance to quality assurance and management programs, research problems of import to nursing practice and health service delivery, collab-

orate with other health professionals and improve the image of the institution.[54]

As nursing advances toward becoming a full-fledged profession of "accountable health care practitioners," faculty practice as a concept will be acknowledged as pivotal to this attainment. Undoubtedly, the time has come for nurse educators to practice and move actively toward tomorrow's nursing world.[55]

UNIFICATION MODELS FOR NURSING EDUCATION AND NURSING PRACTICE

The debate over unification models of nursing education and nursing practice continues to remain an important issue, particularly among nurse educators who question their necessity as a means of uniting nurse educators and nurse clinicians in improving nursing care. Before examining their views, however, a brief historical perspective of this movement, along with several descriptions of unification models and their effectiveness, is presented.

Reviewing the history of nursing in the United States, it is readily observed that nursing education and nursing service were united from the outset. Nursing education and clinical nursing experiences were under the direction of the Superintendent of Nurses. Indeed, it was to nursing's advantage not to separate them in the beginnings of the occupation. However, by the late 1930s, many nursing schools began to organize their own faculties completely independent of nursing service. They provided their own supervision of nursing students in the clinical units of the hospitals and other health agencies. Thus began the so-called split between nursing education and nursing service, with each tending to be isolated from the other, giving nursing educators the status of "guests" to be tolerated in the various health care institutions.

As nursing education moved out of the hospital setting into academia, the presence of faculty no longer practicing in the clinical area became the dominant pattern. Devoid of any authority over nursing service, and eliminating clinical practice from their teaching role, nurse faculty's responsibility for role modeling as expert clinicians was diminished. Yet separation of nursing education from nursing service did assure more adequate learning experiences for students and removed them from the pressing institutional demands for nursing services.

This prolonged separation of nursing education from nursing service continues to create barriers that prevent nurses from actualizing their full professional role. From the 1930s to the 1960s, little or no effort was exerted in implementing a unification model between nursing schools and nursing service. Despite isolated attempts by faculty to improve and update their clinical practice, there was no effort to unite service and education in order to strengthen and advance both areas. However, in 1959, Dorothy Smith, former Dean of the School of Nursing at the University of Florida, established an organization model for unifying nursing practice and education. Smith firmly believed that the nursing school dean should also be the chief administrator for nursing practice, and that nurse clinicians should creatively bring about innovative change in the practice of nursing. Other examples of unification models widely known for their successful endeavors are those at Case Western Reserve University in Cleveland, Rush University in Chicago, and the University of Rochester in Rochester, New York.

The unification model developed by Rozella Schlotfeldt and Jannetta McPhail was funded by the W. K. Kellogg Foundation in 1966, as a five-year demonstration project designed to implement "academic" leadership within all of the various clinical services. This model was implemented at Case Western Reserve. It differs from the other three in that the University and the University Hospitals of Cleveland operate under separate Boards of Trustees. Neither the Dean nor Chief Nursing Administrator direct programs requiring specialized nursing knowledge or competencies. Instead, clinical specialists in nursing education and nursing service are responsible to one administrator, who is responsible for the quality of programs in both areas. In other words, unification of nursing education and nursing service is designed to occur at the clinical department level. Joint appointments by the university and the hospital are the means for further cooperation and collaboration for teaching, practice, and research. To avoid the status of guests, faculty have appointments in nursing service. Chief nursing service personnel hold academic appointments in the school of nursing.

McPhail described three types of joint appointments that were developed: shared appointments for those having responsibilities in both organizations, involving cost sharing on an equal or other basis based on organizational needs; faculty-associate appointment held by full-rank faculty eligible for tenure and having an associate in nursing appointment in the university hospitals with no cost sharing; and clinical appointments for nurses in leadership positions in the university hospitals with salaries paid in full by the hospitals and appointees accountable for a quality of care adequate for student learning.[56] Over twenty years after the conclusion of this demonstration project, which began in 1971, progress continues in improving collaboration and unification between nursing education and nursing service and in meeting the goals of quality nursing care, education, and research.

The Rush University unification model embodies the integration of the full professional role of practice, education, research, and consultation in the hospital setting. The chief academic officer serves as both Dean of the College of Nursing and Vice President of Nursing Affairs at the Medical Center. Associate deans and chairpersons of the clinical departments provide assistance to top administrative leaders. Each chairperson is responsible for the integration of nursing care, education, and practice. Faculty assume practitioner-teacher roles throughout the Medical Center, serving as instructors, consultants, and role models. Rush University uses a matrix model involving decentralization of authority. Each hospital unit determines its staffing requirement and prepares schedules based on the nurses' needs on that particular unit. Practitioner-teachers are supportive of continuing education for staff nurses and for research efforts. They also assist in achievement of goals for each department.

The unification model at the University of Rochester provides for a Dean and Director of Nursing, who is the chief administrator and academic head for all nursing. Introduction of this model occurred in 1971, when a new School of Nursing was established with the assistance of another grant provided by the W. K. Kellogg Foundation. Associate deans and clinical chiefs assist top administration in implementing education-practice programs. Nursing faculty, in addition to their teaching role, update their clinical skills and competencies, either through service or clinical practice. They also collaborate with physicians and other health professionals in improving the quality of patient care.

Throughout the nation, there is strong evidence of nursing educators and nursing service leaders working together to improve nursing care, to provide an excellent learning climate for nursing students, and to prepare more competent practitioners in nursing. The proponents of the unification model are convinced that this is the type of structure nursing should adopt to provide quality nursing care and to bring educators and practitioners together, with each complimenting and profiting from the expertise of each other.

From another viewpoint, there are nurses who do not favor the unification model. They believe it is a demanding and draining one, which frequently leads to "burn out" when energies are expended in too many directions. Several reasons for objecting to the concept of faculty practice are mentioned by nurses who believe it is not in nursing's best interest to accept this plan. These nurses are of the opinion that teaching and clinical practice are weakened under this particular model.

Is unification of nursing service and education under the control of one administration the direction that most nurses leaders will continue to take for the future? Margretta Styles believes that this movement has reached its peak, since less than a handful of such arrangements have occurred in the last decade.[57] She states that "just as joining rather than combining efforts seems to be the mode of the day, collaboration more than unification seems also to be the wave and hope of tomorrow . . . [as it] can be a potent force to achieve our professional aims."[58] This opinion continues to be debated, since advocates of the unification model point to the successes achieved by such an arrangement.

In believing that practicing nurses and nurse educators must be aware of their interdependent roles and direct their united efforts in the accomplishment of common goals, it was concluded that they must be educationally qualified, possess clinical and scientific competence, and demonstrate commitment to a professional career.[59] In the short run, collaboration will be required to achieve this goal. In the long run, nurses may have to blend the major tripartite components of a profession, becoming multiple-function professionals.[60]

IMPACT OF THE CREDENTIALING STUDY ON CREDENTIALING MECHANISMS

The topic of credentialing has been scrutinized since the mid-1970s. Amidst turmoil and confusion, much disunity continues to exist over it. Credentialing may be defined as "the process by which individuals or institutions, or one or more of their programs, are designated by a qualified agent as having met minimum standards at a specified time."[61] In addition, credentialing provides a method whereby standards of education and service are maintained and fostered. It serves further as a stimulant and motivator for self-improvement. More importantly, credentialing provides a means for public accountability. In accepting the principle that the public is protected and served best by credentialing, well-conducted professional credentialing programs provide perhaps the most advantageous means of self-regulating professional services. Another option is regulation by the government.[62]

Licensure, accreditation, and certification are recognized as credentialing mechanisms. They are defined as follows:

> *Licensure,* which is based on statutory law, has as its primary function the protection and safety of the public. Successful completion of a written examination and graduation from a state-approved school of nursing provide evidence that the individual has attained minimal competency to practice in a given occupation. Anyone who practices nursing for compensation must be licensed.
>
> *Accreditation* involves the evaluation and approval of an institution or a program of study as having met specific standards or criteria. The National League for Nursing has served as the accrediting agency for basic and graduate nursing education programs since 1952.
>
> *Certification* is a process by which an association or agency grants recognition to an individual who has met predetermined standards or criteria specified by that association or agency for specialty practice.[63]

Due to the lack of clarity and confusion regarding the definitions of credentialing mechanisms and the resulting financial problems, the ANA awarded a contract of $410,835 to the School of Nursing of the University of Wisconsin-Milwaukee to conduct a twenty-two-month study of credentialing in nursing. Inez G. Hinsvark, Ed.D., was named Project Director of the Committee for the Study of Credentialing in Nursing. Purposes of this study were to determine the adequacy of the current credentialing system including accreditation, certification, and licensure; recommend directions for the future of credentialing in nursing; and suggest means for improving the effectiveness of credentialing mechanisms.

The recommendations and reports of this study, entitled *The Study of Credentialing in Nursing: A New Approach*, were published in 1979.[64] Among other recommendations, this committee suggested that the ANA appoint a task force to study this report further. It also recommended a cost study of credentialing as a basis on which to determine the cost of operating a National Nursing Credentialing Center that would "study, develop, coordinate, provide services for, and conduct credentialing in nursing."[65] These recommendations were presented to the House of Delegates at the June 1980 ANA Convention, and a resolution was passed to facilitate their implementation. Forty-two groups of individuals currently involved in credentialing joined this committee to arrive at a workable solution to the credentialing problem. Thereafter, an independent task force to determine the requirements for forming a viable Credentialing Center was established by the ANA. After several meetings and numerous reports, the task force delineated several models for the proposed Credentialing Center. Unfortunately, the groups involved, with representatives from various nursing organizations, were unable to reach consensus on the proposed models and methods of financing required to maintain and continue their existence.

EFFECT OF THREE NATIONAL NURSING STUDIES

Several significant nursing studies have been conducted since the 1920s on nursing needs and resources and recommendations for the future of nursing and nursing education. Unfortunately, each of these studies and their recommendations remained confined within the pages of nursing's history.

Three important nursing studies of major significance conducted in the early 1980s continue to influence future directions for nursing: the Institute of Medicine Study, the Magnet Hospitals Study, and the National Commission on Nursing Study. These studies are presented chronologically as follows:

Institute of Medicine Study

As a result of conflicting opinions regarding the so-called nursing shortage in the late 1970s, serious debates occurred within the federal government about the need for continued federal aid for nursing education. To bring closure to the debate, Congress mandated in Section 113 of the Nurse Training Act Amendments of 1979 that a study on nursing and nursing education be conducted by the Institute of Medicine (IOM) of the National Academy of Sciences.[66] This two-year study, released early in 1983, contained twenty-one specific recommendations to Congress and continued to form the basis on which nursing policy and funding would be determined throughout the remainder of the 1980s. (The IOM recommendations are listed in the following display.)

Funded by the Department of Health and Human Services for $1.6 million dollars, Congress established four main objectives for the IOM Study: (1) to advise on existing conditions for future federal support of nursing education; (2) to identify why more nurses do not opt for employment in medically underserved areas; (3) to determine if and why nurses do not remain in nursing; and (4) to recommend measures involving the public and private sectors to improve the supply and proper utilization of nursing resources.[67]

Among other recommendations, the IOM Study concluded that because the supply and demand for nurses would be in reasonable balance, no specific federal support for basic nursing education was justified at the time. This "reasonable balance" of registered nurses is attributed to the fact that "nurses, spurred by double-digit inflation in the 1980s as well as by salary increases in 1980 and 1981, reentered the labor force in larger numbers," and general unemployment, resulting in loss of hospital insurance coverage, produced a rapid decline in hospital occupancy rates and a reduction in demand for nurses.[68]

The IOM Study did, however, confirm a continuing shortage of registered nurses prepared for leadership at the graduate level, especially in areas of specialty preparation.

Referring to nurses with graduate preparation as a scarce national resource, the IOM Study requested Congress in 1983 to fund nursing education efforts for this purpose at about $80 million. However, if a tightened job market for the public would have continued, "the profession might want to rethink the size and structure of nursing's educational system . . . [and] whether it is in nursing's best interest to expand the pool of practicing nurses at the rapid rates of the past decade."[69] Ginzberg's warning in 1978 to hold the line on rapid escalation of RN supply to prevent an impending new surplus in the 1980s was given careful consideration.[70] However, nursing shortages continued to occur even during this latter period.

IOM Committee Recommendations

1. Discontinue federal efforts to increase the supply of "generalist" nurses;
2. Give the states funding and technical assistance to plan for generalist nurse education;
3. Maintain federal aid for all kinds of college education so would-be nurses will have access to it;
4. States, cities, hospitals, colleges and insurers to allocate financial aid to generalist nursing education programs;
5. Encourage nurse educators and organizations to attract late-entry and minority students as well as recent high school graduates;
6. End admission barriers that hinder nurses from moving to one educational level from another;
7. Foster closer collaboration between nurse educators and those who are practicing for better "hands-on" training;
8. Expand federal support of fellowships, loans and programs to generate more advanced, specialized nursing degrees;
9. Help alleviate maldistribution of nurses by federal support to demonstration programs designed for educational outreach;
10. Encourage consortia of nurse educators and employers in shortage areas to increase opportunities for minority students;
11. Establish "fair-share" Medicare, Medicaid, state and local payments to pay for care in inner-city hospitals;
12. Increase federal support of geriatric nursing education;
13. Upgrade skills of nursing home staff through federal support of state and local educational programs;
14. Restructure Medicare and Medicaid payment methods to encourage long-term nursing care services in homes and in institutions, moving toward 24-hour RN coverage in nursing homes;
15. End state and local legal barriers to the practices of nurse midwives and nurse practitioners;
16. Encourage employers to improve supply and job tenure by providing career advancement opportunities, reward clinical merit with salary increases, increase wages if there are vacancies, and adapt benefit packages to attract nurses;
17. Improve cost accounting for nursing via hospital-promoted studies;
18. Establish, on a federal level, an organizational entity to place nursing research in the mainstream of scientific investigation;
19. Research nurse competencies at each level of preparation through private and federal sources;
20. Assess and disseminate, from a national level, nursing research results and;
21. Continue federal collection of timely data on national nurse education, supply and practice.

Magnet Hospitals Study

Forty-one "magnet" hospitals were selected by the ANA's American Academy of Nursing as models of nursing practice.[71] Describing the process and criteria used by the Academy in making its selections, McClure, chairperson of the task force directing the project, commented that this study provides information useful to other hospitals in improving their nursing staff.[72] Chosen from a list of 165 hospitals nominated by nurses as attractive places to practice and work, forty-one of these were chosen to participate in this study (see List of Hospitals). The critical issue in this study was good leadership.[73] Designed, conducted, and published in approximately eighteen months, this report "enhances the Academy's posture as an influential body of nursing who have addressed one of today's most critical problems as nursing care in hospitals is provided."[74]

Serving as principal investigators from the task force were Muriel A. Poulin, Ed.D., former Chairperson of the nursing administration program at Boston University School of Nursing (now closed); Margaret D. Sovie, Ph.D., former Associate Dean for nursing practice at the University of Rochester; and Mabel A. Wandelt, Ph.D., former Director of the School of Nursing Center for Research at the University of Texas, Austin. The intent of this study was not to identify all hospitals having high standards of staffing and care, but simply to obtain a "few examples" of such institutions.

Five Academy of Nursing members served as nominators in each of eight regions established by the Bureau of Labor Statistics. Each nominator suggested up to ten names to the task force. These individuals were also invited to join the study. Officials of those hospitals that agreed to participate completed a questionnaire covering areas such as the educational preparation of supervisory nurses and the current status of nurse staffing. In the project's final phase, the task force held group interviews in each region, one for directors of nursing and another for staff nurses of selected hospitals.

Magnet hospital nurses stated that opportunities for professional growth and for practicing professional nursing were two important items. This study clearly documented the significance of the nurse administrator role as a key to improving patient care. Each of these nurse executives used their authority in fulfilling their responsibilities of leadership and in providing valuable service as overall administrative team members.

National Commission on Nursing Study

The National Commission on Nursing, appointed in the summer of 1980 by the American Hospital Association under the directorship of Majorie Beyers, RN, was established to address current nursing-related

These Hospitals Magnetize Nurses

Regions 1 & 2 (Northeast)*

• Beth Israel Hospital; Boston, Mass. • Memorial General Hospital; Union, N.J. • Morristown Memorial Hospital; Morristown, N.J. • Saint Francis Hospital; Roslyn, N.Y. • Strong Memorial Hospital-University of Rochester; Rochester, N.Y. • Worcester Hahnemann Hospital; Worcester, Mass.

Region 3 (Mid-Atlantic)

• Arlington Hospital; Arlington, Va. • Fairfax Hospital; Falls Church, Va. • Franklin Square Hospital; Baltimore, Md. • Henrico Doctors Hospital; Richmond, Va. • Prince George's General Hospital & Medical Center; Cheverly, Md. • Shady Grove Adventist Hospital; Rockville, Md.

Region 4 (South)

• Fort Sanders Regional Medical Center; Knoxville, Tenn. • University Hospital; Augusta, Ga.

Region 5 (Mid & Upper Midwest)

• Evanston Hospital Corporation; Evanston, Il. • Family Hospital; Milwaukee, Wis. • Rochester Methodist Hospital; Rochester, Minn. • St. Joseph's Hospital; Kansas City, Mo. • Saint Michael Hospital; Milwaukee, Wis. • University Hospitals of Cleveland; Cleveland, Ohio.

Region 6 (Southwest)

• Hillcrest Medical Center; Tulsa, Okla. • Charlton Methodist Hospital; Dallas, Texas• Park Plaza Hospital; Houston, Texas• Presbyterian Hospital; Oklahoma City, Okla. • Seton Medical Center; Austin, Texas • Woman's Hospital; Baton Rouge, La.

Regions 7 & 8 (West, Midwest)

• Iowa Methodist Medical Center; Des Moines, Iowa• Lutheran Medical Center; Wheatridge, Colo. • Saint Joseph Hospital; St. Charles, Mo. • VA Medical & Regional Office Center; Cheyenne, Wyo.

Region 9 (West)

• Alta Bates Hospital; Berkeley, Calif • El Camino Hospital, Mountain View, Calif. • Saint Mary's Hospital & Health Center; Tucson, Ariz. • Stanford University Hospital; Palo Alto, Calif. • University of California-San Francisco Hospitals & Clinics; San Francisco, Calif.

Region 10 (Northwest)

• Kaiser Foundation Hospitals; Portland, Ore. • Meridian Park Hospital; Tualatin, Ore. • Sacred Heart Medical Center; Spokane, Wash. • University Hospital; Seattle, Wash. • Valley General Hospital; Renton, Wash. • Virginia Mason Hospital; Seattle, Wash.

problems and nursing education issues in the United States and to make recommendations for the future. Consisting of thirty-one members, including representatives of hospital administration, medicine, business, government, and academia, in addition to seventeen nurses, the Commission issued its final report in the summer, 1983.[75] This report, which included eighteen recommendations, has been generally well accepted by nurses and representatives of other health care organizations.

Consensus on support for the B.S.N. and on nursing involvement in decision making was a positive step forward, despite the varied representation of the group.[76] It should be pointed out, however, that such consensus was reached only after three years of effort that included public hearings in six cities, open forums, testimony, an invitational meeting for representatives of thirty-two hospitals, hospital administrators, and medical directors, and numerous publications. Submitting the final report to intensive review by constituents of the organizations represented on the Commission resulted in several worthwhile comments. Judith Ryan, former ANA Executive Director, pointed out that after all the scrutiny, the Commission continued to support those positions that nursing had already identified as vital to its progress. Both the IOM Study and the Commission report consistently supported nursing's positions on nursing education, nursing practice, and on how nursing services were organized, delivered, and financed.[77]

Leaders among the various constituencies, such as trustees, hospital administrators, physicians, business personnel and educators, reached consensus on beliefs about nursing. They believed that "nursing is a necessary profession, that their clinical practitioners should be well educated, that qualified practitioners should be recognized and adequately paid, and that nursing must have a significant role both in managing and administering institutions where nursing care is an important component of the services offered and in planning for social policy that affects the delivery of those services."[78]

The National Commission on Nursing's Summary Report asked that nurses unite and reach consensus on issues, so that the public could comprehend who nurses were, what they do, and how they were educated and credentialed.[79] If there is a growing consensus about nursing's role on the part of health-care leaders outside of nursing, then it becomes more imperative for nurses to join together to reach agreement on the key issues of standards for nursing education and practice, and resolve the issue of credentialing for nurses in the forseeable future.

The new HHS Secretary's Commission on the Nursing Shortage appointed in 1987 (presented in Chapter 4) made recommendations very similar to those of the 1980 Commission.

PREPARATION FOR POLITICAL INVOLVEMENT FOR NURSES

Another critical issue is nurses' current lack of preparation for political involvement. Health policy planning and development reflect the limited participation by nurses, even though nursing's leaders have repeatedly called for greater involvement.[80] "[N]urses as the major deliverers of health care, must be part of the policy and decision-making processes that determine the type, the setting, the cost, and the quality of health care to be provided."[81]

Only a few nursing schools provide curricula that include coursework to prepare students for involvement in the political process.[82] Many nurse educators agree that such preparation is needed, whether at the undergraduate or graduate level. Most nurses and nursing students are informed about the role of Nurses Coalition for Action in Politics (NCAP), the political arm of the ANA. It is the political voice whose "purpose is to make nurses' viewpoints and votes visible and powerful . . . [and] change misguided health care policies to improve economic equity for women in America."[83] Although the image of nursing on the legislative scene has shown a marked improvement due to greater political activity, nurses both male and female still need to inform and update legislators more frequently on their new roles, their effectiveness in reducing health care costs, and their concern about future health care delivery.

As leaders in the nursing profession, we need to define what essential components of nursing ought to be included in the variety of plans for health care that will be forthcoming from professional planners and those resulting from legislative action. Whether appropriate plans for nursing will be included will depend largely, I believe, on nursing's being able to develop a broadly based constituency. This may be the biggest task ahead of us.[84]

In order to overcome the remaining effects of nurses having been socialized into passive roles, to remove the fear and negative responses that have hindered political development of nurses, and to assist nurses in achieving the goal of becoming "skilled and effective protagonists in a variety of political forums," greater emphasis on political involvement is desirable.[85] Certainly, the future of nursing is far too important to leave the resolution of nursing and health care issues to others, whether they be consumers, politicians, or other health-care providers.[86]

Nurses have begun a political movement targeted to increase the pace of change in health care delivery. Nurse educators are urged to provide knowledge of legislative processes as well as to encourage their students, faculty, and practicing nurses to increase their political activities to improve nursing, nursing education, and health care.

SUMMARY

Entry into practice has been identified as one of the most critical issues currently facing nursing. The ANA position paper on educational preparation for entry into professional nursing and technical nursing still divides nurses, although evidence clearly indicates that circumstances are favoring eventual acceptance of this proposal. Various activities engaged in by the American Nurses Association over a twenty-five-year period and activities by the National League for Nursing and the New York State Nurses' Association indicate continuous progress toward implementing the 1965 position paper. Now that the ANA and the NLN are in agreement on the direction in which to regularize professional nursing, it is hoped that internal confusion and divisiveness may cease.

Another issue of concern to nurse educators involves the need for faculty to engage in clinical practice. The pros and cons of this issue continue to be debated. Ways to enable faculty to include clinical practice in their busy schedules continue to be explored. In considering the issue of unification of nursing education and nursing practice, it is interesting to note that this concept is not new. It has been in evidence since the history of nursing in this country began with educators and practicing nurses serving dual roles until the 1940s. From 1940 to 1960, little effort occurred to reunite nursing education and practice. By the 1970s, the concept of unification was under way in three university schools of nursing. Description of unification models at three highly respected universities, Case Western Reserve, Rush University, and Rochester University, indicates a significant rate of satisfaction with this concept. Despite its success, unification is not favored by many nursing groups. Reasons cited are that the roles of educator and practitioner are equally demanding, and a lack of time and the commitment to many other activities are strong barriers to implementing this concept.

Credentialing in nursing (involving licensure, accreditation, certification) and the related ANA-sponsored study continue to be debated by many nurses. Since no agreement has been reached on a proposed National Credentialing Center, no further action has occurred to date.

Three national nursing studies—Institute of Medicine, Magnet Hospitals, and the National Commission on Nursing—reveal progress being made by nursing, the many problems confronting it, and various recommendations to solve some of these problems and advance nursing's status. Both the IOM and NCON studies support nursing's position on nursing education, nursing practice, and on how nursing should be organized and financed. It behooves nurses to reach agreement on standards for nursing education, nursing practice, and credentialing, since even lay representatives comprising these study groups have been able to reach consensus on nursing's major problems. The need for nurses to become politically active in order to exert leadership in planning for future health care delivery is gaining momentum. Lack of political involvement has prevented nursing from becoming visible in health care arenas where health policies and directions are being established. Faculty in schools of nursing have been urged to include in their nursing curricula coursework on knowledge of the political process in order to prepare nursing students for political activities.

REFERENCES

1. *Education for Nursing Practice in the Context of the 1980s,* Cabinet on Nursing Education (Pub. No.: NE-11 5M 4183). Kansas City, Mo.: American Nurses' Association, 1983, 2.
2. Fagin, C. and McClure, M. "Can We Bring Order out of the Chaos of Nursing Education?" *American Journal of Nursing* 76:1 (January, 1976), 102.
3. Rogers M. "Nursing: To Be or Not To Be," *Nursing Outlook* 20:1 (1972), 42–45.
4. Montag, M. "Looking Back: Associate Degree Education in Perspective," *Nursing Outlook* 28:4 (April, 1980), 250.
5. McClure, M. "Entry into Professional Practice: The New York Proposal," *Journal of Nursing Administration* 6:5 (June, 1976), 93–99.

6. American Nurses' Association. "Resolutions," *American Nurse* 10:9 (September 15, 1978), 9.

7. *Perspectives on Entry into Practice* (Adapted by AORN House of Delegates, March, 1979). Denver: Association of Operating Room Nurses, 1979.

8. American Nurses' Association. "Resolutions Adopted by House of Delegates," *American Nurse* 12:7 (1980), 12–13.

9. *Educational Preparation for Nursing: A Source Book.* Kansas City, Mo.: American Nurses' Association, 1981.

10. *Education for Nursing Practice*, 2.

11. *Ibid.*

12. "Education Task Force Offers Recommendations for Transition," *American Nurse* 15:5 (May, 1983), 3.

13. "Board Adopts Education Proposals, Considers Relocation," *American Nurse* 15:7 (July–August, 1983), 9.

14. *Education for Nursing Practice*, ix.

15. *Ibid.*

16. "ANA '84, Challenging the Choices," *American Journal of Nursing* 84:7 (July, 1984), 915–916.

17. "Board Adopts Education Proposals," 9.

18. Selby, T. "SNA Reps Meet to Develop Education Plan," *American Nurse* 15:8 (September, 1983), 1.

19. "NLN Board Endorses B.S.N. for Professional Practice," *Nursing Outlook* 30:2 (April, 1982), 217.

20. "NLN Statement Stands, B.S.N. for Professional Role," *Convention News*, NLN (June, 1983), 1.

21. "NLN Resolution 3," from the *Report of the Committee on Resolutions to NLN Membership.* New York: National League for Nursing, 1983, 3.

22. Kelly, L. S. "Swords into Plowshares," *Nursing Outlook* 31:5 (September–October, 1983), 261.

23. Williamson, J. "Crisis in Academic Nursing," in N. Chaska (ed.), *The Nursing Profession: A Time to Speak.* New York: McGraw-Hill, 1983, 67.

24. *Ibid.*

25. Schlotfeldt, R. M. *A Brave New Nursing World.* (Pub. No.: 82–83). Washington, D.C.: American Association of Colleges of Nursing, 1982, 18.

26. *Ibid.*

27. *Ibid.*, 9.

28. Baker, C., Boyd, N., Stasiowski, S. and Simons, B. "Interinstitutional Collaboration for Nursing Excellence: Part I, Creating the Partnership," *Journal of Nursing Administration* 19:2 (February, 1989), 9.

29. Styles, M. "Styles To Be Honored with Award," *American Nurse* 22:4 (April, 1990), 31.

30. *Ibid.*

31. Schlotfeldt, R. "Resolution of Issues: An Imperative for Creating Nursing's Future," *Journal of Professional Nursing* 3:3 (May–June, 1987), 149.

32. *Ibid.*

33. Aydelotte, M. "The Evolving Profession" in N. Chaska (ed.), *The Nursing Profession: Turning Points.* St. Louis: C.V. Mosby, 1990, 12.

34. *Ibid.*
35. American Association of Colleges of Nursing. *Essentials of College and University Education for Professional Nursing.* Washington, D.C.: A.A.C.N., 1986.
36. Lindeman, C. "Curriculum Revolution: Reconceptualizing Clinical Nursing Education," *Nursing and Health Care* 10:1 (January, 1989), 24.
37. "How Can Nurses Prepare for Year 2000?" *American Nurse* 19:3 (March, 1987), 10.
38. Infante, M. "Nurse *vs.* Nurse Educator: Conflicting Roles for the Teacher of Nursing," *Nurse Educators Opportunities and Innovations* (March, 1983), 1, 4, 8.
39. Christy, T. "Clinical Practice as a Function of Nursing Education: A Historical Analysis," *Nursing Outlook* 28:8 (1980), 493–497.
40. Ford, L. and Kitzman, H. "Organizational Perspectives on Faculty Practice: Issues and Challenges," in *Structure to Outcome—Making It Work.* Kansas City, Mo.: American Academy of Nursing, 1983, 14.
41. Batey, M. "Structural Considerations for the Social Integration of Nursing," in *Structure to Outcome—Making It Work.* Kansas City, Mo.: American Academy of Nursing, 1983, 43–58.
42. Mauksch, I. "Faculty Practice: A Professional Imperative," *Nurse Educator* 5:3 (May–June, 1980), 23–24.
43. "Resolution on Unification of Nursing Service and Nursing Education," *A.A.N. Newsletter* 1 (Winter, 1979–80), 4.
44. "Statement of Belief Regarding Faculty Practice," *Nursing Outlook* 27:3 (March, 1979).
45. Collison, C. and Parsons, M. "Is Practice a Viable Faculty Role?" *Nursing Outlook* 28:1 (November, 1980), 677–679.
46. Joel, L. "Stepchildren in the Family: Aiming Toward Synergy Between Nursing Education and Service—From the Faculty Perspective," in *Structure to Outcome—Making it Work.* Kansas City, Mo.: American Academy of Nursing, 1983, 43–58.
47. *Ibid.,* 47.
48. "Academy to Sponsor Symposiums on Nursing Faculty Practice," *American Nurse* 15:5 (May, 1983), 16.
49. McCarthy, P. "Faculty Practice Symposium Seeks Way to Make It Work," *American Nurse* 16:2 (February, 1984).
50. Smith, G. "Development of a Faculty Practice Reimbursement Plan," in L. Aiken (ed.), *Health Policy and Nursing Practice.* New York: McGraw-Hill, 1981, 256–267.
51. Smith, G. "Faculty Practice Plans: Latent Obstacles to Success," in J. McCloskey and H. Grace (eds.), *Current Issues in Nursing.* Boston: Blackwell Scientific Publications, 1981, 551–557.
52. Smith, G. "Compensating Faculty for Their Clinical Practice," *Nursing Outlook* 25:11 (November, 1980), 673–676.
53. Smith, G. "Development of a Faculty Practice Reimbursement Plan," 258.
54. Ford, L. and Kitzman, H. "Organizational Perspectives on Faculty Practice," 27.
55. Mauksch, I. "Faculty Practice," 24.
56. McPhail, J. "Implementation and Evaluation of the Case Western Reserve

University, Unification Model," in L. Aiken (ed.), *Health Policy and Nursing Practice.* New York: McGraw-Hill, 1981, 229–241.
57. Styles, M. "Reflections on Collaboration and Unification," *Image: The Journal of Nursing Scholarship* 16:1 (Winter, 1984), 21–23.
58. *Ibid,* 23.
59. Baker, C. "Moving Toward Interdependence: Strategies for Collaboration," *Nurse Educator* 20:5 (September–October, 1981), 31.
60. *Ibid.*
61. Hinsvark, I. "Credentialing in Nursing," in L. Aiken (ed.), *Nursing in the 1980s: Crises, Opportunities, Challenges.* Philadelphia: J. B. Lippincott, 1982, 316.
62. Jacobs, J. "Credentialing Serves Public, Profession Says Keynoter," *American Nurse* 16:6 (June, 1984), 7.
63. *Ibid.*
64. Committee for Study of Credentialing in Nursing. *The Study of Credentialing in Nursing: A New Approach,* Vols. I and II. Kansas City, Mo.: American Nurses' Association, 1979.
65. *Ibid.,* 12.
66. Institute of Medicine, Health Care Services Division, Nursing and Nursing Education Committee, *Nursing and Nursing Education: Public Policies and Private Actions.* Washington, D.C.: National Academy Press, 1983.
67. U.S. Bureau of Health Manpower. Second Report to the Congress, March 15, 1979 (Revised) Nurse Training Act of 1975. (DHEW Publ. No.: [HRA]79-45) Hyattsville, Md.: The Bureau, 1979, Sect. 113(a)(1)., 65.
68. Aiken, L. "Nursing's Future: Public Policies, Private Actions," *American Journal of Nursing* 83:10 (October, 1983), 1441.
69. *Ibid.,* 1444.
70. Ginzberg, E. "Policy Directions," in M. L. Millman (ed.), *Nursing Personnel and the Changing Health Care System.* Cambridge, Mass.: Ballinger Publishing, 1978.
71. American Academy of Nursing Task Force on Nursing Practice in Hospitals, *Magnet Hospitals: Attraction and Retention of Professional Nurses.* Kansas City, Mo.: American Nurses' Association, 1983, 8.
72. "Academy Names 41 'Magnet' Hospitals," *American Nurse* 15:2 (February, 1983), 15, 16.
73. *Ibid.*
74. Ferguson, V. "The President's Message," *A.A.N. Newsletter* 3:1 (Spring, 1983), 1.
75. National Commission on Nursing. *Summary Report and Recommendations.* Chicago: American Hospital Association, 1983.
76. Cole, E. "Commission Earns Points for 'Hearing All Voices, Standing Firm on Basics'," *American Journal of Nursing* 83:9 (September, 1983), 1266.
77. Ryan, J. "Groups Affirm Nursing's Stance—Let's Move Ahead," *American Nurse* 15:7 (July–August, 1983), 4.
78. *Ibid.*
79. *Ibid.*
80. Edwards, L. "Health Planning: Opportunities for Nurses," *Nursing Outlook,* 31:6 (November–December, 1983), 322.

81. *Ibid.*
82. Levinson, K. "Knowledge of Professional Nursing Legislation," *Nursing Times* 73 (1977), 674–676.
83. Montgomery, J. Letter to NCAP Members. Washington, D.C.: N–CAP, ANA, June, 1984, 1–2.
84. Conway, M. "The Impact of Changing Resources on Health Care of the Future," in *The Impact of Changing Resources on Health Policy.* Kansas City, Mo.: American Academy of Nursing, 1981, 17.
85. Archer, S. and Goehner, P. "Acquiring Political Clout: Guidelines for Nurse Administrators," *Journal of Nursing Administration* 11:6 (November–December, 1981), 54.
86. *Ibid.*

SUGGESTED READINGS

"ANA Board Report on Titling: What It's All About," (editorial) *American Nurse* 17:6 (June, 1985), 4, 5, 6, and 16.

"ANA Gears Up New Drive for Entry Level Change: Despite Opposition, Some SNAs See Success Soon," *American Journal of Nursing* 85:2 (February, 1985), 194, 200–201.

Anderson, E. and Pierson, P. "An Exploratory Study of Faculty Practice: Views of Faculty Engaged in Practice who Teach in an NLN-Accredited Baccalaureate Program," *Western Journal of Nursing Research* 5:2 (Spring, 1983), 129–140.

Archer, S. and Fleshman, R. "Faculty Role-Modeling," *Nursing Outlook* 29:10 (October, 1981), 586–589.

Blazeck, A., Clekman, J., Tempe, N., and Wolf, Zane Robinson. "Unification: Nursing Education and Nursing Practice," *Nursing and Health Care* 3:2 (June, 1981), 18–24.

Chickadonz, G., Bush, E., Korthius, and Utz, S. "Mobilizing Faculty Toward Integration of Practice into Faculty Roles," *Nursing and Health Care* 11:9 (December, 1981), 548–553.

Christy, T. "Entry into Practice: A Recurring Issue in Nursing History," *American Journal of Nursing* 80:3 (March, 1980), 485–488.

"Credentialing in Nursing: A New Approach," *American Journal of Nursing* 79:4 (April, 1979), 674–683.

Ford, L. "Closing the Gap Between Service and Education," in I. Mauksch (ed.), *Primary Care: A Contemporary Nursing Perspective.* New York: Grune and Stratton, 1981.

Holm, K. "Faculty Practice—Noble Intentions Gone Awry?" *Nursing Outlook* 29:11 (November, 1981), 655–659.

Langford, T. "Faculty Could Practice If—And Other Myths," *Nursing and Health Care* 4:9 (November, 1983), 515–517.

Mallison, M. "Present Imperfect, Future Tense," *American Journal of Nursing* 85:2 (February, 1985), 121.

McKevitt, R. "Trends in Master's Education in Nursing," *Journal of Professional Nursing* 2:4 (1986), 225–233.

Rothberg, J. "The Growth of Political Action in Nursing," *Nursing Outlook* 33:3 (May–June, 1985), 130–135.

"SNAs Act on Entry Level, Titling, LPN Issues," *American Journal of Nursing* 85:2 (February, 1985), 202.

Scherer, P. "Hospitals that Attract (and Keep) Nurses," *American Journal of Nursing* 88:1 (January, 1988), 34–40.

Snyder, M. "Educational Preparation of the CNS" in A. Hamris and J. Spross (eds.) *The Clinical Nurse Specialist in Theory and Practice.* New York: Grune & Stratton, 1989, 325–342.

Stevens, B. "Does the 1985 Nursing Education Proposal Make Economic Sense?" *Nursing Outlook* 33:3 (May–June, 1985), 124–127.

Warner, F., Ross, M. and Clark, L. "An Analysis of Entry into Practice Arguments," *Image: The Journal of Nursing Scholarship* 20:4 (Winter, 1988), 212–216.

Faculty Governance and Structures in Bureaucratic Organizations

8

INTRODUCTION

The United States economy in the 1990s may ultimately prove to be a boon for nursing education. If for no other reason, it has forced nurse educators to critically evaluate their curricula, budgets, sources of income, recruitment policies, and many other areas vital to their continued existence. Decisions based on sound planning will help nursing become stronger and lead to its legitimate acceptance in society as a recognized professional discipline.

The fact that nursing is predominantly a female profession has been a factor affecting its stature among other health professionals. However, nurses are beginning to achieve professional ideals and to demand greater independence for nursing. Although nursing has existed on college campuses for over sixty years, its history reflects numerous problems involved in moving nursing education from single-purpose, hospital-based programs into institutions of higher learning. Often the philosophy, values, and policies of hospital diploma programs were transferred to faculty in college and university nursing education programs, thus preventing them from reaching true professional status. In many instances, directors of diploma programs became directors and deans of college and university schools of nursing. But neither they nor their faculty were socialized into the realities and responsibilities of life in academia. They simply transferred the diploma model to the campus. Some schools continue to operate on this model even today. "They continue to expect remunerative and promotional rewards more for conscientious fulfillment of assigned responsibilities of teaching and administrative duties than for discovery and transmission of new knowledge."[1]

Unfamiliar values and expectations resulting from changes in organizational structure continue to hamper nursing's quest for acceptance within the academic environment. Now it is time for faculty members to internalize academic values as they strive for greater credibility among their peers and colleagues on college campuses.

> A common expectation is that faculty will be concerned primarily or only with those activities necessary to develop and deliver a curriculum to students. Other activities such as engaging in practice or research, are still viewed by many faculty as peripheral or irrelevant to the function of teaching.
>
> Understanding the source of the value system that says teaching is the only legitimate faculty activity does not, of course, justify its continuation. The past decade has brought increased internal and external pressures for nursing faculty to be more actively involved in research and practice.[2]

Fortunately for nursing, such pressures are resulting in more active participation in research activity. Teaching, for the faculty member, is no longer as central as in previous times because research has assumed more importance.[3]

Faculty members having a professional value system are not confined to university walls. Gouldner, in his landmark study of the orientation and professional commitment of college professors, endeavored to determine whether faculty members were primarily oriented to their role within the university or to their professional discipline. He pointed out that there are two possible roles for the university professor—a cosmopolitan or a local. Locals are oriented to the organization, whereas cosmopolitans are oriented to their profession. They are distinguished by the following characteristics:

Cosmopolitans: Those low on loyalty to the employing organization, high on commitment to specialized role skills, and likely to use an outer reference group orientation.

Locals: Those high on loyalty to the employing organization, low on commitment to specialized role skills, and likely to use an inner reference group orientation.[4]

Generally, most health professionals are inclined to be more cosmopolitan than local. "The local seeks advancement through the organizational hierarchy, wants recognition from superiors . . . exhibits less discontent over organization requirements . . . and identifies with the goals, values, and status system of the organization."[5] The cosmopolitan, on the other hand, is oriented more toward his or her profession, seeks advancement and status in the profession through colleague approval and external recognition.

In the past decade, there has been a trend toward greater cosmopolitanism. As a result, conflict between institutional loyalty and disciplinary loyalty occurs. This tension is reaching an acute phase, particularly in smaller schools and colleges of nursing, when pressures for teaching, administration, and extracurricular services compete with professional concerns and research. Regardless of their particular orientation, the path to prestige and promotion for university faculty is based on research activities. This background of existing affairs in academia may assist in viewing the subject of faculty governance for nursing.

What, then, are the expectations of faculty members as they function within the academic setting? First of all, every faculty member expects that the system of organization and operation in a college or university will recognize the importance of the role of faculty members and provide them with a status of dignity and consideration. Faculty members do not think of themselves as employees of the college or university. In particular they resent suggestions that their relation to a dean, a vice president for academic affairs, and/or a president involve supervisory authority.

Secondly, faculty members expect to be provided appropriate facilities for the practice of their profession and proper remuneration for their services. Thirdly, faculty members expect freedom in which to pursue their profession of scholarship. They expect the academic community to protect their privilege of instructing students and advancing knowledge without external pressure and without the requirement of social approval.[6] The organizational structure of the governance model in which these expectations are met deserves close scrutiny.

BUREAUCRATIC AND PROFESSIONAL MODELS OF GOVERNANCE

In the late 1970s, it was pointed out that "academic decision making in collegiate schools of nursing will reflect the faculty struggle to relate autonomy, scholarship, and accountability."[7] Faculties have begun to change their attitudes toward academic decision making as evidenced in the following statements:

The organizational arrangements through which faculties have traditionally participated in decisions no longer seem to secure the desired degree of participation, and dissatisfaction with what some members of the professoriate view as their increasingly secondary role appears to be growing. . . . The rising status of the professorate and its increasing professionalization are altering the academician's traditional attitudes toward participation in decision making.[8]

The relationship between bureaucratic structures and the professions continues to interest scholars and has produced considerable research. This interest is understandable, given that activities involving both the bureaucratic structures and the professions are becoming more and more interwoven. Professional work is carried out, in many instances, in large, complex organizations, such as schools, hospitals, and research centers. Although the organization usually provides adequate resources for professionals, the bureaucratic rules, regulations, and authority are frequently viewed by professionals as infringing upon their right to act according to their best judgment and beliefs.

Over a decade ago, J. Baldridge analyzed the range of models of faculty governance and described three major models of governance for organizations: bureaucratic, collegial, and political. Baldridge proposed the political model as being most suitable for universities. It focuses on "the process of policy formulation and the dynamics and conflicts of special interest groups" who often influence group decision in their favor. As he points out, in recent years, important decisions affecting the academic organization are being made outside of it—namely, at the federal government level. Thus, environmental pressures, particularly political pressures and external forces, are infringing on and posing serious threats to the organization's autonomy.[9] The difference between the other two more traditional models—bureaucratic and collegial, will be presented for comparative purposes.

In comparing organizations with professions, the former tend to be hierarchically structured, whereas professions tend to place ultimate control over their members in the colleague group. As a result, clashes and conflicts between hierarchical control (bureaucratic) and colleague control (collegial) greatly affect relations between organizations and professions.[10] "Control by professional peers versus control by organizational superiors becomes a critical issue with which institutional governance models must deal."[11] Frequently, administrative and faculty expectations create underlying tensions and the possibility of conflict between professional and work accomplishments.

The bureaucratic, hierarchical model places many constraints on individual faculty members and hinders their active participation in decision making. However, in a collegial organizational model, universities are involved in "government by consensus and voluntary cooperation among groups of independent professional specialists."[12] In this collegial model of shared governance, academic professionals operate "through a dynamic of consensus in a community of scholars."[13] Functioning under this model, they are assured a high level of autonomy and control of the various organizational activities, including peer review. Although the collegial model has been operational in higher education for over a century, many nurse faculty members have yet to internalize and practice this model. One of the impediments to faculty participation in decision making is the rigor of research and the high value placed on it by faculty and administrators alike. Conflicts can arise over research requiring greater loyalty than institutional affairs.

> The demands of research are in a class by themselves as inhibitors of faculty participation in decision making. . . . Research takes precedence over all else; it is the root to professional advancement, disciplinary status, and self-esteem.[14]

As a consequence of the increased importance of research and publication as the marks of professional success and the pathway to promotion and advancement, there has developed an obsessive concern for persistent publication. The "publish or perish" doctrine is real and serves as a strong motivator for faculty to increase their research productivity, thus inhibiting their efforts in academic decision making. Other institutional impediments to decision making, such as growth in size and complexity of the university and greater allegiance to one's discipline than to one's institution, are also possible reasons for lack of faculty participation.

It is interesting to note that the bureaucratic model in organizations is increasingly governed by professional standards. The collegial model is increasingly subject to bureaucratic control. A growing interdependence currently exists between professions and organizations. However, if the orientation to professionalism is stronger, the greater the likelihood that conflict will exist between the professional and the organization. "The dimension of autonomy in the professional environment is manifested in occupational structures which demand that practitioners be free to make their decisions [and] it is particularly at this point that conflict between the environment of professionalization and that of bureaucracy . . . occurs."[15]

If faculty in a sizable number of nursing schools continue to function in a bureaucratic mode and fail to model their beliefs on professionalism, students will not strive for autonomy in their professional lives and will remain confused about the concept of professionalism. If nurse faculty members fail to exert their right to autonomous decision making in areas for which they are responsible, they cannot be considered professional. For example, if faculty members are urged to accept student grade changes that they do not favor but are expected to accept, their autonomy is threatened and inevitably their professionalism as well. Fortunately, this example rarely occurs in nursing schools.

SCOPE OF AUTONOMY
IN ACADEMIC NURSING

In discussing the various characteristics of a profession, the concept of autonomy was defined and elaborated on in Chapter 1. It was pointed out that one of the most important characteristics of a profession is a high degree of autonomy. In fact, Friedson considers it to be the main characteristic of professionals.[16] It is important to understand the scope of autonomy as it relates to faculty functioning in an academic setting. Moreover, autonomy involves the range of decisions and behavior that can be performed at the discretion of the professional group. From this viewpoint, the scope depends on the functions and level of expertise of each profession. Professionals possess autonomy to the extent that they are allowed to use their own judgment. If no independent judgments are required, then no autonomy exists and no profession either. "Autonomy is in effect an ultimate value for self-identified members of an occupational category, and they are extremely unlikely to achieve that goal without having . . . prior qualifications. . . . autonomy builds upon [their] having passed previous selection points."[17]

Autonomy is granted to professions to the extent that society recognizes their specialized knowledge and skill. Since a strong commitment to service typifies professionals, society believes each profession will use its specialized knowledge and expertise in decisions based on the good of the client. In other words, professionals must serve the client's interests above their own personal needs for status or financial gains.

A study was conducted by Grandjean and colleagues to measure the importance and satisfaction associated with twenty-one job characteristics. Special attention was given to aspects of the faculty role as related to professional autonomy. The findings clearly revealed "the importance of a non-directive dean and a high degree of faculty input in determining school of nursing policy."[18] This study confirmed that faculty members regard professional autonomy and the freedom to be self-directed as more important than the extrinsic or material rewards of their position. Any changes in the decision-making structure that would facilitate greater faculty autonomy should be encouraged. Increased faculty morale, productivity, and retention of qualified faculty members occur when faculty functions autonomously in a collegial model of governance.

SOURCE OF AUTHORITY IN ACADEMIA

Nurse faculty in academia have made considerable strides in recent years in assuming authority for decision making. Some faculty groups are somewhat slower than others in exerting their right to determine the directions in which decisions will be implemented. Such slowness might be attributed to a lack of understanding of the concept of authority.

Although authority has been defined as "a relationship in which the subordinate voluntarily surrenders his own judgment and ability to make decisions and bases his actions on the commands of his superior," this relationship is rarely observed in professional organizations.[19] The general idea of authority being vested in position, with the person at one level having authority over individuals at lower levels who are subordinate to those above them, is irrelevant for professionals functioning in professional organizations. Yet, the greatest source of conflict between bureaucracies and professions is in the area of authority relationships. The bureaucratic authority just described is based on executive authority, with the superior in a hierarchical organization having final control over subordinates. On the other hand, "professional authority is based on the demonstration of superior competence."[20]

Independent professionals are expected to use expert judgment in their area of competence and are expected to make their own decisions consistent with professional norms. Colleague authority, shared by members of a work group, results in control being internalized by each individual. Through self-control, adherence to professional norms, and colleague evaluation, professionals are able to achieve integration of their activity into the total organization.

In institutions where there are many professionals at work, the problems of accommodating bureaucratic control and professional control present serious difficulties. A so-called tug-of-war between bureaucratic and professional orientations can be found today in many large organizations.

In the mid-1940s, Max Weber eloquently described bureaucratic authority and how colleague control runs counter to it: "Collegiality unavoidably obstructs the promptness of decisions, the consistency of policy, the clear responsibility of the individual and ruthlessness to outsiders in combination with the maintenance of discipline within the group."[21] In his view, superiors can expedite decisions based on their particular expertise and avoid unnecessary delays resulting from prolonged deliberations over issues. In the contemporary scene, this opinion is unrealistic. Today's professionals are not only competent to fulfill their responsibilities, but they are also expected to do so. Being in command of special knowledge, professionals seek to be free from lay and organizational control. This fact is particularly true in health care institutions, where the medical profession is forceful in substituting its professional authority for that of the organization. How progressive nurse faculty will become in moving toward a professional model of academic decision making remains to be seen.

The source of faculty authority is not based on adequate performance of responsibilities but on power acquired by faculty having superior academic reputations. "Scientists and scholars who command wide respect among colleagues in their discipline and achieve influential positions outside their own academic institutions, are sought after by other institutions, and are needed by their own, since its academic standing depends on them."[22] The power of these cosmopolitans stems from achieving acclaim and prestige from their discipline and from contact with sources of support for scholarship and research.

Burton R. Clark viewed faculty authority as tending to become professional authority. It shifts from protection of collective faculty rights to protection of the autonomy of separate disciplines and individual faculty members.[23] "Thus, professional authority tends to become the dominant form of authority, and collegial and bureaucratic features fall into a subsidiary place."[24] It would appear that nurse faculty members in some schools of nursing are moving rapidly toward assuming professional authority, controlling their work, and achieving prestige and status. These educators are acquiring the rewards that increased power and authority ultimately make available.

STATUS OF ACCOUNTABILITY FOR NURSE EDUCATORS

Accountability may be defined as being responsible for one's actions. To assure that autonomy will not be misused by professionals for their own gain, society expects professionals to exert considerable accountability for their activities. "The irresponsible exercise of professional autonomy is as great an evil as its absence; furthermore, every failure on the part of teachers to fulfill their professional responsibilities weakens their claim to professional autonomy."[25] Claiming to be a professional while disowning accountability for all of one's actions is contradictory to the meaning of professionalism. The demand for accountability should be interpreted into an internalized acceptance of responsibility for the various nurse educator functions as depicted in Fig. 8-1. Reinforcement coincides with the accountability demanded by the organization and the public. To be self-determined, with all that it implies, necessitates a high degree of accountability. To whom, then, and for what is a faculty member accountable?

First, faculty members must be accountable to themselves, to their own sense of what is considered acceptable conduct and idealism. Their conscience should dictate standards of intellectual integrity and scholarship. Second, faculty members are accountable in various ways to their students. They must not only provide effective teaching but also challenge their students to think for themselves, to be analytical in questioning

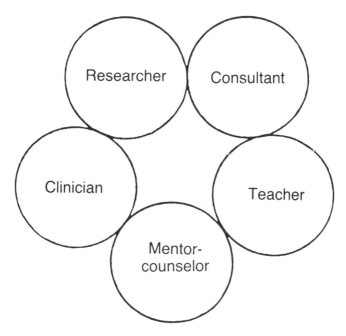

Figure 8-1. Functions of the nurse educator.

faculty views as well as their own, and to use their talents to develop their full potential.

Encouraging a permissive atmosphere in classrooms to foster freedom of expression and a desire to learn for its own sake without the element of fear or reprisal is conducive to good learning. To the extent that faculty members keep abreast in their field, pursue the necessary academic and scholarly credentials, conduct research and publish their findings, engage in clinical practice, and participate in professional organization activity, they will be exercising genuine accountability to students.

However, faculties should prioritize these various responsibilities, realizing that each one of them cannot be undertaken to the same degree during a given time period. At one time, teaching may be all that a faculty member can manage. Whereas at a later period, time can be allocated for research, publications, clinical practice, and service. Moreover, there are developmental patterns in nursing careers, with some nurses engaging in administration while others pursue research or consultation and then changing roles at a future date.

Third, faculty members are accountable to their peers. Collegial evaluations are expressed in several different ways. Appraisal and approval of an individual's research efforts by colleagues frequently become important measures of success. A more formal method of accountability is observed when faculty committees evaluate individual faculty performance in determining appointment, promotion, tenure, or dismissal. A somewhat less frequently used method is observation and evaluation of classroom and clinical teaching by one's peers in order to improve performance.

Fourth, faculty members are accountable to their employing institution and are responsible for assisting it in its mission of teaching, research, and service. Academic freedom must be maintained, and faculty must ensure that the university is intellectually free to accomplish this three-fold mission. Loyalty and dedicated service are expectations for educators as they perform their responsibilities in an accountable manner.

Finally, faculty is accountable to the public it serves. As more and more federal and state funds are awarded to public institutions, faculty becomes more accountable to increasing pressures and demands on its services. Local communities can exert considerable pressure on academics to meet their perceived needs.

Faculty Accountability for Promotion, Retention, and Tenure

Faculty has an opportunity to demonstrate its accountability through promotion, retention, and tenure. Until recently the majority of faculty members in nursing schools were not socialized to understand or appreciate the importance of promotion through effective teaching, scholarly pursuits, research, and publication. Recognition by one's peers and others comes from superior knowledge and research demonstrated through contributions to nursing's scientific base and the authority that such expertise commands. Authority is not derived from position alone.

An objective appraisal of faculty credentials according to the criteria of professionalism in academia does not support the claim that giant strides toward professionalism have been made by nursing in recent years. To believe that the majority of faculties employed in schools of nursing throughout the country are actively engaged in scholarly work would be rather naive. Many faculty members see their chief role as teaching and supervision of nursing students. Perhaps this focus is due to their lack of doctoral preparation. Many of these teachers are also relatively inexperienced within the academic environment. Many faculty members are recent graduates of master's programs. They have expert knowledge and clinical skills but little understanding of the responsibilities inherent in functioning as a productive member in an educational setting. Changing one's role from clinical practice to teaching does not occur easily. Many faculty move rapidly into nursing education positions without a thorough understanding of all that the role requires. Socialization of nurse faculty is a complex process and should be ongoing over a period of several months.

If nursing is to progress as a scholarly, scientific discipline, it is crucial that vast numbers of nurses be prepared at the doctoral level. They can then exert leadership in influencing nursing's future course in the health field. A doctoral degree is a respected credential in academia and is a source of power for faculty. Acquiring a doctoral degree does not automatically produce a scholar, but it does provide the research and statistical knowledge and experience required to facilitate preparation of scholarly work. Many well-known researchers and scholars have begun their scholarly activities on a small scale. Through experience they have secured a remarkable track record of research and publications, which have greatly influenced nursing's growth as a scientific discipline. What is even more remarkable is that some of these individuals consistently publish the results of their research endeavors, while others continue to publish new insights into problems plaguing nursing's professional advancement. As one nurse scholar, busily involved in research commented, "I always have several projects on the fire—some may rest on the back burner, but there is constant shifting from one burner to the other with a new project started as others are completed."

The composition and characteristics of nurse faculty have continued to change considerably over the past twenty years. The results of increased emphasis on scholarship is apparent, particularly faculty capability for meeting promotion and tenure requirements. "Moreover, in today's academic climate, decreased monetary resources and largely tenured departments have made it increasingly difficult to obtain tenure and have thus heightened the need to demonstrate scholarship."[26, 27]

The majority of nurse faculty teaching in collegiate nursing programs should hold an earned doctorate. For example, an examination of faculty statistics provides evidence that in 1970, of 4,887 faculty employed in baccalaureate and higher degree programs, 305 (6.2%) held an earned doctorate; in 1980 these figures increased to 9,531 with 1,278 (13.4%) holding a doctoral degree; and in 1988, of 9,074 faculty, 2,921 (32.2%) held a doctoral degree.[28]

In a sample survey of 841 academicians in six U.S. universities, 366 or 44% of the total faculty contacted responded to the survey.[29] "Teaching effectiveness was selected as an important criterion only by members of the nursing discipline [and] nurses were the only academicians to identify teaching effectiveness as one of the single most important tenure determinants in their present university departments."[30] This is an interesting finding and indicates that nursing should endeavor to meet other criteria as well. In reviewing NLN criteria for accreditation of baccalaureate and higher degree programs, it is readily observed that scholarship and research endeavors are more important for nursing faculty in academia. In a literature review of faculty productivity, fewer studies of faculty research were noted as compared to those describing teaching productivity.[31, 32] These results confirm Moore's findings that nurses apparently place more weight on teaching than on research and other scholarly pursuits.

Motivation, self-discipline, and commitment to scholarship describe those nurses whose productivity should serve to make other nurses desire similar achievements. Currently, there is a growing awareness among the many nurses employed in academia who lack preparation at the doctoral level, that this deficiency prevents them from enjoying equal partnership with faculty from other disciplines or from participation on scholarly, interdisciplinary research teams. Research is the hallmark of a community of scholars. How, then, can faculty in nursing schools continue to fail in meeting this important qualification?

Undoubtedly, it is to nursing's advantage that many colleges and universities are requiring nurses to meet the same criteria for professional advancement required of other disciplines on campus. Formerly, nurse candidates applying for promotion or tenure were granted both although they could not meet standards expected of other collegiate faculty. This assumption is no longer correct. But it did force faculty members desiring to remain in academia to reevaluate their credentials and take positive steps toward improving their status through pursuit of a doctorate and more intense efforts in conducting research and writing for publication.

It is not surprising that many faculty members in schools of nursing remain at either the instructor or assistant professor rank since they lack the education, research, and publications required for promotion to a senior rank. Frequently, nurse faculty have been criticized by other academic and professional disciplines for their inability to adhere to promotion and tenure standards. Nursing's low power position on college campuses is often due to lack of adequate educational preparation, research, and scholarship of its nurse faculty members. Because university professors are expected to contribute to the development of their discipline, nursing can no longer afford to overlook or deny this responsibility.

Faculty should be encouraged to *develop* new knowledge as well as impart it to students. Each individual has a responsibility to achieve this goal. Faculty members in recent years have cooperated with one another to facilitate obtaining such preparation through adjusting teaching schedules and accepting heavier teaching loads in order to release other faculty for sabbaticals for research and manuscript preparation.

Nursing schools that have achieved the goal of having all faculty prepared with doctorates are to be commended, particularly since the number of all nurses in the U.S. with doctoral preparation remains extremely low (2.6 percent). For university nursing schools offering doctoral nursing programs, only prepared faculty with doctorates whose research productivity is firmly established should be permitted to teach and direct doctoral students.

An ever-growing number of nurse faculty are committed to a lifetime of scholarship. Realizing that the doctorate is beginning preparation for scholarliness, they are convinced that through consistent and continuing efforts to improve research capabilities, nursing will achieve recognition as a scholarly discipline in academia and be in the forefront in improving the nation's health. The need for faculty members to assume greater responsibility for their professional role as educators is noted in the following comments.

> Nursing faculties in the 1990s need to consciously and deliberately choose academic maturity as their contribution to professionalization. This involves assuming responsibility for the school's academic enterprise and an active role in the total campus enterprise . . . unless we can demonstrate professional behaviors, students will go elsewhere, and resources will be garnered by politically active faculty from other units. . . . I believe Deans have a right and responsibility to demand . . . academic professionalism from their faculties.[33]

The challenge to promotion and tenure committees in collegiate nursing schools is to evaluate teaching, clinical practice, and service in terms of their scholarliness. Overemphasis on any one of these areas is to be avoided. In general, achievement should be demonstrated by the amount of research accomplished, grants awarded, and publications resulting from such research. It is my belief that nurse faculty members will meet this challenge of accountability and achieve autonomy in their faculty role. By setting realistic goals, the problems they are currently experiencing will, in the foreseeable future, become a part of nursing's long history of struggle to achieve recognition and academic excellence in higher educational institutions.

As a reminder to faculty of its responsibility for accountable behavior, a Code of Ethics for Nurse Educators written by Marlene Merifield Rosenkoetter clearly enunciates what she believes are ethical guidelines for faculty members in their academic role. Believing that the Code of Ethics of the American Nurses' Association and that of the International Council of Nurses fails to address ethical problems of nursing faculty and administrators, Rosenkoetter was convinced that such guidelines were sorely needed in nursing education. Thus in 1982, she developed a version of this code, which is thought-provoking and should be helpful to faculty as they reexamine their rights and responsibilities in fulfilling their teaching role.

A Code of Ethics for Nurse Educators

Preamble

The Code of Ethics for Nurse Educators is based on the premise that each person involved in nursing education is unique and each has the right to have that uniqueness valued. The nurse educator functions as a teacher, clinician, researcher, mentor-counselor, and consultant and is responsible for adhering to ethical principles and established codes of ethics in each of these interrelated roles. The International Council of Nurses and the American Nurses' Association codes are considered basic codes for the practice of nursing and for nursing education.

Nurse educators have a responsibility for maintaining and promoting acceptable standards of nursing care and nursing education without discrimination with regard to race, color, religion, socioeconomic status, nationality, political affiliation, age, or sex. Nurse educators will:

1. Assume responsibility and accountability for their actions in the practice of nursing and in the education of students.
2. Function as advocates for students, clients, and faculty.
3. Strive to promote critical thinking, effective decision making, caring and respect, and excellence in nursing.
4. Facilitate and guide the learning of students in such a way as to reflect credit on nursing and nursing education.
5. Equitably apply standards of performance to students and to themselves.
6. Accept responsibility for contributing to the evolving body of nursing knowledge.
7. Demonstrate respect for confidential matters relating to students, clients, and persons in the academic community.
8. Accept the responsibility of maintaining their own competencies in nursing, in education, and in practice.
9. Endeavor to safeguard the client and the student from incompetent, illegal, or unethical practices by students, faculty, and other health care providers.
10. Assume responsibility and accountability for their own practice of nursing.
11. Deliberately limit their practice and teach within the scope of their own competencies.
12. Participate in professional organizations, attesting to their commitment to the standards of nursing and to nursing education.
13. Be accountable to students, to the academic community, to the profession and to society for fulfilling their academic responsibilities.

14. Demonstrate respect for the rights of students regarding their participation in nursing research.
15. Demonstrate respect for the student as a person and as an individual contributor to the profession and society.

SUMMARY

In discussing the role of faculty in academia, it was noted that conflicts and tension arise when the value system of the organization frequently creates demands that are not part of the expectations that faculty members hold for their positions. Indeed, faculty should be able to internalize academic values as they strive for greater credibility among peers and colleagues within the college or university structure.

Differences in bureaucratic and professional models of governance account for faculty members viewing the former, with its rules, policies, and authority, as infringing upon their professional right to use knowledge according to their best judgment and beliefs. In the collegial model of shared governance, professionals operate through consensus within a community of scholars. A growing interdependence exists between professions and organizations. However, the possibility of conflict is always present when the orientation to professionalism is stronger. In the professional environment, occupational structures demand that practitioners have freedom in making decisions. It is at this point that conflict between the professional environment and the bureaucracy occurs.

Autonomy, or the right to use one's own judgment in professional matters, is not achieved without having met certain qualifications. If no independent judgment is required, then neither autonomy nor a profession exists. The value placed on autonomy is more important to faculty members than the extrinsic rewards of their position. In some schools of nursing, faculty members are exerting professional authority through controlling their work and increasing their power and prestige.

Accountability of faculty members to self, students, peers, employing institutions, and the public they serve indicates the high degree of responsibility they assume in accepting a faculty position in academia. Authority derived from expertise and not from position alone provides recognition from one's peers and colleagues and is far more effective in fulfilling one's responsibilities.

Faculty accountability in relation to promotion and tenure criteria varies from one school of nursing to another. Lack of doctorally-prepared faculty and lack of faculty involvement in research or publications in nursing schools indicate that nurse faculties should acquire these credentials if they are to achieve equal partnership with faculty in other departments of academia. Nurse faculty members are urged to make progress in achieving doctoral preparation and in scholarly research activities.

A Code of Ethics for Nurse Educators provides ethical guidelines to assist nurse faculty members in their efforts to achieve accountable behavior in their teaching role.

REFERENCES

1. Batey, M. "The Two Normative Worlds of the University Nursing Faculty," *Nursing Forum* 8:1 (1969), 15.
2. Jacox, A. "Prerequisite for the Exercise of Professionalism," in *Briefly Noted: Literary Soaps for Deans* Vol. 2, No. 2. Washington, D.C.: American Association of Colleges of Nursing, 1982, 7.
3. Kerr, C. *The Uses of the University.* New York: Harper & Row, 1963, 42.
4. Gouldner, A. "Cosmopolitans and Locals: Toward an Analysis of Latent Social Roles Part I," *Administration Science Quarterly* 2 (December, 1957), 290.
5. Longest, B. *Management Practices for the Health Professional.* Reston, Va.: Reston Publishing, 1976, 54.
6. Millett, J. *The Academic Community: An Essay on Organization.* New York: McGraw-Hill, 1962, 101–103.
7. Pagel, I. *Predicted Trends and Their Impact on Decision-Making—Report of a Study.* Washington, D.C.: American Council on Education, 1968, v.
8. Dykes, A. *Faculty Participation in Academic Decision Making: Report of a Study.* Washington, D.C.: American Council on Education, 1968, v.
9. Baldridge, J. (ed.), *Academic Governance.* Berkeley, Calif.: McCutchan Publishing Corp., 1971.
10. Kornhauser, W. *Scientists in Industry.* Berkeley, Calif.: University of California Press, 1962.
11. Styles, M. *On Nursing—Toward a New Endowment.* St. Louis: C. V. Mosby, 1982, 20.
12. Rice, G. and Bishoprick, D. *Conceptual Models of Organization.* New York: Appleton-Century-Crofts, 1971, 97.
13. Millett, I. *Academic Community.* 235.
14. Dykes, A. *Faculty Participation.* 23.
15. Taylor, L. *Occupational Sociology.* New York: Oxford University Press, 1968.
16. Freidson, E. *Profession of Medicine.* New York: Dodd, Mead & Co., 1970.
17. Moore, W. *The Professions: Roles and Rules.* New York: Russell Sage Foundations, 1970, 16.
18. Grandjean, B., Aiken, L. and Bonjean, C. "Professional Autonomy and the Work Satisfaction of Nursing Educators," *Nursing Research* 25:3, (May–June, 1976), 218.

19. Bucher, R. and Stelling, J. "Characteristics of Professional Organizations," *Journal of Health and Social Behavior* 10:1, (March, 1969), 12.
20. Pavalko, R. *Sociology of Occupations and Professions.* Itasca, Ill.: F. E. Peacock Co., 1971, 189.
21. Henderson, A. and Parsons, T. (eds.), *Max Weber: The Theory of Social and Economic Organization.* New York: Oxford University Press, 1947, 402.
22. Blau, P. *The Organization of Academic Work.* New York: John Wiley & Sons, 1973, 187.
23. Clark, B. "Faculty Organization and Authority," in G. Riley and J. Baldridge (eds.), *Governing Academic Organizations.* Berkeley, Calif.: McCutchan Publishing Corp., 1977, 290–291.
24. *Ibid.*
25. Lieberman, M. *Education as a Profession.* Englewood Cliffs, N.J.: Prentice-Hall, 1956, 91.
26. Moore, M. "Tenure and the University Reward Structure," *Nursing Research* 38:2 (March–April, 1989), 111.
27. Krueger, S. and Washburn, J.. "Tenure and promotion: An Update on University Nursing Faculty," *Journal of Nursing Education* 26:5 (May, 1987), 182.
28. National League for Nursing. *Nursing Data Review, 1988.* (Pub. No.: 19-2290), New York: Division of Research, National League for Nursing, 1989, 105.
29. Moore, M. "Tenure and the University Reward Structure," 112.
30. *Ibid.*, 114, 116.
31. Andreoli, K. and Musser, L. "Faculty Productivity" in H. Werley, J. Fitzpatrick, and R. Tauton (eds.), *Annual Review of Nursing Research* Vol. 4. New York: Springer Publishing Co., 1986.
32. Ostmoe, P. and Sparks, R. "Issues Related to Promotion and Tenure," in J. McCloskey and H. Grace (eds.), *Current Issues in Nursing* 3d ed. St. Louis: C.V. Mosby, 1990.
33. Kritek, P. "Impact of Realities on Faculty Affairs from the Perspective of Deans and Faculty in Nursing Education—A Faculty Member's Perspective," Paper presented at a Dean's seminar entitled *Planning for the Realities of the 80s.* Sponsored by AACN and CBHP–NLN, July 18–21, Fontana, Wis.: The Abbey, 1982, 3.

SUGGESTED READINGS

Abrahamson, M. *The Professional in the Organization.* Chicago: Rand-McNally, 1967.

Baldridge, J. and Kemerer, F. "Images of Governance: Collective Bargaining vs. Traditional Models," in G. Riley and J. Baldridge (eds.), *Governing Academic Organizations.* Berkeley, Calif.: McCutchan Publishing Corp., 1977.

Barley, Z. and Redman, B. "Faculty Role Development in University Schools of Nursing," *Journal of Nursing Administration* 9:3 (May, 1979), 43–47.

Barger, S. and Bridges, W. "Nursing Faculty Practice: Institutional and Individual Facilitators and Inhibitors," *Journal of Professional Nursing* 3:6 (November–December, 1989).

Conway, M. "The Acquisition and Use of Power in Academia: A Dean's Perspective," *Nursing Administrative Quarterly* 6:3 (Spring, 1982), 83–90.

Conway, M. and Glass, L. "Socialization for Survival in the Academic World," *Nursing Outlook* 26:7 (July, 1978), 424–429.

Cook, S. and Finelli, L. "Faculty Practice: A New Perspective on Academia Competence," *Journal of Professional Nursing* 4:1 (January–February, 1988), 23–30.

Dienemann, J. *Power Sharing in Universities: The Case of Nursing.* Doctoral Dissertation, Washington, D.C.: The Catholic University of America, 1983.

Dienemann, J. "Reducing Nursing Faculty Workloads Without Increasing Costs," *Image: the Journal of Nursing Scholarship* 15:4 (Fall, 1983), 111–114.

Fawcett, J. "Integrating Research into the Faculty Workload," *Nursing Outlook* 27:4 (April, 1979), 259–262.

Freeman, L. and Voignier, R. "Clarifying Tenure Requirements," *Nursing Outlook* 33:1 (January–February, 1985), 43–45.

Kelly, J. "Factors Affecting Decision-Making in Academic Nursing from the Viewpoint of Faculty," in *Decision-Making Within the Academic Environment.* (Pub. No.: 15–1719). New York: National League for Nursing, 1978.

Megel, M., Langston, N. and Crowell, J. "Scholarly Productivity: A Survey of Nursing Faculty Research," *Journal of Professional Nursing* 4:1 (January–February, 1988), 45–54.

Perry, S. "A Doctorate—Necessary But Not Sufficient," *Nursing Outlook* 30:2 (February, 1982), 95–98.

Phillips, J. "Faculty Burnout," *American Journal of Nursing* 84:12 (December, 1984), 1525–1526.

Ray, G. "Burnout: Potential Problems for Nursing Faculty," *Nursing and Health Care* 5:4 (April, 1984), 218–221.

Solomons, H., Jordison, N., and Powell, S. "How Faculty Members Spend Their Time," *Nursing Outlook* 28:3 (March, 1980), 160–165.

Spero, J. "Nursing: A Professional Practice Discipline in Academia," *Nursing and Health Care* 1:1 (January, 1980), 22–25.

Sweeney, S. and Ostmoe, P. "Academic Freedom: A Relevant Concept for Collegiate Nursing Education," *Nursing Forum* 19:1 (January, 1980), 4–13.

Williamson, J. "The Conflict-Producing Role of the Professionally Socialized Nurse-Faculty Member," *Nursing Forum* 11:4 (April, 1972), 356–373.

CONTROL OF PROFESSIONAL NURSING PRACTICE

V

Evolving Roles
in Nursing Practice

9

INTRODUCTION

As the health care delivery system in the United States is changing at a rapid pace, nursing continues to strive for a professional model of nursing practice. Achieving increased autonomy and accountability, nursing has begun to change its organizational structure to accommodate new, expanded roles and definitions of the social significance of nursing practice. Changes in the roles of health professionals provide an excellent opportunity for nursing to exert leadership in meeting societal needs.

The majority of nurses agree that their position in the changing health care system can and should be determined by nursing, not by external factors or pressures. This opportunity is particularly true for nurses who agree with ANAs Social Policy Statement (presented in Chapter 3) and the challenges it presents.

One of the purposes of the Surgeon General's Report in 1963 was to alleviate some of the social ills, such as inadequate health care, that burdened society.[1] However, external conditions, societal changes, and unmet health needs are requiring different types of health care services than those needed three decades ago. Currently, disease prevention and health maintenance are emphasized more than the care and cure of illness. The view that health is composed of wellness and illness components agrees with nursing's beliefs about the health needs of the total person. Newer innovations in health care, such as the hospice and home health care movements, technological developments, emphasis on self-care, and an increase in the elderly population are only a few of the factors affecting the scope of nursing's practice. Such factors have created demands for nurses who possess "broader knowledge; wider range of clinical nursing skills; greater awareness of the impact of cultural differences; environmental conditions; socioeconomic factors and family interactions; clearer understanding of values and ethics; and more effective communication skills."[2]

Nursing continues to broaden its evolving role in health care, health promotion, and prevention of illness, and in providing education and interventions that can change behavioral patterns and reduce the risks of serious illness. Providing a preventive type of service that encompasses health education and advice on alteration of lifestyles is one of society's pressing needs.

The critical issue of who will control nursing practice can be resolved, despite external forces impinging on nursing's autonomy, if nurses as a collective body assume more assertive attitudes when voicing their demands for control. It is encouraging to observe that many nurses are implementing their practice responsibilities more independently as well as voicing their demands for clinical decision-making authority and equality with other professionals in health care planning and treatment modalities. If this trend is to continue, however, nurses must build a more adequate power base from which to voice their concerns.

Mowery and Korpman predict that by the late 1990s several significant changes will occur that can either promote or impede the relationship among key primary health care providers: physicians, nurses, and hospital administrators. Among the changes meriting consideration are "the impact of nurse practitioner programs; a physician surplus [in the 1990s]; and the current severe nursing shortage."[3]

Many nurses in a variety of health care agencies continue to be frustrated by the constraints placed on them by bureaucratic, organizational, and physician controls. "To many nurses—frustrated by bureaucratic hassles, long hours, constant stress and lack of advancement—the medical work place has not kept pace with the new academic professionalism of nursing."[4] Because nursing still lacks the power to change this situation, more nurses will, undoubtedly, continue their exodus from the acute care setting and will look for opportunities to develop alternative models for delivering nursing care, particularly ambulatory care. As health services based on health needs of individuals increase, new and exciting nursing roles have developed. An exploration of these roles forms the basis of this chapter.

NURSE PRACTITIONERS AND CLINICAL NURSE SPECIALISTS

Nurse Practitioners

Although almost thirty years have elapsed since the first nurse practitioner program was established in 1965 by Loretta Ford and Henry Silver at the University of Colorado, it is interesting to note that by 1979 there were an estimated 20,000 nurse practitioners available in this country.

In 1973, the ANA defined the nurse practitioner (NP) as a registered nurse having received additional preparation in a specialized educational program. Presently there are two types of nurse practitioners. Some have a two-year associate nursing degree or a nursing diploma, having earned a certificate upon completing a six-week to six- or twelve-month nurse practitioner program. Others have a baccalaureate nursing degree upon entering a nurse practitioner program, which requires two additional years and grants a master's degree in nursing. Eligibility for federal funding now requires that NP programs be at least one year in length.

Many nurse practitioners have become specialized in their particular clinical area. However, in order to become ANA certified, the NP must have a master's degree in a clinical specialty area. Many baccalaureate nursing graduates have been taught physical assessment skills, but they cannot be considered nurse practitioners because they lack graduate preparation for ANA certification.

During the 1984 ANA biennial nursing convention, a proposal was adopted by the House of Delegates calling on the association "to reaffirm its commitment to graduate preparation in nursing for entry into advanced nursing practice as a nurse practitioner by 1990."[5] The proposal charged the state nurses' associations to disseminate information regarding this requirement to their members and to the educational programs preparing nurse practitioners.

Several significant phenomena served as driving forces to augment the nurse practitioner movement in the early 1960s. Severe shortages of pediatricians and family practice physicians, lack of adequate health care for rural areas, nursing's demand for autonomous practice, escalation of health care costs, increased technology, and federal funding of practitioner programs all stimulated growth of the nurse practitioner movement.[6] Initially founded "to test an expanded scope of practice for professional nurses who held a baccalaureate degree in nursing," practitioner programs soon included preparation for "family, adult, school, obstetrics/gynecology, geriatric and perinatal nurse practitioners," as well as pediatric practitioners.[7]

Confusion about this newly expanded role occurred in the 1960s with the emergence of the physician's assistant. Although each of the roles involves performance of similar tasks, the philosophy, licensure, preparation, and practice are very different. Physician assistants (PAs) are dependent upon physicians for their role definition; however, nurse practitioners are functioning within the profession of nursing and are not dependent upon physicians. Due to the possible threat of physician assistants replacing nurses, an effort was made by nursing to obtain legal sanction for its expanded roles. The question of why nursing remained passive while the PA role was developing can be answered by the fact that nurses were predominantly female and lacked power and assertiveness skills to challenge their male colleagues. (PAs are predominantly male.) Controversy over whether nurse practitioners are physician-extenders or whether they abdicate their nursing role continues to the present day.

In the past twenty years, NPs have developed skill in physical assessment, health promotion, and prevention of illness along with legislative skills for political action. During this period, they have become excellent providers of nursing services to the general public. The setting for nurse practitioners varies. Some individuals work in coronary care, renal dialysis, neonatal care, or burn units within hospitals or in doctor's offices. In rural areas, nurse practitioners function autonomously with only indirect collaboration or supervision from physicians.

Changes observed in hospitalized patients are having a definite impact on the role of nurse practitioners. Due to early discharge of patients, the higher level of acuity requiring a variety of complex services has changed nursing practice in the community setting. "Faced with sicker patients and frightened families, nurse practitioners . . . spend a great number of hours merely finding out what was done for the patient in the acute care setting so that services provided will ensure a safe level of care."[8]

In a study conducted by Bleiweiss and Egner in 1976, it was found "that nurse practitioners functioned . . . in individual practice, nurse practitioner groups, private hospitals, group practice of physicians, outpatient or specialty clinics, and health maintenance organizations."[9] Profiles for these nurse practitioners, as the study results indicate, show the existence of two primary groups. One group was characterized as highly nursing-oriented and relatively homogenous in nature. In the other group, a "nurse practitioner" orientation prevailed with the role observed to be a more independent branch of nursing.[10]

H. A. Sultz and colleagues, in a report on the findings of longitudinal studies of nurse practitioners in the United States, provided information on trends in nurse practitioner employment from 1974 to 1982. The report concluded that an integral and viable component of a health care system is the nurse practitioner movement, which now has grown and stabilized.[11] These researchers based their conclusions on evidence that nurse practitioners were providing primary care services particularly to under-served populations and were making improvements in the quality of patient care.[12] Numerous other studies have documented the satisfaction of patients, nurses, and physicians with the high quality of care provided by nurse practitioners.[13–15]

In studies comparing nurse practitioners' and physicians' clinical performances, it was observed that a relatively large number of respondents indicated differences partial to NPs. Despite this favorability for nurse practitioners, Prescott and Driscoll concluded that "even with this wide array of positive findings for nurse practitioners, the most common interpretation was that no differences existed between physician and nurse practitioner performance [and] in one instance, nurse practitioner superiority was attributed to a placebo effect."[16] Their observations are another example of strong support for the NP movement. Although vast amounts of data provide ample evidence of the successful accomplishments of nurse practitioners, obstacles still confront the full utilization of NPs in improving health care and reducing health care costs.

In 1980, four barriers of major importance became more evident: reimbursement, legal constraints, educational support, and under-utilization in practice settings. These barriers stemmed from the predicted excess of physicians by 1990, the anticipated competition in health care delivery, limited federal support for health services, education, and research, and the fear of losing power and control by some professions, particularly physicians.[17] In the 1980s it was observed that, "There is widespread agreement that by 1990 there will be approximately 600,000 physicians in the United States, a projected 41 percent increase over 1980 levels."[18] It is further believed that "physicians will adopt stronger measures to protect their territory from the specialties and from non-physician providers."[19]

The predicted competition resulting from an excess number of physicians by 1990 did not appear so serious. Although there have been federal enticements for medical schools to provide their students with knowledge about primary care, medicine's specialized focus has not been changed, and there has been a leveling off in the number of general and family practice physicians.[20] As technological advances and research increased in the 1940s, the need for physicians to specialize in order to keep pace with these advances was intensified. As a result, health care providers have become increasingly specialized. The statistical information on general practitioners and family practitioners shown in Table 9-1 reflects this growing trend toward specialization rather than general practice or family practice among physicians. Table 9-1 reveals how these two groups of physicians have become relatively stabilized during the early 1980s. From this data, it is readily observed that the number of general practitioners is

Table 9-1. Federal and nonfederal physicians by specialty for selected years

Year	Number	Year	Number
General Practitioners		*Family Practitioners*	
1980	32,519	1980	27,530
1981	29,399	1981	31,195
1982	28,508	1982	33,831
1983	28,202	1983	35,952
1986	25,069	1986	42,618
1988	24,395	1988	44,944

Source: Physician Characteristics and Distribution in the U.S. Chicago: American Medical Association, 1983, 20–21; 1986, 37; 1988. AMA Physician Masterfile, Dept. of Physician Data Services, verified by Primary Sources, unpublished material (phone conversation of May 11, 1990). Reproduced by permission.

on the decline and family practitioners are increasing at a relatively slow pace.[21]

In 1982, similar obstacles confronting nurse practitioners were identified: "differing educational background; limited awareness about NPs among consumers; legal ambiguities; lack of third party reimbursement; and lack of uniformity in goal definition."[22] These major issues facing NPs were on the workshop agenda sponsored by the Executive Committee of the Council of Nurse Practitioner's for its membership in the spring of 1984.[23] Among them, legal constraints or ambiguities have created serious problems for some nurse practitioners in fulfilling their nursing responsibilities.[24]

State nurse licensure laws that have not been revised to include diagnosis and treatment are another major stumbling block to nurse practitioners.[25, 26] Since 1971, thirty-eight states have amended their laws to facilitate expanded nursing roles and authorize nurses to diagnose, treat, and perform functions previously barred to them. Legal changes have also helped nurses establish collaborative and colleague relationships with other health professionals. However, "we in nursing must continue to attend to the issues at hand in reimbursement, legislative matters, educational funding through political processes if the public is to be served well."[27]

It will take money—contributions from nurses in the form of donations and membership dues. It will take unity in nursing . . . It will take new and creative partnerships with consumer and local community groups . . . Finally, it will take the establishment of a common educational base, with appropriate mechanisms for accreditation, certification, and licensure.[28]

In answer to the question "Should all nurses be nurse practitioners?" it has been said that "nurse practitioner probably is a title that will eventually describe all professional nurses, for the practitioner skill should belong to all professional nurses regardless of where they care for people."[29, 30]

Clinical Nurse Specialists

As an outgrowth of the proliferation of nurse aides, licensed practical nurses, and other types of nursing assistants in the 1940s and 1950s, registered nurses were removed from bedside care. They assumed head nurse and supervisory roles to direct and supervise these different groups. Direct patient care by registered nurses was replaced by administrative responsibilities for nursing services. In order to overcome this dilemma and return nurses to bedside care, nurse educators in the 1960s introduced the master's degree curriculum to prepare clinical nurse specialists (CNS) to serve as role models in delivery of high-quality nursing care to patients. At last, well-qualified nurses would be implementing nursing interventions and assuming direct accountability for the nursing care rendered.

Two specialty areas (nurse-midwifery and nurse anesthesiology) had developed in the 1940s. Later impetus from federal funds (available through the expanded Professional Nurse Traineeship Program of the 1960s for the preparation of clinical specialists) made it possible for many professional nurses to seek advanced clinical preparation at the master's level. Since that decade a tremendous increase in the number of master's programs preparing for clinical specialization has occurred, with approximately 213 college and university schools of nursing offering such programs in 1989. In some settings an expanded number of specialist roles have been developed by hospital nurses.

> These have included nurses with expertise in ostomy nursing, working with families, crisis counseling, pain management, discharge planning, teaching for self-care, health promotion activities such as exercise and control of diet, prevention of substance abuse . . . [and serving] as consultants and advisors to other nurses in developing their skills in similar areas.[31]

In many hospitals and other clinical agencies, clinical nurse specialists have greater autonomy than the average registered nurse because they can plan their own schedules around the needs of patients. They also arrange consultation for staff more flexibly than nurses functioning under more rigid schedules and time constraints. In the absence of such freedom, or when their expertise is not utilized sufficiently, an exodus of clinical specialists from these settings usually occurs.

Now that the American Nurses' Association has issued a Social Policy Statement that clearly defines the CNS role, perhaps the heated debate, confusion, and inconsistency over titling and definition of this role (nurse clinician, nurse practitioner, or clinical nurse specialist) may cease. This statement elaborates on specific criteria for the CNS role:

> The specialist in nursing practice is a nurse who, through study and supervised practice at the graduate level [master's or doctorate], has become expert in a defined area of knowledge and practice in a selected clinical area of nursing. Specialists in nursing practice are also generalists, in that they hold a baccalaureate in nursing, and therefore are able to provide the full range of nursing care. In addition, upon completion of a graduate degree in a university graduate program with an emphasis on clinical specialization, a specialist in nursing practice should meet the criteria for specialty certification through nursing's professional society.[32]

In this statement the competencies to be developed are clearly defined by clinical specialists: "ability to observe, conceptualize, diagnosis, and analyze complex clinical or nonclinical problems related to health, ability to consider a wide range of theory relevant to understanding those problems, and ability to select and justify applications of theory deemed to be most useful in understanding the problems and determining the range of possible treatment options."[33] It further notes that as phenomena of concern to nursing are more fully developed, they may ultimately define nursing specialty areas. Margretta Styles, one of two Distinguished American Nurses Foundation (ANF) Nurse Scholars, received a grant from the ANF to research new areas of clinical specialization as yet unidentified, which could be derived from a study of nursing phenomena. Her completed research was published in 1989.

As the role of the CNS in hospitals and other clinical settings is further developed and utilized and as their cost effectiveness is demonstrated and validated more thoroughly, greater utilization should occur. Quality nursing care would thus be assured. This development should signal that nursing has come of age and matured as a full-fledged profession. By the end of this century or shortly thereafter, preparation for clinical specialization at the master's or doctoral level may become the recognized "entry into practice" level for professional nursing.

Although preparation for generalist nursing practice was originally conceived to be at the baccalaureate level, the majority of master's nursing programs now prepare generalists. However, some nurse educators have recommended that specialization for clinical practice be offered in Doctor of Nursing Science programs.[34–36]

PRACTICE OF NURSING OR EXTENSION INTO MEDICAL PRACTICE

From the outset of the nurse practitioner movement, concern persisted over whether this practitioner role was more closely associated with the practice of nursing or with the practice of medicine. In the early 1970s, Martha Rogers waxed eloquent about how NPs had abdicated their nursing role and joined the ranks of physician-extenders. She believed that nurses have the privilege of making a choice for either role. They should, however, make intelligent choices, fully aware of the consequences of their decision. In other words, they should either remain with nursing or leave the profession to assist medicine with its functions. Rogers also believed that those leaving nursing were not entitled to identify themselves as nurses.[37] Other nurses held similar views, believing that the NP who opted for primary care had defected and was adversely affecting nursing.

It is interesting to note that many NPs see themselves as practicing or implementing functions essential to medicine and nursing. Now that nursing has more clearly defined its focus as that of disease prevention, promotion of health, and health maintenance, while medicine continues to focus on pathology or cure of disease, there is a need for nursing to utilize both orientations in fulfilling its mission to society. In the case of NPs, however, using techniques, functions, and technology identical to medicine does not mean they have become physicians' assistants. Doctors and NPs observe patients from different vantage points and as a result, see different problems. Research and studies conducted on NPs found them to be closely identified and oriented to nursing, viewing their expanded role as a means to advance nursing and assure its place in the forefront of health care planning.[38,39]

Undoubtedly, "it is the different therapies that distinguish nursing from medicine, for there is much that is shared in the gathering of data."[40] For example, the use of a stethoscope by both physician and nurse for data collection has been described. But the former relates findings to medical treatment or surgical intervention, and the latter utilizes findings for planning therapy involving positioning, ambulation, diet modification, and monitoring intake and output. "Nursing and medicine need each other to provide the best and most appropriate health care [but] the need for nursing to find an identity cannot compromise the need for closeness with medicine [since] autonomy does not mean isolation."[41]

The future of the nurse practitioner movement will largely depend on how this role is developed. If this role is practiced as purely a substitute for medical practice, the anticipated glut of physicians in the 1990s would probably eliminate the practitioner role, or at least reduce its effectiveness substantially.[42] On the other hand, if the present functions of the NP continue to emphasize health education, maintenance, and promotion, the future for expanding this role is promising. If legal barriers are removed, direct reimbursement for services occurs, and greater autonomy is achieved, then NPs can anticipate a successful future.

Although nurse practitioners were one of the first nursing groups to set up an independent practice (IP), today numerous opportunities exist for nurses to establish this type of nursing practice. Third-party reimbursement through legislation has made IP more attractive and attainable. As more nurses assume independent practice, more and more health policy makers will be made aware of the significance of nursing's contribution to the health and welfare of society. With health care costs escalating, independent practice based on fee for service may not be one of the preferred choices of third party payors. Instead, they seem to favor models of managed care with nurses playing a key role in providing more economical systems due to increasingly limited resources.

INDEPENDENT PRACTICE OR INTERDEPENDENT PRACTICE

Independent Practice

One of the well-known proponents of independent nursing practice, Lucille Kinlein, had written extensively about her experiences as a provider in this type of practice.[43–45] Introduced by her in 1971, the concept of independent practice involved a close, one-to-one nurse-patient relationship. Opening her office in the community of Hyattsville, Maryland, she began offering health services—health teaching and counseling, assessment of health status, and assisting with implementation of a medical regimen—emphasizing wellness-oriented care. Viewing illness as episodic, Kinlein believed physicians should be needed only on an intermittent basis, whereas health was ongoing, and the primary NP would be needed over an entire life span.

For nurses eager to increase their professional status and expand their service opportunities, independent practice as described by Kinlein will, in the future, probably attract only a relatively small group of practitioners. Sometimes referred to as "solo practice," it requires stamina and a high degree of emotional maturity because support or colleagueship from other health team members is lacking on a regular basis. Moreover, since primary health care involves responsibility and accountability for each patient on an around-the-clock basis seven days a week, independent practice can be a very demanding and exhausting experience, regardless of the number of referrals made.

Other opportunities for independent practice are occurring in nursing homes, nursing clinics, and ambulatory health care centers, where support services are more readily available. Despite the fears of some physicians, who view nurse practitioners as threats to their economic status, it appears that the doctor-nurse relationship is improving and a more collaborative practice is slowly developing. Most health planners seem to agree that nursing's health care focus will involve all nurses to a greater extent in health care delivery in the future.

Interdependent Practice

Ingeborg Mauksch, a strong advocate for nursing autonomy, recognizes the interdependent role of the nurse practitioner when she asserts that the NP "practices nursing by applying the nursing process, accounts to herself and the consumer for her services, behaves as a decision maker and risk taker, and delivers care interdependently with other health professionals."[46] To function in an interdependent role, nurses must be mature and self-confident about their knowledge base, and fully cognizant that alone they are insufficient to meet the health needs of their clients, families, and community. Physicians and nurses must learn to accept their own deficiencies and collaborate with one another to improve the quality of health care.

Unfortunately, there are few nurses willing to fight for autonomous practice and willing to use their power base to change the existing health care system. Perhaps one reason is the fact that the majority of nurses practicing in the acute care setting have graduated from diploma and associate degree programs, whose curricula lack preparation in assertiveness, community health nursing experiences, and a health care orientation. Taught to be docile and obedient in fulfilling their responsibilities, they assumed dependent, subservient behaviors that are still evident today. While medicine gradually increased its status and power within hospitals, nursing slowly became dominated by these institutions. To be professional and dependent is, indeed, contradictory since the mark of the true professional is autonomous practice.

To move from dependency to a scientifically based independent practice and finally, to interdependent practice requires significant changes in attitudes, educational preparation, and professional goals. Today, a majority of nurses (approximately 68% working in hospital settings) neither desire nor plan to make extensive changes in their present method of functioning or in their long-range goals. However, the winds of change are slowly affecting sizable numbers of these individuals, as they become better informed regarding the possibility of professional advancement and greater independence in their day-to-day activities.

Nurses who have achieved a high level of professional maturity and are confident of their expert nursing knowledge and skill, function very effectively with other health team members and enjoy greater satisfaction and acceptance in their role. Recognized by others for their nursing competence and abilities, they experience close collaboration, cooperation, and a level of autonomy that many other nurses never realize in their practice settings.

NURSING'S ROLE IN PRIMARY CARE

Nursing's continued resistance to recognizing primary care as an outgrowth of nursing's historical development, along with outside pressures for nurses to concentrate solely on illness, have delayed its development and growth since the mid-1960s. Today, however, nursing literature frequently refers to the necessity for nursing to command a vital influence on primary care delivery. "Only if nurses, by organization, by design, and with unity of purpose, lend the considerable weight of their influence and numbers to the fight for a preventive, wellness-oriented health care system will the profession achieve its full potential to upgrade the quality of health care as well as the quality of life for millions of Americans."[47]

Since many of the health problems that plague the well are not of great interest to the disease-oriented medical profession, it appears likely that primary care will become the major jurisdiction of nursing in the future. Preventive services, such as health education, advice on changing behavioral patterns, and choosing alternative lifestyles, along with psychosocial dimensions of care, are areas that generally have not been stressed in most medical education programs. Moreover, many physicians are unwilling to deal with problems of a nonmedical nature.

Included in the 1971 report of the Secretary of Health, Education, and Welfare's Committee to study the expanded role of the nurse was a definition of primary care described as "first contact care during an episode of illness; continuous care which is comprehensive and family-centered."[48] Since that time, many nurse practitioners have suggested that primary care be moved from concentrating solely on screening activities and first contact care to responsibility for providing comprehensive, continuous, family-centered care.

However, "until the health care system develops the capacity to assess the health of populations and to deliver care to those who may not come but who may be at the greatest risk of serious illness, the system will remain illness oriented."[49] Targeted population groups that nursing should seriously consider for better health care programs are "school children, the elderly, workers, and college students" because as segregated groups they would be most receptive to primary care.[50]

Nurse practitioners, with their background of humanistic concern and sensitivity to patient health needs along with clinical knowledge and expert skills, seem uniquely qualified to redirect the present focus of primary care. In addition, the setting for primary care provides opportunities for autonomous practice without the bureaucracy and more structured relations within hospitals. "The provision of an alternate type of career opportunity, in which the nurse has more responsibility and authority, may attract nurses who may otherwise be lost to the profession because they fail to gain satisfaction in other areas of nursing."[51]

It appears that the current supply of labor resources cannot meet the increased demand for ambulatory health care services in the United States. Health professionals prepared in primary care are few in number compared with physicians and nurses available for secondary or tertiary care.[52] Rather than create new levels of health care personnel to meet health care's needs, logic dictates that well-qualified nurse practitioners could and should alleviate this problem.

If NPs are a bridge between nurse and physician, their importance in the area of preventive health services will be the key to refocusing the health care system. Thus, nursing must encourage more nurses to prepare for a primary care role in order to greatly improve the health status of the American public. Primary care forms the groundwork for the entire health care system, and physicians, aware of its importance, seem determined to control access to it.

FUTURE FOR GERONTOLOGICAL NURSING

Home Health Care

Profound changes in the health care industry, particularly within Home Health Care (HHC), are having an impact on the employment of registered nurses. The number of home care agencies has grown tremendously over the past few years, due primarily to an increase in the elderly population and the cost-containment issue necessitating early discharges from hospitals. More nurses will have to be recruited to meet this growing demand for home care services. "A high acuity case mix of clients in the home requires technologically advanced nursing skills and more detailed documentation for reimbursable services."[53]

By the year 2000, the percent of older Americans will be approximately 17 percent of the total population. Americans 85 years and older are the fastest growing group, with their numbers expected to double by the year 2000. By 2050, one in twenty-nine Americans will be over 85 years of age.[54] Whether there will be sufficient numbers of registered nurses to meet the ensuing home health care explosion remains uncertain. Evaluation of present health care strategies should be given serious consideration to determine whether they can meet the need for diversified home care programs providing continuity of care. Home health care is another waiting opportunity for nursing to exert leadership in providing quality care for this relatively new and growing health service industry.

Home health care continues to gain prominence. Due to prospective payment of the 1980s resulting in earlier discharge of patients from acute care institutions, a tremendous demand for health care in the home and community has shifted many nurses from hospital walls to health care centers and home health services.[55] Pressure from third party payors for an alternative model of health care delivery has resulted in home health professionals now treating more acutely ill patients in their homes. "Today registered nurses are administering blood transfusions, antibiotic therapy, pain management, and chemotherapy via central and peripheral lines, plus managing various types of parts and pumps—all in the home setting."[56]

In 1989, the home health care market was estimated to be $15.9 billion. Predictions were that total health care costs would increase to $812.6 billion in 1993, with home care costs totalling $23.2 billion.[57] As expected, some authors stress that home health care is at a critical transition point. Nurses are uniquely qualified to demonstrate and assume responsibility for delivering high-quality, cost-effective home health services. As a result, they should take advantage of the extraordinary opportunity to be on the cutting edge of health care policy reform to enhance access to and the quality of home health care.[58] Increasing longevity and advances in health care technology have placed great stress on the health care system. Thus, the trend from institutional care to home care continues to be well-documented.[59, 60]

The NLN Board proclaimed 1990 as the year of the Community Health Accreditation Program (CHAP) at their February 1990 meeting.[61] CHAP, representing a private accreditation program to improve the quality of home care, became an independent subsidiary of NLN in 1987.[62] With the appointment of a new administrator of Health Care Financing Administration (HCFA), it was anticipated that "deemed status" under Medicare from HCFA would allow CHAP to determine eligibility of home health care agencies for participation in the Medicare program and for certifying their eligibility for Federal Medicare reimbursement. CHAP continues to work with consumer groups such as the American Association of Retired Persons (AARP) to provide information about quality health care, since "one of the biggest gaps in the delivery and financing of health care is the fact that there is no organized plan to provide long-term supportive care."[63] Assuring quality and shaping care standards for home care provides nurses with the opportunity to voice their opinions on the quality of home care standards.

An exciting, innovative project was developed in 1980 at Creighton University School of Nursing in Omaha, Nebraska. It involves the establishment and operation of a university-sponsored home care agency as a clinical sight for baccalaureate nursing students in community health nursing. Referred to as the Creighton Home Health Care Agency, it involves cooperation between the Community Health Division of the School of Nursing and the Family Practice Division of the School of Medicine of Creighton University.[64] Recognizing that health services were not adequately meeting the needs of certain sectors of the community, nursing faculty, with the cooperation of physicians functioning in an inner-city ambulatory family practice clinic, were able to obtain numerous physician referrals to provide quality nursing care to low-income, minority families in their homes. Similar examples of interdisciplinary, cooperative efforts in home health care between university schools of the health sciences can be found throughout the United States, such as the Rush Home Health Services at Rush Presbyterian-St. Lukes Hospital in Chicago.

A proposal submitted by the California Nurses' Association and adopted by the House of Delegates at the June 1984 ANA Biennial Convention requested the ANA to:

> revise its standards for the practice of community health nursing to emphasize the changes in practice, particularly in home health care; to formulate a strategy for implementation of these standards including identification of the educational preparation for the home health care nurse; to explore mechanisms for direct reimbursement to the registered nurse as a provider of home health care; to recommend development of nursing diagnoses as a basis for home health care reimbursement; and to recommend that the registered nurse be authorized to determine and certify a plan of care for home health.[65]

In October, 1982, the first annual meeting of the newly established National Association for Home Care convened in Atlanta, Georgia, drew more than 800 Home Health Agency representatives. At this historic meeting, Florida Congressman Claude Pepper, the keynote speaker (now deceased), presented a "forceful argument for in-home care as a humane and cost-effective alternative to institutionalization."[66]

Nursing Homes

According to figures obtained from a National Nursing Home survey conducted in 1977, seventy-three percent of the nursing homes in this country lacked twenty-four-hour registered nurse coverage.[67] Critical of the available health care currently provided in the nation's nursing homes, H. A. Sultz asserted that "elderly citizens, who are caught in the political and economic crossfire associated with Medicaid and Medicare regulations and the nursing home industry, are frequently placed in facilities that provide little or no medical nursing care."[68] Sultz believes that "the routine employment of geriatric nurse practitioners to supplement or, in some cases, to replace disinterested or overworked physicians, who perform perfunctory checks of nursing home patients, could do much to bring humane and competent health care to that segment of the population unfortunate enough to survive to the age of dependency."[69]

Believing that nursing could play a major role in efforts to solve the nation's nursing home scandal, it was pointed out that

> by assuming leadership in the development of standards in the provision of professionally managed care to those who are now 'warehoused' in the country's nursing homes, nursing could make a unique contribution to the nation's well-being. Clearly there must be a full-time health professional presence in these institutions, for despite all efforts to regulate the quality of care, there is little accountability for maintaining reasonable standards.[70]

An excellent example of cooperative effort between universities and nursing homes is that of the Teaching Nursing Home Program, sponsored by the Robert Wood Johnson Foundation and the American Academy of Nursing in 1982. The program provides "demonstrations [that] offer a testing ground for professional care and management innovations that will influence national policy decisions."[71] Located in eight states and the District of Columbia, the eleven sites include six public and six private education institutions. Through affiliation agreements between the university school of nursing faculty and the nursing home, these demonstration sites are beginning to confront some of the major social issues involved in the care of the elderly.[72]

Another example of the cooperation between ANA Councils concerned with gerontological nursing is the merger of the ANA Council (formerly Division) on Gerontological Nursing Practice and the Council of Nursing Home Nurses to form the Council on Gerontological Nursing.[73] A new model to improve the long-term care of older adults, originally created by a task force established by the ANA Division on Gerontological Nursing Practice, has been field-tested and further developed by the Council on Gerontological Nursing. It is hoped that this new model will serve as a guide to all nurses working with older people so that they will all be heading in the same direction.[74] This model applies to a variety of health care settings.

NURSE-MANAGED CENTERS

The decade of the 1980s introduced another innovation in primary care—nurse-managed centers. Recognizing nursing's importance in this latest development in health care delivery, the ANA believes that nurses are central in their role as coordinators, managers, and providers of health care services.[75] The ANA views these centers as a way for nursing to show its "ability to meet the health care needs of unserved and underserved populations, demonstrate the long-term and short-term benefits of good nursing care, offer an alternative to traditional health care, show the good things that happen when nurses control their practice, and do it all cost-effectively."[76]

Currently there are over 150 nursing centers known to exist throughout the country. Of this number, three in particular have become nationally known: The Erie Family Health Center in Chicago, Illinois; The University of Wisconsin-Milwaukee Nursing Center; and The Nursing Consultation Center of the Department of Nursing, College of Human Development, Pennsylvania State University, University Park, Pennsylvania. The University of Wisconsin-Milwaukee Nursing Center has as its main purpose to provide opportunities for undergraduate nursing students to learn about health promotion. The Nursing Consultation Center at Pennsylvania State University, located ninety miles from the nearest medical center, does not collaborate with any medical facility. Such isolation has resulted in a unique perspective on health care and autonomy for their School of Nursing.[77]

Opportunities for representatives from nurse centers throughout the nation to meet biennially to discuss problems such as legislation to create a federal payment mechanism for the centers has occurred since 1982. The recurring theme at all these meetings revolves around the need for control of nursing practice by nurses and the financial viability of nurse-managed centers. Two other universities that have described their nurse centers in the literature are the University Family Health Center, University of Wisconsin, Madison, and the Georgetown University Community Health Plan, Washington, D.C.[78, 79]

Bills to provide coverage of Community Nursing Centers under Medicare and Medicaid, developed with ANA assistance, were introduced in the Senate and House in 1983 and 1984. "The principal focus of the Community Nursing Center legislation is to provide for ambulatory care through independent nursing centers as a real alternative to high cost institutional care."[80] Interestingly, it is the nurse and not the physician who controls access to services at community nursing centers.[81] However, the nurse submits a care plan to the client's physician, who may recommend changes or disapprove of the plan. In addition, an independent committee must review the care plan. Thus, a health care delivery system as significant as health maintenance organizations, which began with federal assistance, can be developed by nurses managing nursing centers.[82]

It is refreshing and exhilarating to see the progress being made by nurses in their expanded role in health care delivery. More and more individual nurses and groups of nurses in primary care are working to achieve control of nursing practice and reimbursement for their services. No longer willing to serve in a dependent role, many nurses are demanding autonomy and the right to provide their clients with high-quality nursing care. Assuming accountability for the delivery of nursing care through peer review and collaborative efforts, nurses are reaching out for professionalism. Undoubtedly, with such enthusiasm and determination they will achieve it.

SUMMARY

To keep pace with the rapidly evolving health care system, nursing has begun to require a professional model of nursing practice. Achieving increased autonomy has necessitated changes in organizational structures to accommodate new, expanded roles for nurses. Unlike any other time in its history, nursing is asserting its demands for clinical decision-making authority and equality with other health professionals.

Over thirty years, new and exciting roles have been developed. For example, the nurse practitioner movement, which currently numbers over 20,000 members, has grown substantially. It has become an important component in the existing health care system. By providing needed primary care services, particularly to under-served populations in rural areas, NPs are making a vital contribution to health care. Barriers to the success of this movement include lack of direct reimbursement, legislative constraints, lack of educational support, and under-utilization in the practice arena. Concern over the anticipated glut of physicians in the 1990s and its possible effect on NPs has been voiced continually, but it is difficult to predict how serious this problem may later become.

Data available on the number of general practitioners and family practitioners in medicine show a strong decline in the former and stabilization of the latter in the early 1980s and 1990s. Several nurse authors have concluded that the expanding functions of NPs will eventually belong to all professional nurses, regardless of the setting in which health care is provided. Clinical specialists prepared for advanced clinical practice in nursing specialty programs that grant a master's degree in nursing have provided role models in the delivery of high-quality nursing care to patients. Since these specialists function under less rigid schedules than the average staff nurse, they can be more flexible in arranging for staff consultation or in meeting patient needs. Now that the ANA has clearly defined the CNS role in their Social Policy Statement, the confusion over definition of this role and titling may be ended.

Although some nurses view NPs as having abdicated their nursing role and are no longer entitled to be called nurses, others believe nursing should be oriented to care and cure in order to fulfill its societal mission. Nursing and medicine need each other, and although nursing seeks its own identity, it cannot isolate itself from medicine or other health workers in order to achieve autonomy. Evidence indicates that the future looks bright for nurse practitioners and clinical specialists, especially if health education, maintenance, and promotion continue to be emphasized. If legal barriers are removed, direct reimbursement is made available, and greater autonomy is acquired, these expanded roles should move nursing forward in its quest for professionalism.

Independent practice and interdependent practice for the majority of practicing nurses will continue to be a goal. Unless significant changes occur in attitude, educational preparation, and professional goals, most nurses will continue to function in a dependent mode. Nursing's role in primary care is serving to redirect the present focus of health care, stressing health rather than an illness orientation. Satisfaction derived from providing primary care retains nurses who might otherwise be lost to nursing due to dissatisfaction with other types of nursing care.

The impact of the Home Health Care industry on the total health care system is only recently receiving attention from legislators, third-party payors, and nurses interested in providing this type of care. Problems involving nursing homes, particularly the lack of adequate physician and RN coverage, must be rectified if a large percentage of elderly patients are to receive competent and humane care in these institutions.

Nurse-managed centers are a new innovation in health care, with over 150 nursing centers currently in existence throughout the United States. Legislation introduced to promote nursing centers recommends them as an alternative to high-cost institutional care. Each of these evolving roles provides nursing with exciting opportunities to become more autonomous and accountable, as nurses collaborate with one another to provide high-quality independent nursing care.

REFERENCES

1. U.S. Public Health Service. "Toward Quality in Nursing: Needs and Goals," in *Surgeon General's Consultant Group on Nursing* (Pub. No.: 992). Washington, D.C.: U.S. Government Printing Office, 1963.
2. Carroll, M., Fischer, L. and Frericks, M. "Education Must Adapt to Changing Health Care System," *American Nurse* 12:3 (March, 1980), 5.

3. Mowry, M. and Korpman, R. "Hospitals, Nursing, and Medicine" *Journal of Nursing Administration* 17:11 (November, 1987), 16.
4. "For 'New Nurse': Bigger Role in Health Care," *U.S. News and World Report* 88:1 (January 14, 1980), 60.
5. "Summary of Proposals Adopted by A.N.A. House," *American Nurse* 16:7 (July–August, 1984), 15.
6. Silver, H. and Ford, L. "The Pediatric Nurse Practitioner at Colorado," *American Journal of Nursing* 67:7 (July, 1967), 1443–1444.
7. Ford, L. "Nurse Practitioners: History of a New Idea and Predictions for the Future," in L. Aiken (ed.), *Nursing in the 1980s: Crises, Opportunities, Challenges.* Philadelphia: J. B. Lippincott, 1982, 233, 235.
8. Whitney, F. "Nurse Practitioners: Mirrors of the Past, Windows of the Future," in N. Chaska (ed.), *The Nursing Profession: Turning Points.* St. Louis: C.V. Mosby, 1990, 364.
9. Bleiweiss, L. and Egner, B. "The Nurse Practitioner Role: Issues for the Future," in M. Miller and B. Flynn (eds.), *Current Perspectives in Nursing: Social Issues and Trends.* St. Louis: C. V. Mosby, 1980, 92.
10. *Ibid.,* 90–91.
11. Sultz, H., Henry, O. Bullough, B., Baskin, G. and Kinyon, L. "Nurse Practitioners: A Decade of Change—Part IV" *Nursing Outlook* 32:3 (May–June, 1984), 163.
12. *Ibid.*
13. Winterton, M. "Evaluation of Nurse Practitioner Effectiveness: An Overview of the Literature," *Evaluation and the Health Professions* 1:1 (Spring, 1978), 69–81.
14. Sultz, H., Cielezny, M. and Gentry, J. *Longitudinal Study of Nurse Practitioners Phase III* (Pub. No.: HRA 80–2). Hyattsville, Md.: Department of Public Health, 1980.
15. Lewis, C. and Resnick, B. "Nurse Clinics and Progressive Ambulatory Patient Care," *New England Journal of Medicine* 277 (1967), 1236–1241.
16. Prescott, P. and Driscoll, L. "Nurse Practitioner Effectiveness: A Review of Physician-Nurse Comparison Studies," *Evaluation in the Health Professions* 2:4 (December, 1979), 414.
17. Ford, L. "Nurse Practitioners," 244.
18. Ellwood, P. and Ellweiss L. "Physician Glut Will Force Hospitals to Look Outward," *Hospitals* 55:2 (January 16, 1981), 83.
19. *Ibid.*
20. Diers, D. and Molde, S. "Nurses in Primary Care—The New Gate Keepers?" *American Journal of Nursing* 83:5 (May, 1983), 745.
21. *Physician Characteristics and Distribution in the U.S.* Chicago: American Medical Association, 1983, 20–21; 1986, 37; 1988 (Phone conversation, May 11, 1990).
22. "Nurse Practitioners Develop Strategies," *American Nurse* 16:5 (May, 1984), 6.
23. *Ibid.*
24. Mallison, M. (ed.), "A Tale of Two Coalitions," *American Journal of Nursing* 84:1 (January, 1984), 7.
25. Bullough, B. *The Law and the Expanding Nursing Role.* New York: Appleton-Century-Crofts, 1975.

26. Bullough, B. "Nurse Practice Acts: How They Affect Your Expanding Role," *Nursing 77* 2:78, 1977.
27. Ford, L. "Nurse Practitioners," 245.
28. *Ibid.*
29. Mundinger, M. *Autonomy in Nursing.* Rockville, Md.: Aspen Systems Corp., 1980, 196.
30. Kalisch, B. "The Promise of Power," in E. Hein and N. Nicholson (eds.), *Contemporary Leadership Behavior.* Boston: Little, Brown & Co., 1982, 175.
31. Jacox, A. "Role Restructuring in Hospital Nursing," in L. Aiken (ed.), *Nursing in the 1980s: Crises, Opportunities, Challenges.* Philadelphia. J. B. Lippincott, 1982, 91.
32. *Nursing: A Social Policy Statement.* (Pub. No.: NP-63). Kansas City, Mo.: American Nurses' Association, 1980, 23.
33. *Ibid.*
34. Andreoli, K. "Specialization and Graduate Curriculum: Finding the 'Fit,' " *Nursing and Health Care* 8:2 (February, 1987), 65–69.
35. Snyder, M. "Educational Preparation of the CNS," in A. Hamric and J. Spross (eds.), *The Clinical Nurse Specialist in Theory and Practice.* New York: W. B. Saunders Co., 1989, 325–342.
36. Styles, M. *On Specialization in Nursing: Toward a New Empowerment.* Kansas City, Mo.: American Nurses Foundation, Inc., 1989.
37. Rogers, M. "Nursing: To Be or Not To Be," *Nursing Outlook* 20:1 (1972), 42–45.
38. Flynn, B. "Study Documents Reactions to Nurses in Expanded Role," *Hospitals* 49 (1975), 81–83.
39. Bleiweiss, L. and Egner, B. *Nurse Practitioner Role,* 93.
40. Mundinger, M. *Autonomy in Nursing,* 9.
41. *Ibid.,* 11.
42. Billingsley, M. and Harper, D. "The Extinction of the Nurse Practitioner: Threat or Reality," *Nurse Practitioner* 7:9 (October, 1982), 22–30.
43. Kinlein, M. *Independent Nursing Practice with Clients.* Philadelphia: J. B. Lippincott, 1977.
44. Kinlein, M. "Independent Nurse Practitioner," *Nursing Outlook* 20:1 (January, 1972), 22–24.
45. Kinlein, M. "Point of View on the Front: Nursing and Family and Community Health," *Family and Community Health* 1 (April, 1978), 57–68.
46. Mauksch, I. and Rogers, M. "Nursing is Coming of Age . . . Through the Practitioner Movement," *American Journal of Nursing* 75:10 (October, 1975), 835.
47. Sultz, H. "Nurse Practitioners Can Change the Focus of Primary Care," in M. Miller and B. Flynn (eds.), *Current Issues in Nursing.* Vol. 2. St. Louis: C. V. Mosby, 1980, 85.
48. U.S. Health, Education and Welfare Department. *Extending the Scope of Nursing Practice: A Report of the Secretary's Committee to Study Extended Roles in Nursing.* Washington, D.C.: U.S. Government Printing Office, 1971.
49. Aiken, L. "Primary Care: The Challenge for Nursing," *American Journal of Nursing* 77:11 (November, 1977), 1832.
50. Sultz, H. "Nurse Practitioners," 85.
51. Lewis, C. and Resnik, B. "Nurse Clinics," 1240.

52. Millis, J. "Primary Care: Definition of and Access to . . . ," *Nursing Outlook* 25 (1977), 444.
53. Oda, D. "Home Visits: Effective or Obsolete Nursing Practice," *Nursing Research* 38:2 (March–April, 1989), 121.
54. Duffy, M. "Needed: New Models for Professional Nursing Education," in N. Chaska (ed.), *The Nursing Profession: Turning Points*. St. Louis: C.V. Mosby, 1990, 84.
55. Michaels, C. "Information—A Key to Nursing's Future," in *Nursing's Vital Signs: Shaping the Profession for the 1990s*. Battle Creek, Mich.: W.K. Kellogg Foundation, 1989, 67.
56. Stainton, M. "Home Health Care Comes of Age," *American Nurse* 22:2 (February, 1990), 4.
57. Selby, T. "Home Health Care Finds New Ways of Caring," *American Nurse* 22:2 (February, 1990), 1.
58. Kent, V. and Hanley, B. "Home Health Care," *Nursing and Health Care* 11:5 (May, 1990), 240.
59. Stainton, M. "Home Health Care Comes of Age," 4.
60. Somers, A. "The Changing Demand for Health Services: A Historical Perspective and Some Thoughts for the Future," *Inquiry* 23:2 (Winter, 1986), 395–402.
61. "NLN Board of Governors Meet in February," (NLN Perspective) *Nursing and Health Care* 11:4 (April, 1990), 211.
62. *Ibid.*, 212.
63. Newman, M. and Autio, S. *Nursing in a Prospective Payment System Health Care Environment*. Minneapolis: University of Minnesota, 1986, 16.
64. Herman, C. and Krall, K. "University Sponsored Home Care Agency as a Clinical Site," *Image: The Journal of Nursing Scholarship* 17:3 (Summer, 1984), 71–75.
65. "Summary of Proposals Adopted by A.N.A. House," *American Nurse* 16:7 (July–August, 1984), 15.
66. "Home Care Providers Join Forces as First NAHC Meeting Convenes," *American Journal of Nursing* 82:12 (December, 1982), 1905.
67. National Center for Health Statistics. *National Nursing Home Survey: 1977* (DHEW Pub. No.: (PHS) 79–1794). Washington, D.C.: U.S. Government Printing Office, 1979.
68. Sultz, H. "Nurse Practitioners," 82.
69. *Ibid.*
70. Aiken, L. "Nursing Priorities for the 1980s: Hospitals and Nursing Homes," *American Journal of Nursing* 81:2 (February, 1981), 329.
71. Mesey, M., Lynaugh, J., and Cherry, J. "The Teaching Nursing Home Program," *Nursing Outlook* 32:3 (May–June, 1984), 146.
72. *Ibid.*, 150.
73. "Board Takes Action on Council Recommendations," *American Nurse* 16:7 (July–August, 1984), 7.
74. "Task Force Will Create, Test New Model of Long-Term Care," *American Nurse* 15:5 (May, 1983), 11.
75. Selby, T. "Nurse-Managed Centers Show Their Potential," *American Nurse* 16:5 (May, 1984), 1.
76. *Ibid.*

77. *Ibid.*, 10.
78. Aradine, C. and Hansen, M. "Nursing in a Primary Health Care Setting," *Nursing Outlook* 27:4 (April, 1979), 45–46.
79. Chickadonz, G., Burke, M., Fitzgerald, S., and Osterweis, M. "Development of a Primary Care Setting for Nursing Education," *Nursing and Health Care* 4:2 (February, 1982), 83–87, 92.
80. "Nursing Centers Bill Introduced in Senate by Inouye, Packwood," *American Nurse* 15:3 (March, 1983), 2.
81. Dayani, E. "Nursing Centers Bill Lets Us Show What We Can Do," *Nursing and Health Care* 5.5 (May, 1983), 4.
82. *Ibid.*

SUGGESTED READINGS

American Academy of Nursing. *Primary Care by Nurses: Sphere of Responsibility and Accountability.* Kansas City, Mo.: The American Nurses' Association, 1976.
Balassone, P. "Territorial Issues in an Interdisciplinary Experience," *Nursing Outlook* 29:4 (April, 1981), 229–232.
Bedrosian, C., *Home Health Nursing.* Norwalk, CT: Appleton & Lange, 1989.
Bullough, B. "State Certification of the Nursing Specialities: A New Trend in Nursing Practice Law," *Pediatric Nursing* (March–April, 1982), 121–124.
Choi-Wolcott, M. "Nurses as Co-Providers of Primary Health Care," *Nursing Outlook* 29:9 (September, 1981), 519–524.
Cooke, M. "Taking Charge of Change in Hospital Nursing Practice," *American Journal of Nursing* 81:3 (March, 1981), 541–543.
Department of Health and Human Services. *Study of Nurse Practitioners* (Pub. No.: (HRP) 0904775;cb.) Springfield, Va.: The National Technical Information Service, 1984.
Grimes, D. and Stamps, C. "Meeting the Health Care Needs of Older Adults Through a Community Nursing Center," *Nursing Administrative Quarterly* 4:3 (Spring, 1980), 31–40.
Hagopian, G., Gerrity, P. and Lynaugh, J. "Assessment Preparation for Nurse Practitioners," *Nursing Outlook* 38:6 (November–December, 1990), 272–274.
Hamric, A. and Spross, J. *The Clinical Nurse Specialist in Theory and Practice.* New York: Grune and Stratton, 1983.
Hazard, M. and Kemp, R. "Keeping the Well-Elderly Well," *American Journal of Nursing* 83:4 (April, 1983), 567–569.
Hegyvary, S. *The Change to Primary Nursing: A Cross-Cultural View of Professional Nursing Practice.* St. Louis: C. V. Mosby, 1982.
Holt, F. "A Theoretical Model for Clinical Specialist Practice," *Nursing and Health Care* 5:8 (October, 1984), 445–449.
"Home Health Care Should Be the Heart of a Nursing-Sponsored National Health Plan," *Nursing and Health Care* 10:10 (December, 1989), 300.
Mershon, K. and Wesolowski, M. "The Business of Community Health and Human Care," *Nursing and Health Care* 6:1 (January, 1985), 33–35.

Milio, N. *Primary Care and the Public's Health.* Lexington, Mass.: Lexington Books, 1983.

"Nursing Homes Hardest Hit by Shortage," *American Nurse* 22:6 (June, 1990), 30.

Ramsey, J., McKenzie, J., and Fish, D. "Physicians and Nurse Practitioners: Do They Provide Equivalent Health Care?" *American Journal of Public Health* 73:1 (January, 1982), 55–57.

"Rep. Ron Wyden Introduces Nursing Center Bill," *The American Nurse* 16:3 (March, 1984), 2.

Reisch, S., Felder, E. and Stander, C. "Nursing Centers Can Promote Health For Individuals, Families, and Communities," *Nursing Administrative Quarterly* 4:3 (Summer, 1980), 1–8.

Ropka, M. and Fay, F. "Clinical Nurse Specialist—Alive and Well?" *American Journal of Nursing* 84:5 (May, 1984), 661–662, 664.

Selby, T. "Nurse Practitioner Groups Form Coalition," *American Nurse* 17:6 (June, 1985), 1, 16.

Economic Issues Affecting Nursing Practice

10

INTRODUCTION

Among the goals that nursing hopes to attain by the end of this decade, a more equitable economic base for its practitioners continues to be of high priority. Undoubtedly, the state of the economy plays a major role in affecting the economic status that nursing desires to achieve. Since the American Nurses Association in issuing a Social Policy Statement has defined the nature and scope of nursing practice and as more nurses are demonstrating their competence, it is time for nurses to claim their rightful rewards. These rewards should not only be intrinsic to nurses' work performance but also provide status and adequate compensation equal to the contributions nurses make to health care delivery.

The major concern throughout the past decade, and currently, is the institutional byword of cost containment. This issue, plus the nation's slow economic growth, continues to have an adverse effect on nursing's efforts to obtain improved financial status for its members. Because the United States' economy cannot be ignored, it would seem that the time is propitious for nursing to demonstrate its cost effectiveness and to demand appropriate reimbursement for its role in advancing the health status of Americans. Escalating health care costs have combined with the public's increasing demand for quality health care services to create tensions within the health care delivery system that will, ultimately, affect the general welfare of nurses.

Pressure from the federal government to control health care costs is forcing hospital administrators to reduce their numbers of nursing personnel. For nursing to prevail against severe budget cutbacks, the majority of nurses must be organized and knowledgeable about collective bargaining activities. Through a united front on collective bargaining, nursing can best serve the public's need for high-quality nursing care.

COLLECTIVE BARGAINING AND THE NURSING PROFESSION

Over forty years have elapsed since delegates to the thirty-fifth convention of the American Nurses' Association unanimously endorsed a national economic security program enabling state and local nurses' associations to engage in collective bargaining for their members. Several issues remain to be solved if nurses are to improve their economic status and continue to elevate the standards for nursing practice.[1] A brief review of certain labor laws and their amendments reveals some highlights that have greatly affected nursing's ability to negotiate for economic and professional improvements in the work situation.

In 1935, the National Labor Relations Act (NLRA) required hospitals to engage in bargaining activities with their employees. The American Nurses' Association, through its Economic Security Program in 1946, granted state nurses' associations the right to successfully engage in collective bargaining.[2] However, the passage of the Taft-Hartley Act in 1947 excluded private, nonprofit health care institutions from the legal obligation of bargaining with their employees. This act provided legal authority for nonprofit employers to disregard improving the economic status of their employees, including nurses. Without any legal jurisdiction to safeguard their rights, registered nurses were hindered from negotiating contracts with their employers.

The Taft-Hartley Act placed nursing in a weakened position and contributed to the slow rate of progress in improving wages and working conditions for nurses. In an effort to strengthen professionalism and the ideal of service, the ANA approved a "no strike" policy in 1950.[3] As a result of the Taft-Hartley Act and ANA's determination to avoid strikes, nurses' bargaining power was reduced substantially. The continued pressure from nurses to improve their economic status led the ANA House of Delegates to rescind its "no strike" clause in 1968.[4] From 1969 to 1974, state nurses' associations were successful in obtaining sound bargaining contracts for their members. However, the number of strikes by nurses increased markedly during this period, as a result of nursing's inability to otherwise negotiate economic issues effectively with its employers.

Fortunately for nursing, a major breakthrough occurred with the passage of amendments to the Taft-Hartley Act by Congress in 1974. By means of these amendments, nonprofit hospitals were no longer exempt from bargaining with their employees over increasing wages, improving working conditions, and achieving more realistic staffing patterns. Sanction of strikes by the ANA provided the impetus for nurses to resort to such means when other tactics produced no positive results. Some important concerns about collective bargaining center on questions such as: "Is collective bargaining professional?" "Who will represent *nurses* in bargaining negotiations?" "Who will represent *nursing?*" and "Who will have control over nursing practice?" Many nurses consider strikes unprofessional.[5] Yet, some of these individuals often reap the benefits resulting from such efforts. Other nurses, confident that collective bargaining poses no threat to their professional status, view it "as a method by which to achieve greater control over patient care decisions, staffing levels, and the management of health care facilities."[6]

Numerous articles have appeared debating the pros and cons of collective bargaining and its compatibility with the ideal of professionalism. In reality, this question no longer seems relevant, since thousands of nurses employed in hospitals work under contracts negotiated either by state nurses' associations or by labor unions. The focus of such negotiations is frequently as much on issues of professional practice as on economics.

In many instances, improvement in salaries, benefits, and control over practice has resulted from work stoppages, strikes, or mass resignations when bargaining sessions with employers proved ineffective. The successes of collective bargaining through the professional association to improve compensation and employment conditions is well documented in reports published in the *American Journal of Nursing*. These reports attest to successful negotiating efforts by nurses in obtaining improved contracts from hospital employers through collective bargaining. Thus,

> . . . in skillful hands collective bargaining becomes a resource for the actual achievement of goals. Timely threats of work stoppages, knowledgeable give and take with hospital administrators, and the use of mandatory membership and other goals won through strong and unified nursing organizations represent ways collective bargaining can be used to create further power resources. Thus, collective bargaining appears—at this moment—to be the most viable strategy nurses have at their command.[7]

Moreover, collective bargaining is beneficial in that "it provides for elected spokesmen, for freedom of expression, for joint decision making, and enforceable agreement in ways not possible within the bureaucracy."[8]

WHO SHOULD REPRESENT NURSES?

The question of who will represent nurses depends on which issue is the most important to be addressed—economic, professional, or both. Improvement in salary and benefits alone convinces some nurses that an industrial union type of organization would be more appropriate in achieving the goal of improved economic status. However, experience indicates that economic issues cannot be separated from professional issues, since one greatly affects the other.

A current question is whether the professional association (ANA) can most effectively represent nurses, or whether an industrial labor union or a labor organization controlled by nurses might be more advantageous for nursing. Charges that the ANA, in addressing economic and general welfare problems, has abdicated its responsibilities for professionalism and become a "trade union" are unwarranted. Professional issues continue to consume much of ANA's time, financial resources, and energy.

By establishing a separate labor organization, the persistent charge that the professional association is manager-dominated by supervisory members and cannot be classified as a labor organization would no longer be relevant. Actually this charge should have been finally "put to rest" by the National Labor Relations Board decision in 1979, which affirmed the right of state nurses' associations to act as legitimate labor organizations. And yet, the fact that many nursing administrators withdrew their membership in ANA continued to cause dissension.

The withdrawals were due to the fact that these nurse administrators refused to be associated with what, in their view, was a labor union. Since some of the dues for ANA are directed toward supporting the Economic Security Program, these nurse administrators were indirectly supporting a labor union (ANA) when labor laws constrained them from either interfering or dominating local units. As a result, pressure from some hospital administrators for withdrawal from ANA continued. Since nurse administrators were not allowed to participate in the ANA's economic and general welfare programs, though a portion of their dues supported them, many of them discontinued their membership in the association. Currently, no specific suggestions for remedying this situation have been provided. Apparently misunderstanding still exists over this issue.

In a separate labor organization, nurses would be in control of directing their future, not simply backing into it with neither autonomy nor status. Moreover, they would speak with a unified voice for all nurses in determining salaries, flexible scheduling, and other work improvements. On the surface, such reasoning appears quite appropriate. However, the problems involved in establishing a separate nurse union raise several questions that make its existence questionable. Presently the courts are obtaining evidence that does not appear to justify separate nurse labor units.[9] Another related problem, which some nurses might overlook, is the extent of the resources required to organize a labor union. Because no collective bargaining would occur during the organizational phase, no economic gains or personal advancement would result during that time.[10]

> Resources expended on convincing potential members to join, creating consensus and forming a bureaucracy will present sunken costs. Additional resources will then be needed to maintain the organization and to campaign for organizational goals.[11]

If nurses choose the industrial union as the organization to represent them, how effective will it be in resolving economic and professionalization issues confronting the profession? Presently, a tremendous interest exists on the part of organized labor unions, such as the AFL-CIO and the American Federation of Teachers, to recruit registered nurses into their organizations.[12] Can these unions speak for *nursing* as well as for nurses?

Many feel strongly that only the professional association can adequately represent nursing's economic and professional concerns. Although some raise questions about the ANA's ability to provide sufficient staff and financial support for collective bargaining endeavors, others believe that the only alternative to nurses from an "ethical, professional, and pragmatic standpoint" is for them to unite in efforts to make their collective bargaining agent that of the national, state, and local nursing organizations.[13] "No other organization replaces or duplicates what the ANA does and should continue to do for nurses [because] it is the voice of the profession on both national and state levels [and] it is within the power of the professional organization to make this economic and general welfare program its primary commitment."[14]

If the ANA fails to expand its collective bargaining efforts and simply stands by while other groups organize nurses, the professional association and its federation of constituent state nurses' associations will undoubtedly lose over one-half of its membership. The ANA cannot conduct its collective bargaining functions as it did previously and still continue to be a competitor in the labor relations field.[15]

As nurses become more attuned to the power generated through their collective activity, they will become more involved in the collective bargaining process. To fail to act judiciously in supporting collective bargaining activities and in choosing the ANA as *the* bargaining agent, nurses and nursing may remain at a semiprofessional level. Thus, society will be deprived of quality nursing care.

DIRECT REIMBURSEMENT FOR NURSING PRACTICE

The issue of reimbursement for nursing practice becomes more urgent as nurses strive for professional autonomy and a more just distribution of economic rewards. Since the late 1940s, nurse leaders have pressed for a change in reimbursement practices. Currently, reimbursement for nursing services involves three options: "fee-for-service payment [paid directly by a client to a nurse engaged in private practice], receiving reimbursement from government and private third party payors, and reallocation of existing resources to pay for nursing services."[16]

Nurses should continue their efforts to remove the current restrictions and constraints that exist in some state regulations regarding direct reimbursement for nurses. Removal of restraints preventing consumers from access to alternative health providers should occur also. Until such reimbursement is obtained, however, competition will not create any significant problems. "Without direct third-party reimbursement for all licensed professional providers, entry into the health care system is restricted and true competition is impossible."[17] To seek reimbursement for the services provided, nurses must document the outcomes of such services and their ability to provide them at much lower costs.

> . . . the most sensible approach for nursing at present is to seek reimbursement for services that will substitute for those currently being provided . . .
>
> . . . not to convert nurses to doctors but to generate for nurses the revenues to which they are entitled and that will enable them to offer consumers an alternative to expensive traditional medical services. In recognition of fiscal restraints, services to be reimbursed must be substitutive rather than supplementary.[18]

Third-party reimbursement for nurses is recommended to increase the possibility of nursing being included in any competition at the federal level. Currently, the movement toward competition in health delivery should be grasped as an opportunity to promote the legitimization of nursing's roles and the realization of its potential.[19]

Reimbursement for nursing services is currently centered on treatment modalities of acute illness and primary care services. It does not provide for health promotion, health education, or counseling. By obtaining third-party reimbursement, nurses would become a force that is accepted and recognized in the development and implementation of methods for advances in these three areas.[20] Data are needed to determine the particulars of nursing practice that deserve reimbursement. Several pertinent questions to be asked are: "What are the outcomes of spending more time? Is the health problem altered favorably as a result of teaching? Are certain problems prevented, is life preserved or prolonged, and are hospitalizations and episodes of illness reduced by specific nursing interventions?"[21]

Some nurses in expanded nurse roles have achieved fee-for-service reimbursement. From the standpoint of legislation, however, this method is still in an infancy stage. To obtain additional fee-for-service recognition will depend on nurses demonstrating that customary physician roles may be replaced by nursing specialties.[22]

It is encouraging to note that several state nurses' associations have been successful in obtaining changes in reimbursement for nursing services. In 1981, Maryland nurses succeeded in having legislation passed that changed insurance laws to specify that services for which others are reimbursed should be reimbursable when nurses provide them.[23] In West Virginia, Governor Rockefeller in 1983 signed into law a bill that required health insurers to provide reimbursement for primary health care services if these services were reimbursable when provided by other health care practitioners. The law defines primary health care services as "nursing care rendered by a nonsalaried duly licensed registered professional nurse engaged in private practice or partnership with other health care providers within the lawful scope of practice."[24] In 1983, Minnesota nurse-midwives and nurse anesthetists became eligible for third-party reimbursement under a law requiring health insurers to cover such services. This represented one step toward a long-range goal of third-party reimbursement for all Minnesota nurses.[25]

The New York State Nurses' Association, after a ten-year campaign, met with success when the state assembly passed a bill in 1984 providing third-party reimbursement to registered nurses providing services outside of institutions. Limitations are that "reimbursed services must already be covered by an insurance policy and that the client must request a nurse as provider."[26] Third-party reimbursement for New Jersey nurses in private practice also began after legislation was passed in 1984. Those eligible were nurse entrepreneurs owning their own practice as well as nurses in private practice in ambulatory care and other primary settings.[27]

The concept of reimbursement for nursing services has shown considerable growth in the past ten years. Congress directed state Medicare programs in November 1989 to directly reimburse pediatric and family nurse practitioners, regardless of whether or not they receive physician supervision. At least three states (Ohio, Illinois, and West Virginia) placed third party reimbursement on their legislative agendas in 1990.[28] In Virginia, the legislature passed the first RN reimbursement bill ever introduced in the state in February 1986. It qualifies clinical specialists in psych./mental health for direct third party reimbursement.[29] Progress was evident in enactment of laws in other states for third party reimbursement also.

In April 1990, Medicare coverage was granted to nurse practitioners for their services to residents in Medicare or Medicaid certified nursing facilities. Under this Medicare provision, nurse practitioner services covered by the Medicare law involved those that are "reasonable and necessary for the diagnosis or treatment of an illness or injury or to improve the functioning of a malformed body member."[30] A twenty percent co-payment must be paid by the Medicare beneficiary and the NP's employer bills the beneficiary for the co-payment. This new legislation allows NPs to provide essential medical treatments and affect changes in patient care plans.

From these examples and others occurring in several other states, it is observed that nurses are convincing legislators of their economic worth as essential health care providers. Nurses as a collective body should diligently increase their pursuit of this goal until third-party reimbursement is made available in all states.

Some nurses believe that since nurse entrepreneurs are slowly leaving private practice and fee-for-service is becoming nonexistent, basing the cost of nursing services on this type of payment may not be a wise decision in the long run. Only time will prove the correctness of their belief.[31, 32]

Escalation of health care costs in the United States over the past two decades has caused those responsible for health care funding in the federal government to seek means to reduce these expenditures. According to statistics from the Department of Health and Human Services, the total bill for health care in 1982 was $322.4 billion, or 10.5 percent of the gross national product.[33] As a part of the Social Security Amendments of 1983, signed into law (P.L. 98-21) by President Reagan on April 20 of that year, Title VI—prospective reimbursement—provided a new payment method for hospitals to control escalating costs of Medicare. This plan, mandated by Congress and made effective on October 1, 1983, provides a flat payment to hospitals based on a patient's diagnosis. Rates were established in advance by the Health Care Financing Administration (HCFA) for each of 467 diagnosis-related groups (DRGs). Data for each group were based on diagnosis, age, sex, treatment procedures, and discharge status. If the actual cost of patient care is less, hospitals retain the excess amount. However, if the actual cost is higher, hospitals absorb the loss.

Under prospective reimbursement, early discharge from hospitals is encouraged, because hospitals are paid a fixed rate by the government for treating patients with specific diagnoses. Length of stay has no influence on this payment. In the previous cost-based system no incentive for controlling costs existed and no rewards were provided for efficient management. Hospitals now have an economic incentive to cut costs and deliver services in a cost-efficient way. This incentive was lacking when payment was made after care was already provided. The new payment system was phased in over three years with one set of uniform rates for urban areas and another for rural areas. Hospitals are currently reimbursed solely by the federal rate. Studies have been under way by the Department of Health and Human Services to determine the feasibility of utilizing prospective reimbursement for skilled nursing facilities, home health agencies, and for payment of physicians for services to Medicare patients. HCFA officials are developing prospective plans for these areas.

Margaret Heckler, former Secretary of Health and Human Services, speaking to the 1984 ANA House of Delegates, stated that Medicare's prospective reimbursement system

> will require your direct involvement and judgment and will therefore bring you directly into the hospital's decision-making process. We believe this is necessary and proper, not only in the interest of better patient care, but in the interest of more equitable status for your profession.[34]

Another nurse leader, Carolyne Davis, former Administrator of HCFA, shares similar views on nursing's role in cost containment when she asserts that "this transition in reimbursement policy, with its shifting forces, offers nursing and nurses the choice opportunity to increase control over their professional practice."[35] Although prospective reimbursement may somewhat alleviate the rise in health care costs, the Congressional Budget Office predicted that Medicare insurance funds would be threatened with bankruptcy by 1988 unless more drastic cost-cutting measures were taken. A DHHS fifteen-member advisory council, chaired by former Governor of Indiana, Otis Bowen, M.D., looked into "more radical surgery to save the ailing system."[36] Further measures would have to be severe, according to Dr. Bowen.

HOSPITALS REACT
TO COST-CUTTING MEASURES

Despite the need for greater efficiency in the nation's hospitals, many nurses fear that hospitals will continue to respond to the prospective payment system by cutting nurse staffing and lowering standards of care. "Many key hospital officials have made public statements regarding the potential cost savings that would accrue from using cheaper labor in lieu of registered nurses."[37]

State Nurses' Associations in Washington and Massachusetts sued their Rate-Setting Commissions in 1983 for "putting a disproportionate burden on nurses by their new rate-setting laws."[38] Efforts of hospitals in Minneapolis-St Paul to lay off nurses in 1984 resulted in a bitter strike of 6,300 nurses that lasted almost six weeks. As a result of decrease in census, some hospitals have responded by closing units and laying off staff.

Although many hospitals are threatened by the possibility of bankruptcy due to low census and the impact of the DRG system, most seem to weather these challenges reasonably well. However, David Talbot of Drexel Burnham Lambert "predicts that attrition [of hospitals] will be drastic enough to produce 'a shortage of well-located, efficient, and well-financed hospitals' and an 'oligopoly' for the investor-owned chains."[39]

With more hospitals forming a corporation type of administrative structure and with the prediction that the number may increase to 100 percent, nursing may soon find itself functioning in a very different hospital administrative structure. Names of for-profit health care corporations, such as Health America, U.S. Health Care Systems, Humana, Inc., Surgicare, and National Health and Care Enterprises, were virtually unheard of a decade ago.[40] Hospitals that will survive in times of cost restraint are those that can be characterized as well organized and managed as successful business operations.

GOLDEN OPPORTUNITY FOR NURSING'S COST EFFECTIVENESS

If nursing is to assume a more visible role in decision making in health care, data on the cost effectiveness of nursing care must be produced. "Sophisticated clinical nursing is the ingredient that will make nursing fiscally successful under Medicare's prospective payment mechanisms [and] nurses must be prepared to show through documentation that therapeutic programs were initiated one minute after admission."[41]

The nursing component is essential in a prospective payment system. Nurses must be able to generate data that will specify what is required for delivering quality nursing care in each of the DRGs determined by HCFA. They must use computers to track data, check early discharge information, and be alert to spot a need for intervention. Moreover, they must isolate the real costs of quality nursing care. Also, nurses must be visible and vocal in asserting nursing's chief role in health care delivery. If nursing can continue to exert effort through improved organization and management techniques, it could greatly expand its role and responsibility for health care in this country.

Carolyne Davis, in 1983, indicated that "a milestone in the history of our nation's health care financing system [would occur, and] if . . . there were a time for the nursing profession to reach its maturation, that time is now."[42] For "never has the opportunity been greater for nursing to assert itself. . .the moment to act is now—let us seize that moment."[43]

IDENTIFICATION OF NURSING CARE COSTS

Nursing administrators have been concerned for over a decade with the payment methods used for nursing services in health care institutions. With the advent of DRGs, they continue to experience pressure for greater operational efficiency. Moreover, they have recognized the need to isolate nursing costs from "bed and board" and other per diem cost figures:

> . . . nursing service costs, as well as certain other service costs, have traditionally been lumped in the multipurpose category of operating costs of institutions. This practice has prevented true cost accounting, hampered the development of a financially responsive health care system, and prevented consumers from evaluating the services received in relation to their costs.[44]

Nursing costs must be identified and then allocated appropriately among patients before they can be controlled. Systems developed to identify these costs are referred to as *variable billing*. This type of billing is defined as "billing for specific aspects or levels of nursing care, which vary from patient to patient."[45] A strong data base is needed to document the revenue generated from nursing staff's contributions to patient care. Until all hospitals show nursing care charges as a separate item on patients' bills, the public will remain largely ignorant of nursing's significant role. Nurses should negotiate with top institutional administrators to remedy this situation and allow nursing to be recognized for its essential services.

A significant improvement in the cost-benefit ratio could be observed by removing the costs of professional nursing care to patients from the daily room charge. A separate billing should be provided for these services.[46] However, the problem of how to determine nursing care costs will remain unanswered until the practice of concealing costs and revenues from nursing care, is abandoned.

> Indeed, the time is long overdue for a more extensive study of the costs of nursing care. . . . If nursing in acute care hospitals and other health care facilities is ever to be recognized and reimbursed as an essential professional service, the time for working toward these goals is now.[47]

It is encouraging to note that a New Haven, Connecticut, hospital is the first in that state to have separate listing for nursing services on patient's bills.[48] In June 1983, a resolution calling for identifying nursing costs was passed by the delegates attending the National League for Nursing biennial convention:

RESOLUTION 1: IDENTIFYING NURSING COSTS
    WHEREAS, The consumer has a better understanding of the costs and

value of health care when these are communicated plainly and are easy to identify; and

WHEREAS, This is the age of the computer, which enables rapid and simple communication of data, especially quantitative data; and

WHEREAS, The present system of communicating the costs of nursing services does not permit a separate itemization of these costs on the customer's bill or account; therefore, be it

RESOLVED, That the National League for Nursing promote a policy that supports the establishment of billing and accounting systems which identify nursing costs separately from room, board, and other consumer charges.[49]

This resolution was timely and appropriate because the delegates were aware of the impending DRG system and the impact it would have on nursing's budgetary allotments.

The ANA conducted a survey of selected hospitals in October 1983 to ascertain what implications the DRG system may have on organized nursing services. The results showed that ninety-three percent are making an effort to determine the actual costs connected with providing nursing services and listing them separately on hospital bills.[50] The ANA was charged by the 1984 House of Delegates to investigate other methods of determining nursing costs and connecting patient classification systems to financial systems to assure that nursing services receive recognition in all types of financing systems.

"The need to determine the cost of nursing services, to price nursing services, and to determine productivity is imperative if nursing is to compete successfully for limited resources."[51] Fagin comments that "it should be nursing's uppermost pursuit in the years ahead to gain financial control over nursing practice . . . without it, our future as professionals seeking to fulfill our contract with society is a very tenuous one."[52]

DEVELOPMENT OF CLASSIFICATION SYSTEMS FOR PRACTICE

Now that the DRG prospective payment is operational, the need for nursing to establish classification systems to achieve adequate reimbursement for care provided is of major importance. An eight-member ANA committee sponsored by the Cabinets on Nursing Practice and Nursing Research in 1982, referred to as the Steering Committee on Classifications for Nursing Practice Phenomena, established four major goals: "recommending policy to the ANA Board of Directors through the Cabinet on Nursing Practice in matters that relate to classification systems; monitoring the state of the art; working with the divisions on practice and the ANA councils around classification issues; and maintaining a collaborative relationship with the North American Nursing Diagnosis Association (NANDA)."[53] In 1983 this new association replaced the National Group for Classification of Nursing Diagnosis. Composed of approximately 400 American and Canadian nurses, this association has identified over fifty nursing diagnosis categories.

The Sixth International Conference on Classification of Nursing Diagnosis was held in St. Louis, Missouri, in April 1984. Major topics considered included "taxonomic issues, . . . the nature of nursing diagnosis; clinical decision making; reimbursement for health services, and quality assurance."[54] Since that time over eight conferences have been held by NANDA. The current NANDA list of nursing diagnoses has been generated from work accomplished by the National Conference Group on the Classification of Nursing Diagnosis since 1973.[55-57] Gebbie and Lavan, early leaders in this movement, described in 1974 the identification of diagnostic categories that nurses believe they are capable of treating adequately.[58]

Another of the pioneers in efforts to identify diagnostic categories, Marjory Gordon, defined nursing diagnosis as actual or potential health problems that nurses are capable and licensed to treat as a result of their education and experience.[59] For nurses to accept the concept of nursing diagnosis they must be willing to accept responsibility and accountability for autonomous nursing practice—the mark of the true professional. According to Callista Roy, nurse theorist and educator, expanding nursing's role means that a part of nursing's efforts to expand its knowledge and skills will be that of involvement in the nursing diagnosis process.[60]

FUTURE OF NURSE CORPORATIONS

To date very little has been written about the topic of nurse corporations. Why is there not more interest in exploring this challenging concept? If nursing is determined to achieve autonomy for its members, then it would seem that establishing nurse corporations would be a relatively rapid way to accomplish this goal. To some, it may seem premature for the collectivity of nurses; yet, many nurse entrepreneurs have set up corporations in which to function as independent professionals. What, then can be learned from existing literature on this topic?

As a result of prospective payment, new models of patient care are developing and nursing services may be delivered by means of contractual agreements through nurse corporations. "Shifts in payment will be observed with third party payors moving to direct contracting, health insurance, and integrated health plans."[61]

According to Beercroft, "contracting of nursing services is a choice that offers more flexibility for the professional nurse [as the] contracting nurse functions as an independent practitioner."[62] Reimbursement by contract on the basis of salary rather than by time cards and hourly wages as hospital employees would enable nurses to act more independently in providing nursing care.

In a contract model of nursing practice developed in 1981 at Johns Hopkins Hospital in Baltimore, "the form of reimbursement was changed from hourly wage to salary."[63] Higher levels of job satisfaction were noted among contract unit nurses as they assumed responsibility for determining staffing levels, scheduling, and assuring coverage. " . . . Compensation practices consistent with a professional approach to delivering nursing services" were an important element in achieving a positive outcome from this model.[64]

Although contracting for services by a group should be encouraged, it is not something to be practiced by the bulk of nurses today. Under contract law, nurses could group together "and form partnerships or corporations to contract with health service institutions for providing nurses services in specific areas for the institution as a whole."[65]

Some interesting role changes for nurses have been suggested that would provide more autonomy for nursing in delivering nursing services. For example, there is the possibility of professional nurses contracting, as private practitioners, for providing the type and amount of nursing services prescribed by physicians for clients.[66] If and when these suggestions become a reality, the nursing service department as presently organized would no longer be necessary. If this sounds unrealistic, consider that nurse entrepreneurs forming corporations were unheard of less than a decade ago. Some foresee the time when professional nurses will no longer be employed by hospitals, but will belong to professional corporations rendering nursing services on a fee-for-service basis to clients. If nursing is to survive as a profession, "such a change in the nature of the social contract is necessary."[67]

In the early part of this century, private duty nurses were reimbursed directly by clients. Although some nurses in private practice are remunerated in this way today, it appears that nurse corporations would be the more appropriate agent for most nurses in the future. Because many ancillary services are provided on a contract basis to hospitals (dietary, laundry, housekeeping, etc.) and because many physicians are contracted through corporations providing medical services, nurse corporations may become the means to solve existing collective bargaining problems that currently beset nursing. What is needed is a courageous, and knowledgeable group of nurses who would begin to experiment with the possibilities of such a creative venture.

SUMMARY

Achieving a more equitable economic base for nurses continues to have high priority among nursing's major goals. The issue of whether collective bargaining for professional nurses is unprofessional no longer concerns the majority of nurses. However, the issue of who will represent nurses and nursing at the bargaining table continues to be debated. Whether the ANA will most effectively represent nurses or whether an industrial union or labor organization controlled by nurses will be more effective is central to this issue. Individual nurses and groups of nurses throughout the country are confronting this serious concern. Problems associated with nurses establishing a separate labor organization are numerous, and presently the courts are obtaining evidence that lacks justification for separate nurse labor units. On the other hand, many nurses are convinced that the ANA should be fully supported as the collective bargaining agent for all nurses.

Concern for cost containment has led to increased competition in health care delivery, and as a result, nurses have an excellent opportunity to work toward a more legitimate role in health care. Certainly, direct reimbursement for nursing practice would provide greater visibility and autonomy for nurses. However, before direct reimbursement can be accomplished, nurses need to demonstrate that their services are cost-effective so that they can challenge the customary physician roles.

Introduction of the DRG prospective reimbursement system is providing nurses with an opportunity to increase control over their clinical practice. Although designed to provide an incentive for hospitals to cut costs and deliver services in a more cost-efficient manner, it is feared that hospitals will decrease nurse staffing and lower standards of care. Also, nurses are greatly concerned that the low patient census in many hospitals has resulted in decreased staffing and closing of clinical units. Since the nursing component is vital to the success of a prospective payment system, it is important that nurses provide data indicating the requirements for delivering quality nursing care for each of the DRG categories.

It is encouraging to note that some hospitals are beginning to list nursing care charges separate from other hospital charges on patients' bills. And yet, until all hospitals show separate billing for nursing services, the public will continue to be unenlightened about nursing's significant role.

Classification systems to help nursing receive adequate reimbursement have been generated by the National Conference on the Classification of Nursing Diagnosis since 1973. Ten years later, the North American Nursing Diagnosis Association (NANDA) replaced this conference group and identified over fifty nursing diagnostic categories.

An innovation that may eventually affect the traditional nursing department is that of nurse corporations, which would contract for nursing services through the organized group efforts of nurse entrepreneurs. Whether this will become an acceptable means of assuring nurse autonomy in the future and of solving nursing's collective bargaining problems, can only be determined if a group of courageous nurses begins to experiment with this concept.

REFERENCES

1. Flanagan, L. *One Strong Voice: The Story of the American Nurses Association.* Kansas City, Mo.: American Nurses' Association, 1976.
2. *Ibid.*
3. *Ibid.*
4. *Ibid.*
5. Colangelo, M. "The Professional Association and Collective Bargaining," *Supervisor Nurse* 11:9 (1980), 29.
6. Eldridge, I. and Levi, M. "Collective Bargaining as a Power Resource for Professional Goals," *Nursing Administrative Quarterly* 6:2 (Winter, 1982), 32.
7. *Ibid.*
8. Conta, L. "Bargaining by Professionals," *American Journal of Nursing* 72:2 (February, 1972), 312.
9. Bumpass, M. "Appropriate Bargaining Units in Health Care Institutions: An Analysis of Congressional Intent and Its Implementation by the National Labor Relations Board," *Boston College Law Review* 20:5 (1979), 913.
10. Eldridge, I. and Levi, M. "Collective Bargaining," 36.
11. *Ibid.*
12. "Unions Intensify Organizing Effort Among Nurses," *American Journal of Nursing* 80 (1980), 185.
13. Colangelo, M. "The Professional Association," 32.
14. *Ibid.*
15. Cleland, V. "Nurses' Economics and the Control of Nursing Practice," in L. Aiken (ed.), *Nursing in the 1980s: Crises, Opportunities, Challenges.* Philadelphia: J. B. Lippincott, 1982, 391.
16. Aiken, L. "Primary Care: The Challenge for Nursing," *American Journal of Nursing* 77:11 (November, 1977), 1831.
17. Griffith, H. "Competition in Health Care," *Nursing Outlook* 31:6 (September–October, 1983), 264.
18. Fagin, C. "Nursing's Pivotal Role in American Health Care," in L. Aiken (ed.), *Nursing in the 1980s: Crises, Opportunities, Challenges.* Philadelphia: J. B. Lippincott, 1982, 468–469.
19. *Ibid.*, 471.
20. Jennings, C. "Nursing's Case for Third Party Reimbursement," *American Journal of Nursing* 79:1 (January, 1979), 113.
21. Fagin, C. and Lambertsen, M. "Nurse-Physician Collaboration: Evaluation of a Nursing School—Medical School Joint Practice," in L. Aiken (ed.), *Health Policy and Nursing Practice.* New York: McGraw-Hill, 1981, 276–277.

22. Powell, P. "Fee-for-Service," *Nursing Management* 14:3 (March, 1983), 15.
23. Goldwater, M. "From Legislator: Views on Third-Party Reimbursement for Nurses," *American Journal of Nursing* 82:3 (March, 1982), 411–414.
24. "West Virginia Law Requires R.N. Reimbursement," *American Nurse* 15:5 (May, 1983), 19.
25. "Minnesota Ok's Reimbursement for CNMs," *American Journal of Nursing* 83:9 (September, 1983), 1269.
26. "New York Wins Third-Party Reimbursement for All," ANA (News) *American Journal of Nursing* 84:8 (August, 1984), 1052.
27. "New Jersey Nurse Entrepreneurs Now Eligible for Third-Party Reimbursement," *American Journal of Nursing* 84:3 (March, 1984), 377.
28. "SNAs Face Legislative Issues," *American Nurse* 22:1 (January, 1990), 34, 35.
29. "RNs Gain in Battle for Direct Reimbursement," *American Journal of Nursing* 89:6 (June, 1989), 862.
30. Mittelstadt, P. "Reimbursement Extended to NPs," *American Nurse* 22:5 (May, 1990), 2.
31. Joel, L. "The Economics of Health Care: Trends and Problems," Keynote Address at the Scientific Session of the Twelfth Annual Meeting of the American Academy of Nursing, Atlanta, December 10, 1984.
32. Lockhart, C. "Nursing's Future in a Shrinking Health Care System," Paper presented at the Scientific Session of the Twelfth Annual Meeting of the American Academy of Nursing, Atlanta, December 10, 1984.
33. U.S. Health and Human Services Department. *Health—United States, 1983* (DHHS Pub. No.: PH8 84-1232). Washington, D.C.: U.S. Government Printing Office, 1983, 177.
34. "6,000 Enjoy Convention '84," *American Nurse* 16:6 (July–August, 1984), 20.
35. Davis, C. "Nursing and the Health Debates," *Image: The Journal of Nursing Scholarship* 15:3 (Summer, 1983), 67.
36. Wallis, C. "Putting Lids on Medicare Costs," *Time* 122:16 (October 10, 1983), 56.
37. "The World According to DRGs," *Public Policy Bulletin.* New York: National League for Nursing, 1983.
38. "The DRG Revolution Gets Rolling; Hospitals Already Cutting Back," (News) *American Journal of Nursing* 83:11 (November, 1983), 1607.
39. "The Big Business of Medicine," *Newsweek* (October 31, 1983), 73.
40. *Ibid.*, 66.
41. "Sophisticated Clinical Nursing Key Under DRG Plan, says Joel," *American Nurse* 16:1 (January, 1984), 1.
42. Davis, C. (ed.), "Nursing and the Health Care Debates," *Image: The Journal of Nursing Scholarship* 15:3 (Summer, 1983), 67.
43. "Nursing Leaders Sight Danger, Opportunity in Switch to DRGs," *American Journal of Nursing* (News) 83:12 (December, 1983), 1707.
44. Fagin, C. "Nursing's Pivotal Role," 469.
45. Higgerson, N. and Van Slyck, A. "Variable Billing for Services: New Fiscal Direction for Nursing," *Journal of Nursing Administration* 12 (June, 1982), 20.
46. Walker, D. "The Cost of Nursing Care in Hospitals," in L. Aiken (ed.), *Nursing in the 1980s: Crises, Opportunities, Challenges.* Philadelphia: J. B. Lippincott, 1982, 142.

47. *Ibid.*
48. "Connecticut Hospital Bills Separately for Nursing," (News) *American Journal of Nursing* 85:1 (January, 1985), 96.
49. National League for Nursing. "Resolution 1. Report of the Committee on Resolutions to N.L.N. Membership," New York: National League for Nursing, 1983, 1.
50. "Hospitals Identifying Nursing Care Costs, A.N.A. Study Reveals," *American Nurse* 16:8 (September, 1984), 1.
51. Johnson, M. "Perspectives on Costing Nursing," *Nursing Administrative Quarterly* 14:1 (Fall, 1989), 65.
52. Fagin, C. and Maraldo, P. "Feminism and the Nursing Shortage: Do Women Have a Choice?" *Nursing and Health Care* 9:7 (September, 1988), 68.
53. "Committee Monitors Development of Classifications for Practice," *American Nurse* 15:7 (July–August, 1983), 3.
54. Woods, M. (ed.), *Nursing Diagnosis Newsletter* 11:2 (September, 1984).
55. Gebbie, K. and Lavin, M. (eds.), *Summary of the First National Conference on Nursing Diagnosis.* St. Louis: C. V. Mosby, 1973.
56. Kim, M. and Moritz, D. *Classification of Nursing Diagnosis: Proceedings of the Third and Fourth National Conference.* New York: McGraw-Hill, 1982.
57. Kim, M., McFarland, G. and McLare, A. (eds.), *Proceedings of the Fifth National Conference on Classification of Nursing Diagnosis.* St. Louis: C. V. Mosby, 1983.
58. Gebbie, K. and Lavin, M. "Classifying Nursing Diagnosis," *American Journal of Nursing* 74:2 (February, 1974), 250–253.
59. Gordon, M. "Nursing Diagnosis and the Diagnostic Process," *American Journal of Nursing* 76:8 (August, 1976), 1298.
60. Roy, C. "The Impact of Nursing Diagnosis," *Nursing Digest* 4 (Summer, 1976), 67.
61. Colle, R. *The New Hospital: Future Strategies for a Changing Industry.* Rockville, Md.: Aspen Systems Corp., 1986.
62. Beercroft, P., "A Contractual Model for the Department of Nursing," *Journal of Nursing Administration* 18:9 (September, 1988), 22.
63. York, C. and Fecteau, D. "Innovative Models for Professional Nursing Practice," *Nursing Economics* 5:4 (July–August, 1987), 163.
64. *Ibid,* 166.
65. Cleland, V. "Nurses' Economics," 389.
66. Froebe, D. and Bain, R. *Quality Assurance Programs and Controls in Nursing.* St. Louis: C. V. Mosby, 1976, 134.
67. Sills, G. "Letter to the American Nurses Association Board of Directors," March 26, 1979 (Unpublished).

SUGGESTED READINGS

American Nurses' Association. *Third-Party Reimbursement for Services of Nurses.* Monograph 7 (Pub. No.: D-72G). Kansas City, Mo.: American Nurses' Association, 1983.

American Nurses' Association, *Collective Bargaining and the Nursing Profession.* Monograph 5 (Pub. No.: D-72D). Kansas City, Mo.: American Nurses' Association, 1983.

American Nurses' Association, *Economics and Employment Issues for Registered Nurses.* A Ten Volume Monograph Series. (Pub. No.: D-72). Kansas City, Mo.: American Nurses' Association, 1983.

Brewer, C. "Variable Billing: Is It Viable?" *Nursing Outlook* 32:1 (January–February, 1984), 38–41.

Brider, P. "The Struggle for Just Compensation," *American Nursing* 90:10 (October, 1990), 77–78, 80, 83–84, 86, 88.

Congress of the United States. Congressional Budget Office. *Containing Medical Care Costs Through Market Forces.* Washington, D.C.: U.S. Government Printing Office, 1982.

Curtin, L. L. "Determining Costs of Nursing Service per DRG," *Nursing Management* 14:4 (April, 1983), 16–20.

Curtin, L. L. (ed.), *DRGs: The Reorganization of Health.* Chicago: Nursing Management Books, 1984.

Donabedian, A. "Quality, Cost, and Cost Containment," *Nursing Outlook* 32:3 (May–June, 1984), 142–145.

Eisenhauer, L. and Cleland, V. "Is Collective Bargaining the Solution?" *Nursing Outlook* 31:3 (May–June, 1983) 150–153.

Fagin, C. "Nursing as an Alternative to High Cost Care," *American Journal of Nursing* 82:1 (January, 1982), 56–60.

Grandbouche, A. "Nursing's Cash Value: How It's Hidden: Why It Must Be Revealed," *RN* 45 (May, 1982), 83–84.

Holzemer, W. "Quality and Cost of Nursing Care: Is Anybody Out There Listening?" *Nursing and Health Care* 11:8 (November, 1990), 412–415.

"Hospitals Identifying Nursing Care Costs, A.N.A. Study Reveals," *American Nurse* 16:8 (September, 1984), 1.

Lubic, R. "Reimbursement for Nursing Practice: Lessons Learned, Experiences Shared," *Nursing and Health Care* 6:1 (January, 1985), 23–25.

McCarty, P. "Nurses Eligible for Direct Payment in 13 States," *American Nurse* 15:6 (June, 1983), 1.

"New Nurse Role Will be Vital to DRG Success, says HCFA's Davis," *American Journal of Nursing* 84:1 (January, 1984), 112.

"NY Law Allows Third-Party Reimbursement to all RNs," *American Journal of Nursing* 85:2 (February, 1985), 198–199.

"New York Wins Third-Party Reimbursement For All," (News) *American Journal of Nursing* 84:8 (August, 1984), 1052.

Nursing Centers: Meeting to Demand for Quality Health Care. New York: National League for Nursing, 1989.

Ponak, A. "Unionized Professionals and the Scope of Bargaining: A Study of Nurses," *Industrial and Labor Relations Review* 34:3 (March, 1981), 396–406.

Shaffer, F. *DRG's: Changes and Challenges* (Pub. No.: 20-1959). New York: National League for Nursing, 1984.

Governance and
Self-Regulation
of Nursing Practice

11

INTRODUCTION

The recurring theme throughout previous chapters of this book has been nursing's need for a scientific body of knowledge and for control over its education and practice. If nursing is to be a full profession, then nurses should control their own professional practice. Without this control, professionalization of nursing cannot occur. Until nursing openly confronts the issue of control over nursing practice, it will remain at a semiprofessional level and continue its present course of subservience to other health professions, while depriving society of the quality of service it desires. Now is the time to remedy the problems facing staff nurses in their practice.[1]

Working conditions that prevent effective service to clients include "improper utilization of nurses and other staff; too few or an improper balance of qualified nurses in decision making regarding delivery of services; assignment of non-nursing duties; lack of professional support system; . . . inadequate supplies and equipment . . . and unsafe and hazardous conditions."[2] The lack of autonomy in clinical practice frequently is found heading the list of unsatisfactory conditions.

It is only quite recently that nurses began what can be legitimately described as *professional* practice. Nurses engaged in such practice are free to function autonomously in independent decision making and assume authority for the nursing care provided. In addition, they are held accountable for the outcomes of such care.

Ingeborg Mauksch raises several significant questions surrounding the issue of control.

> Is it possible for an occupation whose members are primarily employees to practice autonomously within the framework of an institutional employment setting? Can an occupation strive toward excellence in institutional practice without exerting the control necessary for that occupation to be sufficiently autonomous? Will tomorrow's nurses engage in autonomous practice within a variety of employment settings, assuming the responsibility to control their practice and exhibiting accountability for quality of care delivered?[3]

Answers to these questions will not be found in nursing service settings where minimal attention is paid to meeting nurses' needs for professional practice. If service is all that is expected of nurses, then the present organizational structures that are essentially in control are adequate. But these structures do not nurture practice that is professional in character. In fact, they frequently threaten autonomy and the ideal of quality service. Ultimate authority exerted by nonprofessionals or by supervisors with less educational preparation or experience has created tension and conflict among professional workers. In many hospitals, nurses are corrected or reprimanded by doctors and by head nurses. But such supervision is unlike the type observed in full-fledged professions.[4]

Doctors and lawyers function under professional norms that have been internalized. The expert knowledge they possess allows them a degree of autonomy not found in less prestigious occupations. In contrast, social work, education, and nursing, are controlled by authority figures and bureaucratic rules and policies that hinder control over their practice. "In most acute care hospitals control over nurses' work by physicians and administrators remains firm and pervasive."[5] Admittedly there are exceptions in several hospitals throughout the country, but they are far from numerous. The situation first described is far more typical of what is occurring in many of today's health care institutions. Fortunately, times are changing, and a trend toward allowing nurses to function in hospital environments that are conducive to independent practice is becoming more apparent. Organizational structures that facilitate and encourage professional practice are characterized by decentralized decision making and an atmosphere of openness, accountability, inquiry, and autonomy (freedom to be self-directing).

To ensure nursing's advance toward professionalism in the 1990s, nurses should endeavor to assume a greater role in governance and to acquire increased knowledge and skills in the delivery of nursing care.[6] Governance is defined here as "the establishment and maintenance of social, political, and economic arrangements by which nurses maintain control over their practice, their self-discipline, their working conditions and their professional affairs."[7]

If autonomy, authority, and accountability for nursing practice are essential for improved patient care, certain organizational conditions are necessary to foster them. These conditions are described as "decentralization of authority and responsibility in the nursing department; identification of professional nurses as peers rather than as supervisor and supervisees; consensus of philosophy and objectives of nursing care; . . . and responsibility and answerability for all care given to the patient over a 24-hour day, 7-day week span of time."[8]

A decided change in nurses' attitudes toward their work environment has occurred, particularly over the past decade. The nurse of yesterday who accepted work hours that were inconvenient, was patronized by individuals on the job, and made an inadequate salary while simultaneously being loyal to the hospital and its physicians is quickly disappearing from the scene.[9] In an interesting article entitled "Rebellion Among the Angels: Nurses Are No Longer Content To Be the Doctor's Handmaiden," it was pointed out that in addition to being concerned about their working conditions, nurses want professional advancement.[10] The cry for more autonomy is echoing through the halls of many present-day health care institutions.

SCOPE OF AUTONOMY IN NURSING PRACTICE

A review of nursing literature on autonomy reveals that most nurses believe in their right to control nursing practice and to implement it. Implied in this belief is the freedom to make decisions about client or patient care without pressure or external control from administrators, physicians, or other non-nurse members of the field. Professional people are privileged in enjoying freedom from outside controls.[11] Three claims justify this privilege.

1. Professional work involves such a high degree of skill and knowledge that nonprofessionals are not equipped to evaluate or regulate it.
2. Professionals are responsible and can be trusted to work without supervision.
3. The profession can be trusted to undertake proper action when an individual fails to perform with competence and ethical behavior.[12]

For nursing to achieve full professional status, the concept of autonomy must be understood and diligently sought by all professional nurses. If
autonomy is *power*, then nursing should continue its struggle to achieve it.
Only recently has nurse power begun to demonstrate strength in pursuing
professional rights and privileges for its practitioners.

Autonomy is defined as freedom to make prudent and binding
decisions consistent with the scope of one's practice. It is also freedom to
implement those decisions.[13] As true professionals, nurses must fulfill
their right to practice autonomously and to be responsible and accountable
for their clinical decisions and the outcomes of those decisions. It has been
defined also as a "measure of the freedom an employee has to define his or
her own tasks or projects, the method or procedures used to accomplish
those tasks . . . and how exceptions will be handled and the means used to
evaluate performance."[14] If nurses carry out treatment modalities that
require the physician's legal authorization in caring for patients, such
activities cannot be considered autonomous nursing practice. On the other
hand, autonomous nursing practice occurs when nurses use their self-
directed authority in diagnosing and treating phenomena of concern to
nursing.

For over sixty years nurses have been admonished to strive for
autonomy in fulfilling their nursing role. Yet, even today, nursing has not
acquired the degree of autonomous functioning indicative of full professional status. Among the various reasons given for this limited degree of
autonomy is the fact that the public does not believe that nurses can claim
the specialized knowledge granted to legitimate professional workers.

Some authors point out that since semiprofessionals are predominantly female, autonomy is granted by the public less willingly to women
than to men.[15] As products of the prevailing culture, despite the extensive
efforts of the women's movement, many nurses have accepted societal
expectations of women as inferior and obedient to men—the ideal female
role. However, a growing number of nurses are becoming more assertive in
expressing their demands. Still, their efforts to date have not made substantive changes in organizational structures. The issue of male versus
female prerogatives cannot be overlooked, as it has continued to surface
throughout most of nursing's efforts to achieve parity with other health
professions.

Since the majority of nurses are employed by organizations, their
status as employees in a bureaucratic structure limits their independent
decision making. Unfortunately for nursing, many health care settings do
not encourage the development of autonomous nursing practice. It is not
unusual to find departments of nursing whose organizational structure is
highly centralized and consists of numerous layers of hierarchical control.
Thus, "the conflict in nursing resides in its treatment as a task-oriented
industrial model unit rather than a professional clinical unit, with its own

professionals who possess content and logic and who are accountable and autonomous in practice."[16]

That conflicts and tension occur when professionals attempt to resist bureaucratic rules and regulations is documented frequently in the literature on organizations.[17, 18] It is presumed that professionals are persons who derive their goals and methods of operation from a professional body. They engage in independent work and command the right to determine what and how the work should be done.[19] But if bureaucrats are persons performing specialized though somewhat more routine activities under the supervision of hierarchical officials, then the average nurse working in today's hospital also fits this definition.[20]

Professional autonomy for nurses functioning in bureaucratic organizations is difficult to achieve. Nurses are subject to the power structure of physicians and administrators, and there is little evidence to demonstrate that this situation will change markedly over the next decade. As long as either group can authoritatively refuse to sanction nursing's request for additional budgetary allotments or involvement in decision making, true autonomy will be nonexistent.

In a few hospitals nurse administrators are members of hospital boards. They are accountable to the hospital administrator for the nursing practice. A study was conducted of ninety-three hospitals by the HHS Inspector General's Office at the request of the Secretary's Commission on Nursing. It concluded that 60% of the CNOs report directly to their CEOs; one-third attend governing board sessions; and one-half are members of hospital-medical staff committees.[21] In contrast, doctors are self-governing and directly responsible to hospital trustees for their medical practice. Physicians' power and autonomy are granted as an exclusive right of their profession to determine who will practice and how such practice should be implemented. Evaluation by others outside of the profession is considered intolerable and is not allowed.

Nursing has undertaken a massive public relations campaign to inform the general public about the significance of nursing's contribution to the health care of this country. One must realize that professions are not granted autonomy automatically, nor are they chosen "spontaneously" from among other occupations. By virtue of having the protection of an elite group of society, who are convinced that special value is found in its work, a profession achieves and retains its position.[22] The political and economic influence of the elite group—an influence that requires others to be subordinated to it—is what secures its position.[23] Until such time as society is persuaded of nursing's special value in advancing the nation's health, little or no increase will be evidenced in the level of nursing's autonomy.

On a more positive note, control of nursing practice by nurses is on the increase in several institutions. Within these individual organizations and nursing as a whole, the emergence of interest in and commitment to change is evident.[24] "In fact, nurses are reassessing their role as members of the health care team, and after carefully evaluating their contributions to health care, they are convinced that opportunities for service and independent action could be greater for them than at present."[25]

In fact, some nurses believe that professional autonomy will be a very important issue in the 1990s. Others feel strongly that "professional recognition will be as important to staff nurses in the 1990s as salary and staff retention."[26] Is nursing exemplifying more of the characteristics that distinguish a profession from that of an occupation? Some authors would answer in the affirmative, emphasizing that nursing has issued statements on the scope and goals of practice, set standards for nursing service and practice, and set standards for nursing education, along with a code of ethics and a viable professional association. Moreover, they acknowledge that nurse practitioners and clinical specialists are being given the opportunity to enlarge and expand their clinical responsibilities.[27, 28]

Still others note that the efforts of occupations to achieve professional status (i.e., university education and creation and development of theory, code of ethics, and licensing or registration), are insufficient to arrive at professionalism. In fact, occupations persistently fail to achieve full autonomy in developing their training and licensing standards and in the performance of their work.[29] They achieve only a partial autonomy because it is limited by a dominant profession. It is this irreducible criterion that retains them as paraprofessions in spite of their being successful in achieving many of the institutional attributes of professions.[30] As long as nursing's work remains medical in character, it cannot gain autonomy. To achieve professional autonomy, the occupation must control a *distinct* area of work that can be differentiated from medicine and can be practiced without routinely contacting or being dependent on medicine.[31]

If professionalism involves the right to make one's own decisions and control one's practice, why do many health care organizations fail to believe that nurses are professional and capable of governing and managing their practice the same as other professionals? Invariably the whole issue of nursing's professionalism has to be addressed if changes in organizational structure and management for nursing practice are to occur. On the other hand, if the "status quo" continues without resolution of nursing's professional status, nurses' practice will remain at a technical level despite efforts by those seeking to professionalize nursing. Moreover, if this issue is not resolved, efforts to remove economic and political barriers to autonomous nursing practice will be hindered. The conflict and unhappiness experienced by many nurses in the workplace will continue to exist. The best recruitment campaign, including the NCNIP and Ad Council project, can never replace the enthusiasm resulting from nurses' being challenged and satisfied with their autonomous nursing role.

Some authors observe that the doctor-nurse relationship is one of dominance of the doctor over the nurse. In this view the doctor assumes full responsibility for all decisions affecting patient care. Such an outlook assumes that the body of all health care knowledge is subsumed under medical knowledge and that all other health care workers are dependent on the decisions of doctors relative to patient care.[32] In the contemporary scene, however, health care professionals make decisions on patient care far more frequently after consultation with intraprofessional peers and interprofessional colleagues.[33] Thus, professional autonomy can be redefined as decision making related to practice that is independent and interdependent, based on complex knowledge and skills. Such autonomy recognizes the professional's changing role.[34]

Actually, it would be difficult to determine how many practicing nurses engage in independent or interdependent practice. Highly qualified nurses, knowledgeable about nursing theory and phenomena reflective of patient's responses to health problems, probably seek interdependent consultation more frequently than the typical nurse. As more nurses acquire advanced educational preparation in nursing, the number who consult others should increase substantially. It should be stated, however, that some nurses believe there are no interdependent functions in nursing. When consultation is sought it does not make the nurse interdependent but simply a professional colleague of the consultant contacted.

COLLABORATION WITH PHYSICIANS AND OTHER HEALTH PROFESSIONALS

In the future it is likely that health care delivery will be provided by groups of health professionals utilizing a team approach. Such an approach is occurring in several health centers across the country. Collaborative practice implies information sharing, a respectful attitude for others' skills, and knowledge of the important contribution that each member has to make.[35] As nurse autonomy increases, nurses will internalize a sense of their own worth and abilities and, with the utmost self-confidence, demonstrate the value of their work to patients and to other health team members. Collaboration rather than competition should describe the relationship between physicians and nurses. And yet, if the physician must still authorize a nurse to receive third-party payment, the situation can hardly be referred to as a collaboration between equals.

Efforts at collaboration are rather difficult for many nurses because they have not been socialized for such roles early in their preparation. However, nurse educators have started to include assertiveness training, improved communication skills, and respect for other health disciplines in their nursing curricula. Nursing students today are more knowledgeable about their role in health care than are those of previous decades. Many young physicians are also more receptive to recognizing the contributions of nurses to health care. "Many professionals and patient care issues in hospitals and other health care institutions result from the lack of early collaboration between nurses and physicians."[36] The process of learning about each other's roles "must begin during the formal years of educational preparation . . . (and) new collegial roles must be stressed during the students' formative years and realized in the postgraduate years."[37]

One example of nurse-physician collaboration occurred in 1979, when the School of Nursing at the University of Pennsylvania and the Department of Medicine, Presbyterian Hospital/University of Pennsylvania Medical Center opened a collaborative health care practice staffed by a nurse clinician and a physician intern. Claire Fagin, former Dean of the Nursing School, believed "the demonstration is necessary for student learning, faculty skill maintenance, demonstrating nursing to and with members of other disciplines, developing a faculty-clinician role, and nursing research."[38] In this particular situation, the fact that nursing and medicine shared a value (that by collaboration between nurses and medicine, there would ultimately be improvement in health care) became the most important variable.[39]

Another more recent example of a collaborative program was initiated by New York University Division of Nursing and the Medical School in 1989. This program aimed at "building an effective basis of cooperation between the two professional schools and their students, with the objective of affecting professional practice long after graduation by the participants."[40]

Nursing care is greatly enhanced when joined with the contributions of other health professionals. The ultimate goal is a health team, with members having autonomy within their own discipline and equal authority for patient-care decisions as collaborative roles evolve. For this to occur, changes in the attitudes and behavior of physicians toward nurses must be forthcoming. In order to collaborate and allow nurses to have a shared role and authority in decision making for health care, physicians must view professional nurses as colleagues and co-workers in patient care delivery. This change of attitude toward nurses presents serious problems for many doctors who are unwilling to admit that nursing and nurses have unique contributions to make to patient care. For these individuals, collaboration with nurses is nonexistent. Unfortunately, their attitudes are not likely to change in the immediate future.

That collaboration was a concern of the Department of Health, Education, and Welfare Secretary's committee to study extended roles for nurses is evidenced in its report published in 1971. The report pointed out that nursing practice will be extended only as collaboration between physicians and nurses occurs. As nurses assume expanded roles, major adjustments will be required by both professions in their orientation and practice.[41]

Two key questions that the collectivity of nurses must address in the 1990s are:

> Will professional nurses, the largest and potentially the most influential group of health professions, continue to fulfill work roles defined by others and to practice within constraints imposed upon them by a tradition of performance? Or will nurses emerge as collaborators with other professional health-providers and decision-making leaders in developing and maintaining a system of health care which will assure all citizens essential services at reasonable cost and realistic accessibility?[42]

Unless the second question is answered with a resounding "yes," nursing will continue to play a subordinate role by simply providing services that are delegated by medicine and other health disciplines. Changes are sorely needed in order to develop this collaboration among health professionals. New arrangements for clinical decision making must be worked out between nurses and physicians who recognize the knowledge and expertise of one another. Institutional models that acknowledge only physicians as having the right to make professional decisions about patients result in nurses being wastefully underutilized.[43]

Lundeen recognizes that a truly collaborative interdisciplinary practice model for nurses and physicians is possible only for disciplines that are operating from bases of equal power and mutual respect.[44] She believes that interdependence of health professionals must be preceded by independence and that demonstration of "independent practice models" should form the basis for collaborative practice models.[45] "With the complexity of modern societal and health issues and with the knowledge explosion and concomitant escalation of specialization and fragmentation, interdisciplinary collaboration and teamwork will take on ever-increasing importance in the years ahead."[46]

PARTICIPATIVE DECISION MAKING THROUGH SHARED GOVERNANCE

Control of the decision-making process distinguishes the professional from the ordinary layman or semiprofessional worker. It is this process that professional people are unwilling to relinquish, as it connotes power and the authority to function without the approval of individuals at higher levels in the organizational structure. Without the power emanating from the right to make independent decisions involving one's practice, no professional person can function as a true professional.

Nursing literature has many examples of nursing's efforts to obtain shared governance through decentralizing the nursing department. Involving professional nurses in decision making assures that their knowledge and expertise are more effectively utilized in delivering quality patient care. Whether decisions pertain to responsibility and accountability for nursing practice, working conditions, staff privileges, standards of practice, or other areas of concern to the nursing staff, the key word for success is autonomy. Professional nurses must be held accountable and responsible for their clinical judgment and practice in implementing the care process. Their knowledge and competence should be recognized, and the opportunity for peer collaboration and consultation should be increased.

In the past, some nurses had grave reservations about the role of the professional nurse in a hospital setting. An article appearing in 1972 stated that "the professional nurse who practices in a hospital setting will probably function below her professional capacity at a semiprofessional or technical level . . . [since] in the hospital milieu, professional and technical nurses share a common subservience and hearken to a common master."[47] Such comments are useful for comparing existing hospital conditions with those of the past.

Recently, nurses have begun to feel strongly that professional nurses can practice autonomously and participate actively in patient care decisions and outcomes.[48, 49] They agree that, although the patient seeks medical care primarily, the opportunity to practice professional nursing is not only available but desperately needed in today's hospitals. Actually, the delivery of professional nursing service is neither compromised nor limited by the setting or the legitimate presence of other professionals.[50] Although care is provided by other professions, carrying out dependent functions requested by another profession is insufficient. The provision of autonomous nursing care should also occur.[51]

Shared governance models that address the nurse's need for autonomous practice require the support and efforts of every member of the nursing staff if successful outcomes of quality nursing practice are to occur.[52] Undoubtedly, "shared governance builds on trust—trust in the commitment to high-quality nursing care, trust in the belief that all nurses in the organization constantly seek the very best for their patients and for the profession and trust in the manager's commitment to keeping the resources, tools, and supports essential for good nursing care in place."[53]

Role of the Professional Association

In order to promote the well-being of its members, most occupations have recognized the need to organize for this purpose. A review of the history of evolving professions reveals that as a profession emerges, its practitioners, moved by the recognition of common interests, form a professional association.[54] Their aim is to require all practitioners to meet minimum qualifications for admittance to the association and to encourage all practitioners to join it. Implied in this aim is the ideal of having all competent practitioners as members of the association, thus promoting societal recognition of its practitioners. Enforcing rules of honorable conduct (codes of ethics) is another objective, in addition to raising qualifications of practitioners to at least minimal standards. Professional groups must have an orderly procedure for setting standards for entrance into and exclusion from the profession, for promoting high standards of practice, and for raising their social and economic status. The machinery required to implement these related functions is provided by the professional organizations.[55]

Toward the close of the nineteenth century nurse leaders were fully cognizant of the need to organize their ranks and to strive for professional status. As a result, the Nurses Associated Alumnae of the United States and Canada was established in 1896 to obtain control over nursing and to provide recognition for nurses and upgrade educational standards. With the withdrawal of the Canadian nurses to form their own organization in 1911, the name of the original organization was changed to the American Nurses Association (ANA). Since one of the characteristics of a profession is the establishment of a professional association, the existence of ANA helps convince nurses of the legitimacy of their chosen profession.

Since its inception, this association has been in the forefront of efforts to advance the professionalization of nursing. Although the ANA is only one among many nursing organizations, it is the one professional association that members refer to as *the* professional association. It seems appropriate to concentrate on this professional association, the ANA, in discussing the topic of professionalization of nursing, since it is directly related to *nurses* and all that concerns their needs in striving for true professionalism.

Among its various accomplishments, the ANA has developed a code of ethics for professional practice, promoted nursing research and nursing legislation, established standards for nursing education and nursing practice, articulated and clarified a meaningful statement on the scope of nursing practice, and worked diligently to promote the economic and general welfare of nurses.

Due to the high percentage of nurses employed by hospitals, it is appropriate that the ANA should continue to strive for economic goals, despite the objections of nurses who argue that such activity is unprofessional and resembles the work of labor unions. Until such time as nursing's economic base is strengthened and compatible with other health professions, the goals of professionalism for nursing will not be achieved. Only by means of a strong, cohesive, professional association, with nurses pursuing goals collectively, will nursing be able to generate the power to compete in the highly competitive arena of health care delivery.

Despite the ANA's accomplishments, there is still divisiveness over the entry into practice issue, thus preventing nursing from achieving standardization of nursing education. Support of legislation for funding nursing education and lobbying efforts to strengthen nursing's position at national and state levels should intensify. In addition, a single credentialing mechanism (to remove the excessive competition among organizations active in credentialing nurses) is still to be created.

Reimbursement for nursing services should be given high priority in the ANA's agenda, and continued efforts to encourage and endorse legislation to achieve third party payment for all nurses should also be pursued. Continued recruitment of new nurse members into the association through the federation of constituent state nurses' associations should be a strenuous, ongoing activity engaged in by ANA members in order to strengthen its economic base and viability at the local, state, and national levels.

With increased numbers, the association can more effectively influence trends impinging on the delivery of quality nursing care. "The professional association must continue to speak out for nursing and doing that job will require resources, both human and financial."[56] If in unity there is strength, then it is time for all professional nurses to support the ANA through active membership and participation in the association through this federation.

Modification of Nurse Practice Acts

The history of licensing in nursing parallels that of other recognized professions. As professions developed over the decades, they sought the protection of registration acts to control their right to practice and to prevent unauthorized persons from attempting such practice. North Carolina became the first state to pass a nurse registration bill in 1903, followed by New York and New Jersey. By 1923 all of the states had passed legislation regulating the practice of nursing. Nurse practice acts assured the public that licensed practitioners were minimally competent to practice nursing.

Bullough divides nursing licensure in the United States into three major phases. In the first phase, from 1900 to 1923, nurse practice acts were concerned solely with registration of trained nurses. During the second phase, from 1938 to 1955, the goals were to define the scope of nursing functions of registered nurses and practical nurses, condense educational standards, and prevent unlicensed individuals from practicing nursing. The current phase, which began around 1971, centers on amendments to nurse practice acts to allow diagnosis, prescription, and treatment for the expanded role of nurses in delivering health care.[57] In addition, professional accountability and clarification of the definition of nursing are emphasized.

In 1938, for example, the first mandatory practice act restricted nursing practice to registered and practical nurses. Scope of practice had to be defined and included in legislation, so violators of mandatory acts could be identified. To facilitate passage of mandatory nurse practice acts throughout all the states, the ANA adopted a model definition of nursing, which defined professional practice as:

> . . . the performance for compensation of any act in the observation, care, and counsel of the ill, injured, or infirm, or in the maintenance of health, or prevention of illness of others, or in the supervision and teaching of other personnel, or the administration of medications and treatments as prescribed by a licensed physician or dentist; requiring substantial specialized judgment and skill based on knowledge and application of the principles of biological, physical, and social sciences. (The foregoing shall not be deemed to include acts of diagnosis or prescription of therapeutic or corrective measures.)[58]

In the years that followed, due to an increase in the number of independent nurse practitioners engaged in diagnosis and treatment, this ANA definition of nursing became too limited, although it is still in effect for some states. By 1977, seventeen states had adopted amendments to the 1955 statement, enlarging the scope of nursing practice and allowing nurses to function in an expanded role.

Since 1977, at least thirty-five states have rewritten the 1955 ANA definition of nursing to allow for greater flexibility in defining the expanded role. "Probably the ideal nurse practice act would include an expanded scope of functions for all nurses as well as special provisions for specialists including nurse practitioners, nurse midwives, nurse anesthetists, and clinical specialists."[59]

Disappearance of restrictions on the nurse's right to diagnose and provide treatment opens the way for registered nurses to expand and further refine their clinical practice. An example of nurse practitioners' success in broadening their field of nursing practice occurred in 1983, when a ruling that restricted the practice of registered nurses in Missouri was overturned by the Missouri Supreme Court.[60] The judge believed that Missouri's 1975 Nurse Practice Act allowed a broader spectrum of nursing functions than the previous act. Two certified nurse practitioners employed by a family planning service were accused by the State Board licensing physicians of practicing medicine without a license. Their responsibilities included "performing breast and pelvic examinations, dispensing medications and contraceptives, and providing birth control information, all under physician standing orders and protocol."[61] The successful outcome of this case verifies for nurses that the expanded role is a legitimate part of nursing practice.

SOURCE AND STRUCTURE OF AUTHORITY IN NURSING PRACTICE

Authority as defined by Max Weber, an expert in organizational analysis, is "legitimated power." It is derived from two principal sources: position and expert knowledge. Within an "ideal-type" bureaucracy, "authority of position and authority of competence coincide with each other."[62] Weber's definition, however, does not refer to conflicts arising between these two types of authority when subordinates perform complex, highly technical tasks.

For the past several decades, nursing's lack of authority over its practice resulted from being under the control of a more dominant profession. Lacking well-qualified professionals to engage in professional practice, nursing has been unable to overcome this dominance, except in specialized nursing roles. Thus, the degree of conflict occurring over the last sixty years has not been noticeable. Now, however, many nurses have increased competence and capabilities for making intelligent nursing decisions. Conflicts arising between nursing and other health professions, particularly medicine, have increased substantially.

To the consumer of nursing's services, practicing nurses are perceived as having a subordinate role to medicine and lacking in the authority they believe necessary to treat their clients' health problems. Consumer opinion surveys continue to indicate that nurses are primarily responsible for carrying out "doctors' orders" and are presumed to have little authority.

> . . . in deciding what will be done for the client and how it will be done, the salaried professional has potentially reduced authority. Aspects of his work are likely to be strongly influenced by organizational policies. In addition, other professions in the organization may claim authority to determine and provide some of the services to be rendered the client. In nursing, both these sources of constraint to nurses' professional autonomy operate simultaneously and extensively.[63]

Physicians' legitimate authority, derived from their expert knowledge and expertise, is recognized and delegated to them by society. It is the authority that gives them the right to "order" care and services. Hospital nurses are faced with serious and frustrating problems as a result of the present ambiguous concept of nursing authority.[64] Most nurses agree that authority is necessary in determining patients' needs, supporting their life processes, preparing them to maintain their health after hospital discharge, and providing an environment that will permit such actions.[65] Clear-cut authority to practice within the full scope of their preparation and competence is sought by hospital nurses.[66] Whether nurses will ultimately be granted the degree of authority that will allow them to use their judgment in making decisions and issuing directives to other health personnel, can be answered only at some future date.

Decentralization of Organizational Structures

In considering the changing role of nurses in hospitals, F. E. Katz, a sociologist, made the following observation:

> The new professional aspirations, . . . with their focus on the nurse as a scientific colleague of the physician, hold the promise of making personalized care of patients increasingly sophisticated. But hospitals will have to develop adequate arrangements for translating the new sophistication of nurses into workable organizational patterns.[67]

Restructuring of traditional organizational patterns is occurring in some nursing service settings. What was once considered a complete departure from the traditional organization of nursing service departments is now observed more frequently as the preferred pattern—a decentralized nursing department. Decentralization refers to dispersing decision-making authority. Unless decentralization is clarified by means of an organizational chart that explains the lines of authority, conflicts will result. Loss of control through excessive decentralization cannot be tolerated, since goal achievement and the very existence of the organization may be threatened. However, if there is a proper balance between what is centralized and what is decentralized, effective organizational functioning should occur.

Traditionally, nursing service departments have been organized in a pyramid fashion, with the Director of Nursing at the top of the hierarchical structure controlling the decision-making process. Although the Director of Nursing is given more autonomy from hospital administration, in many institutions, decision making at the unit level does not occur.

Although nurse administrators are supportive of decentralized structures, they cannot abdicate their responsibility for the nursing services provided by their department. Delegating authority implies that individuals accepting it will exercise responsibility in fulfilling their roles. This delegation does not, however, free the nurse administrator from ultimate responsibility for the nursing care rendered. Proper feedback should be obtained to assure that the authority exercised by practicing nurses is used to promote the goals and productivity of the department.

Decentralized decision making in clinical units could occur if experienced nurse clinicians were in charge of each service. "Given the autonomy to manage their own units, experienced clinicians could vastly improve recruitment and retention of nurses by serving as clinical role models, by forging collegial relationships with physicians and by developing strategies for the provision of 24-hour coverage" to meet nurses' needs and patients' needs.[68]

Fortunately, role restructuring in hospitals is slowly providing for self-governance models, allowing greater freedom for nurses to control their clinical practice, to make decisions about patient care, to restructure the work environment, and to influence the quality of care provided. Decisions about working conditions, such as salary, benefits, and opportunities for advancement, are also becoming a part of nurses' decision-making role. "Direction and empowerment mean we should give our staff the right to make decisions, the right to make mistakes and the right to give us some of the best information and direction for our organization that we could ever have."[69]

PROFESSIONAL NURSING PRACTICE MODELS

With nursing moving toward becoming a more mature, independent profession, professional nursing practice models are developing in hospitals throughout the country. An excellent example of the professional practice model used at Beth Israel Hospital in Boston, Massachusetts, was presented by Joyce Clifford and Lynn Cavaliero in the keynote address for the 70th Biennial Convention of the Illinois Nurses Association in Chicago on November 30, 1989.[70] Entitled "Empowerment within Nursing," they presented their perspectives on a model that describes nurse empowerment as flowing from the adoption of a clear mission which values the actual practice of nursing. In this model the nurse/patient/family relationship is at the center with organization decision-making made in support of this relationship. Primary nursing, decentralized nursing administration, competitive salaries and nurse-physician collaboration, are among the reasons why this hospital experienced no shortage of nursing personnel.[71]

A differentiated practice geared toward professionalizing nursing and providing autonomy and control should be of top priority for nursing service directors. A problem continues to exist because "there is no clear distinction within the present structure of nursing practice between the roles of the nursing professional and the nursing technician."[72]

The problem is one of a mismatch of education with the expectations of the position. The expectations of the staff nursing position are for a highly skilled technician. The education needed for the position is technical education . . .

Programs of professional education in nursing emphasize the development of critical thinking, decision-making, and independent judgment.[73]

Need for Differentiated Practice

". . . Nursing service directors should develop staffing patterns truly differentiating professional and technical nurses and commensurate roles and establish a practice climate and reward system to foster recruitment into professional nursing."[74] Aydelotte points out that "the knowledge base for each type of graduate nurse must be sufficiently differentiated so that the practice of each resides upon a different base and the exchange or substitution of one type of practitioner is not possible."[75] Furthermore, "it is critical that role expectations change as a nurse's role changes within any system of differentiation and that salary and benefits are tailored to recognize these levels of personal growth and accomplishment."[76]

An example of a position-differentiated registered nurse practice model has been in existence since February 1988 at Maryvale Samaritan Medical Center in Phoenix. Here "experienced nurses select the case manager or case associate role based on their knowledge and skill. This facility is one of four hospitals in Arizona participating in a "Differentiated Group Professional Practice" project sponsored by the University of Arizona."[77]

Among the sixteen remedies for the nursing shortage proposed by the Commission on Nursing in its final report (February 1989), one in particular emphasized that "staffing patterns should take account of RNs different levels of education and experience" and that salaries should reflect different levels of experience and performance.[78] Recognizing the importance of differentiation in practice, the American Academy of Nursing at its fall 1990 meeting entitled "Differentiating Nursing Practice: The Twenty-First Century" stressed the importance of clearly pointing up differences in levels of education, experience, and performance among the various categories of nursing personnel and the need to establish salary scales commensurate with these differences. Specific questions about the present and future of such practice were addressed.

Appointment of Nurse Administrators to Top Levels in the Administrative Hierarchy and External Agencies

Nursing's role in hospitals since the 1930s has never been visible for its power, influence, or autonomous decision making in matters vital to the welfare of the institution. Historically, nurses were never included in the decision-making structure of the hospital.

Currently, a promising development in role restructuring of nursing service departments is the appointment of Directors of Nursing to major policy-making roles, such as membership on boards of trustees of hospitals. In addition, many of these directors have been promoted to Vice-President for Nursing Affairs, Assistant Administrator, or other similar titles. These changes not only provide greater visibility for nursing within the overall hospital structure but also give greater autonomy to nursing. Having direct access to board members to acquaint them with the nursing department needs for quality patient care and nursing's contribution to health care can only add strength to the nursing administrator's role.

Placing the nursing department head on the same level with other top-level administrators provides "clout" for the nurse administrator. For example, assigning the opportunity to defend budgetary, capital, and staffing needs to a top administrator, rather than to an assistant administrator at a lower level in the organizational structure, has many advantages. In dealing with ancillary service departments that affect nursing, nurse administrators at a higher level will experience fewer problems than in the former structural arrangement.

Appointment of nurse administrators to top-level committees of the hospital (where strategic planning and goal setting for the entire institution occurs) is beginning to happen but not as frequently as desired by many nurses. Ideally, nurse administrators and practicing nurses should be represented on all major committees that involve planning and establishing priorities for the hospital. Interestingly enough, physicians are frequently called on to chair important committees affecting both present and future plans of the institution. Although some nurses may serve on quality assurance, research, or evaluation committees, they are rarely appointed to committees having responsibility for budget, capital expenditures, or long-range goals.

Hospital administrators should be made aware of the significant contributions that nurses make to the successful operation of the hospital. To continue to overlook the talents, ability, and commitment that nurses could bring to the influential committee structure of hospitals denies the significant input from this knowledgeable group of professionals at the expense of the patients.

In addition to active roles in the committee structure of hospitals, nurses should be vigorously involved in external activities affecting their clinical practice. "Nurses and their interests must be effectively represented at decision-making and policy-making levels in local, state, and national government; in private and public institutions; and in societies related to health."[79] Examples of how this can occur are the appointment of nurses on boards of directors of organizations and agencies concerned with health-related issues, advising governmental groups, and election of nurses to fill positions of public office.[80] Health maintenance organizations and local health planning groups are reflecting a more active nurse membership.

Nursing and Hospital Staff Privileges

If professional nursing practice is to become more visible in the delivery of health care, particularly in hospitals, then qualified nurses should be permitted to admit patients to these institutions. The Joint Commission on Accreditation of Hospitals (JCAH), concerned about pressures from antitrust suits, recommended in 1982 that nonphysician providers such as nurse-midwives, nurse practitioners, nurse anesthetists, podiatrists, and psychologists be allowed to admit patients to hospitals.[81] The American Hospital Association supported this recommendation, but strong opposition from the American Medical Association delayed its implementation. The AMA House of Delegates, at its June 1983 meeting, opposed the term "organized staff" as a replacement for "medical staff." After several revisions of a fourth draft, JCAH commissioners approved a compromise in December 1983 that "broadens access to staff privileges while keeping control in the hands of a medical staff executive committee that must include a majority of physician members."[82]

A new law opening up staff privileges in the District of Columbia hospitals, allowing nurse practitioners, nurse-midwives, and nurse anesthetists to apply for staff privileges in D.C. hospitals became effective on January 1, 1984. It is noteworthy that Washington Hospital Center in the District of Columbia granted its first admitting privileges to a nurse-midwife in conjunction with this new legislative mandate. Also included in this new law are hospital admitting privileges for podiatrists and psychologists.[83] If hospitals deny privileges to one of these providers, they must provide evidence that the individual's credentials were evaluated and nondiscrimination was applied.[84] Close observation of this trend and its impact on the future of professional nursing practice is warranted. Due to the physician glut, however, it seems highly likely that the medical profession will strongly discourage expanding hospital staff privileges to include non-medical health care providers.

SUMMARY

Lack of nursing autonomy or lack of control over nursing practice is cited frequently by many nurses as contributing to unfavorable working conditions. If professional people are free from control by outsiders, then nurses should exert their right to practice autonomously and to be accountable for the decisions affecting their patients.

The fact that most nurses function in bureaucratic organizations limits independent decision making. This situation will continue to exist for nursing throughout the coming decade because nurses in many hospitals are subject to the power structure of physicians and hospital administrators. Although nursing is determined to change its public image, lack of autonomy will continue until society values nursing's ability to improve and advance the health of its citizens. Changes in attitudes of nurses and physicians regarding the need for a collaborative relationship between them has been documented in the literature. To continue to disregard the contributions that nursing makes to health care and to deny its right to have a shared role in decision making is to drastically underutilize nursing's knowledge and expertise.

Despite the accomplishments of the ANA, nursing's professional association, several unresolved issues, such as entry into practice, credentialing, reimbursement for nursing services, and the need to recruit new members into the association, should receive high priority if nursing is to effectively influence the delivery of health care. Revision of nurse practice acts is allowing for an expanded scope of functions for all nurses and further refinement of their clinical practice. The successful outcome of court cases involving nurse practitioners verifies that nursing's expanded role is a legitimate part of nursing practice.

Now that more nurses have increased competence and capability for decision making in nursing care, conflicts are arising between nursing and other health professions. Unlike physicians, nurses lack the authority to "order" care and services. Whether nurses will be granted full authority to use their judgment in making decisions and in issuing directives to other health personnel remains to be seen. Decentralizing organizational structures permits the dispersing of decision-making authority to the unit levels where direct action actually occurs. Such restructuring in hospitals involves a self-governance model that allows freedom for nurses to control their practice and favorably influence the quality of care provided.

As a part of this role restructuring, appointment of nurse administrators to the position of Vice-President for Nursing Affairs, Assistant Administrator for Nursing, or other similar titles is providing greater visibility and autonomy for nursing. Appointment to top-level committees within the hospital and externally within organizations and health-related agencies, such as HMOs and local planning groups, is increasing nursing's power base and reflecting an active nurse membership.

The broadening of staff privileges for nonphysician providers (nurse-midwives, nurse practitioners, and nurse anesthetists) to allow them to admit patients to hospitals is yet another factor that will strengthen nursing's opportunity to increase its autonomy, status, and power.

REFERENCES

1. Hassenplug, L. "Nursing Can Move from Here to There," *Nursing Outlook* 25:7 (July, 1977), 435.
2. "A.N.A. Monograph Examines 'Professional Collectivism,' " *American Nurse* 16:5 (May, 1974), 7.
3. Mauksch, I. "Attaining Control over Professional Practice," in B. Stevens (ed.), *Focus on Professional Issues*. Wakefield, Mass.: Contemporary Publishing, 1975, 3.
4. Etzioni, A. *The Semi-Professions and Their Organization*. New York: The Free Press, 1969, xiv.
5. Jacox, A. "Role Restructuring in Hospital Nursing," in L. Aiken (ed.), *Nursing in the 1980s: Crises, Opportunities, Challenges*. Philadelphia: J. B. Lippincott, 1982, 86.
6. Aydelotte, M. "Governance, Education Are Watchwords for the 80s," *American Nurse* 12:4 (March, 1980), 4.
7. *Ibid.*
8. Maas, M. "Nurse Autonomy and Accountability in Organized Nursing Services," *Nursing Forum* 12:3 (March, 1973), 252.
9. Jacox, A. "Role Restructuring," 97.
10. "Rebellion Among the Angels: Nurses Are No Longer Content To Be the Doctor's Handmaiden," *Time* 114:9 (August 27, 1979), 63.
11. Freidson, E. *Profession of Medicine*. New York: Dodd, Mead and Co., 1970, 83.
12. *Ibid.*
13. Batey, M. and Lewis, F. "Clarifying Autonomy and Accountability in Nursing Service: Part I," *Journal of Nursing Administration* 12:9 (September, 1982), 15.
14. Allen, D., Calkin, J. and Peterson, M. "Making Shared Governance Work: A Conceptual Model," *Journal of Nursing Administration* 18:1 (January, 1988), 40.
15. Simpson, R. and Simpson, I. "Women and Bureaucracy in the Semi-Professions," in A. Etzioni (ed.), *The Semi-Professions and Their Organization*. New York: The Free Press, 1969, 200.
16. Schlotfeldt, R. *A Brave New Nursing World* (Pub. No.: 82-N3). Washington, D.C.: American Association of Colleges of Nursing, 1982, 5.
17. Hall, R. "Professionalization and Bureaucratization," *Administrative Science Quarterly* 33 (February, 1968), 92–104.
18. Kornhauser, W. *Scientists in Industry: Conflict and Accommodation*. Berkeley, Calif.: University of California Press, 1962.
19. Bucher, R. and Stelling, J. "Characteristics of Professional Organizations," *Journal of Health and Social Behavior* 10:1 (March, 1969), 13.
20. Scott, W. "Professional Employees in a Bureaucratic Structure: Social Work," in A. Etzioni (ed.), *The Semi-Professions and Their Organization*. New York: The Free Press, 1969, 82.
21. "Top Nurse Execs Are Gaining Clout," (Newscaps) *American Journal of Nursing* 89:3 (March, 1989), 414.
22. Freidson, E. *Profession of Medicine*, 72.

23. *Ibid,*
24. Nehls, D., Hansen, V., Robertson, P. and Manthey, M. "Planned Change: A Quest for Nursing Autonomy," *Journal of Nursing Administration* 4:1 (January–February, 1974), 23.
25. *Ibid.*
26. "RNs Strive to Improve Working Conditions," *American Nurse* 22:3 (March, 1990), 16, 17.
27. Baer, C. "Nursing Diagnosis: A Futuristic Process for Nursing Practice," *Advances in Nursing Science* 6:1 (January, 1984), 91.
28. Nehls, D. "Planned Change," 23.
29. Freidson, E. *Profession of Medicine,* 76.
30. *Ibid.*
31. *Ibid.,* 69.
32. McKay, P. "Independent Decision Making: Redefining Professional Autonomy," *Nursing Administrative Quarterly* 7:4 (Summer, 1983), 23.
33. *Ibid.,* 23, 26.
34. *Ibid.,* 26.
35. De Tornyay, R. *Teaching-Learning Strategies for Baccalaureate Nursing Education.* (Pub. No.: 15-1622). New York: National League for Nursing, 1976, 12.
36. Barnum, B. "At New York U., the Division of Nursing Develops a Model for Nursing and Medical School Collaboration," *Nursing and Health Care* 11:2 (February, 1990), 89.
37. Mowry, M. and Korpman, R. "Hospitals, Nursing, and Medicine," *Journal of Nursing Administration* 17:11 (November, 1987) 21.
38. Fagin, C. and Lamberton, M. "Nurse-Physician Collaboration: Evaluation of a Nursing School-Medical School Joint Practice," in L. Aiken (ed.), *Health Policy and Nursing Practice.* New York: McGraw-Hill, 1981, 268.
39. *Ibid.*
40. Barnum, B. "At New York U., the Division of Nursing Develops a Model for Nursing and Medical School Collaboration," 189.
41. Department of Health, Education, and Welfare. *Extending the Scope of Nursing Practice: A Report of the Secretary's Committee to Study Extended Roles for Nurses.* Washington, D.C.: DHEW, 1971.
42. Crawford, A. "The Second Century: Collaboration or Continuing Conformance," *Journal of Nursing Administration* 4:2 (March–April, 1974), 24.
43. Aiken, L. "Hospital Changes Urged to End Nurse 'Shortage,' " *American Nurse* 13:2 (February, 1981), 4.
44. Lundeen, S. "Nursing Centers: Models for Autonomous Nursing Practice," in J. McClosky and N. Grace (eds.), *Current Issues in Nursing.* (3d ed.), St. Louis: C.V. Mosby, 1990.
45. *Ibid.*
46. Marians, C. "The Case for Interdisciplinary Collaboration," *Nursing Outlook* 37:6 (November–December, 1989), 288.
47. Sheahan, S. "The Game of the Name: Nurse Professional and Nurse Technician," *Nursing Outlook* 20:7 (July, 1972), 442.
48. Aiken, L. "Hospital Changes," 4.
49. Christman, L. "The Autonomous Nursing Staff in the Hospital," *Nursing Digest* 7 (1978), 71–75.

50. Mundinger, M. *Autonomy in Nursing.* Rockville, Md.: Aspen Systems Corp., 1980, 197.
51. *Ibid.*
52. Jones, L. and Ortiz, M. "Increasing Nursing Autonomy and Recognition Through Shared Governance," *Nursing Administrative Quarterly* 13:4 (Summer, 1989) 16.
53. Porter-O'Grady, T. "Shared Governance: Reality or Sham?" *American Journal of Nursing* 89:3 (March, 1989), 351.
54. Carr-Saunders, A. "Professions," in H. Vollmer and D. Mills (eds.), *Professionalization.* Englewood Cliffs, N.J.: Prentice-Hall, 1966, 4–5.
55. Lieberman, M. *Education as a Profession.* Englewood Cliffs, N.J.: Prentice-Hall, 1956.
56. Cole, E. (ed.), "Nurses Will Consider Important Issues at Convention," *American Nurse* 16:6 (June, 1984), 4.
57. Bullough, B. "The First Two Phases in Nursing Licensure," in B. Bullough (ed.), *The Laws and the Expanding Nursing Role.* New York: Appleton-Century-Crofts, 1975.
58. "A.N.A. Board Approves a Definition Nursing Practice," *American Journal of Nursing* 55:4 (April, 1955), 1474.
59. Bullough, B., Bullough, V. and Soukup, M. *Nursing Issues and Nursing Strategies for the Eighties.* New York: Springer Publishing, 1983, 284.
60. Selby, T. "Court Overturns Ruling Restricting NPs Practice," *American Nurse* 16:1 (January, 1984), 3.
61. *Ibid.*
62. Weber, M. *The Theory of Social and Economic Organization.* A. Henderson and T. Parsons (trans.) and T. Parsons (ed.), Glencoe, Ill.: The Free Press, 1947, 333–334.
63. Jacox, A. "Collective Action and Control of Practice by Professionals," *Nursing Forum* 10:3 (March, 1971), 250.
64. Nehls, D. "Planned Change," 23.
65. *Ibid.*
66. *Ibid.*
67. Katz, F. "Nurses," in A. Etzioni (ed.), *The Semi-Professions and Their Organization.* New York: The Free Press, 1969, 76.
68. Aiken, L. "Hospital Changes," 4.
69. Ripple, N. "Capitalizing on the New Economics: Nurse Executives as Catalysts for Action," *Nursing Economics* 6:2 (February, 1988), 70.
70. Clifford, J. and Cavaliero, L. "Empowerment Within Nursing," Keynote Address of Illinois Nurses Association 70th Biennial Convention, Chicago. *CHART* 87:1 (January, 1990), 5.
71. *Ibid.*
72. Newman, M. and Autio, S. *Nursing in a Prospective Payment System Health Care Environment.* Minneapolis, Minn.: University of Minnesota, 1986, 14.
73. *Ibid.,* 14, 15.
74. Styles, M., and Holzemeyer, W. "Educational Remapping for a Responsible Future." Paper presented at the AACN/AONE Conference on Nursing in the 21st Century, Aspen, Colo., July 9–11, 1985, in *Journal of Professional Nursing* 2:1 (January–February, 1988), 67.

75. Aydelotte, M. "The Evolving Profession," in N. Chaska (ed.), *The Nursing Profession: Turning Points.* St. Louis: C.V. Mosby Co., 1990, 13.
76. Joel, L. "Changes in the Hospital as a Place of Practice," in J. McCloskey and H. Grace (eds.), *Current Issues in Nursing* (3d. ed.) St. Louis: C.V. Mosby, 1990, 79.
77. Mulloch, K. and Milton, D. "Practice Models Succeeds in Phoenix," *American Nurse* 22:5 (May, 1990), 32.
78. "The Commission's 16 Remedies for the Shortage," *American Journal of Nursing* 89:2 (February, 1989), 278.
79. Aydelotte, M. "Governance, Education Are Watchwords," 14.
80. *Ibid.*
81. "JCAH is Weighing Wider Access to Staff Privileges in Hospitals," (News) *American Journal of Nursing* 83:9 (September, 1983), 1260.
82. "Non-MDs Can Join Medical Staffs, says JCAH," (News) *American Journal of Nursing* 84:3 (March, 1984), 382.
83. "D.C. Law Gives Nurses Hospital Staff Privileges," *American Nurse* 16:1 (January, 1984), 8.
84. "In Brief" Newscaps *American Journal of Nursing* 85:1 (January, 1985), 94.

SUGGESTED READINGS

Aiken, L. (ed.), *Health Policy and Nursing Practice.* New York: McGraw-Hill, 1981.
Aiken, L. "Charting the Future of Hospital Nursing," *Image: the Journal of Nursing Scholarship* 22:2 (Spring, 1990), 72–78.
American Nurses' Association. *Issues in Professional Nursing Practice.* Kansas City, Mo.: American Nurses' Association, 1984.
"The Doctor-Nurse Game Revisited," *New England Journal of Medicine* 322:8 (February 22, 1990), 546–549.
Griffith, H. "Direct Third Party Reimbursement of Nursing Services: A Review of Legislation and Implementation," *Nursing Administrative Quarterly* 12 (1987), 19–23.
Hinshaw, A., Smeltzer, C. and Atwood, J. "Innovative Retention Strategies for Nursing Staff," *Journal of Nursing Administration* 17:6 (June, 1987), 8–16.
Jacox, A. "Determining the Cost and Value of Nursing," *Nursing Administrative Quarterly* 12:1 (1987), 7–12.
Jamieson, M. "Block Nursing: Practicing Autonomous Nursing in the Community," *Nursing and Health Care* 11:5 (May, 1990), 250–253.
Manion, J. *Change from Within: Nurse Entrepreneurs as Health Care Innovators.* Kansas City, Mo.: American Nurses Association, 1990.
McCloskey, J. "Implications of Costing Out Nursing Services for Reimbursement," *Nursing Management* 20:1, 44–49.
McCloskey, J. "Two Requirements for Job Contentment: Autonomy and Social Integration," *Nursing Outlook* 22:3 (Fall, 1990), 140–143.
Mechanic, D. and Aiken, L. "A Co-Operative Agenda for Medicine and Nursing." *New England Journal of Medicine* 307 (1982), 747–750.
Pinch, W. J. "Ethical and Moral Dilemmas in Nursing: The Role of the Nurse and

Perceptions of Autonomy." Doctoral Dissertation, Boston University, May 1983.

Porter-O'Grady, T. and Finnigan, S. *Shared Governance for Nursing: A Creative Approach to Professional Accountability.* Rockville, Md.: Aspen Systems Corp., 1984.

Porter-O'Grady, T. *Reorganization of Nursing Practice: Creating a Corporate Venture.* Gaithersburg, Md.: Aspen Publishers, Inc., 1990.

Porter-O'Grady, T. *Creative Nursing Administration: Managing Participation into the 21st Century.* Gaithersburg, Md.: Aspen Publishers, Inc., 1990.

Prescott, P. and Bowen, S. "Controlling Nursing Turnover," *Nursing Management* 18:6 (June 1987), 60–66.

Ripple, H. "Capitalizing on the New Economics: Nurse Executives as Catalysts for Action," *Nursing Economics* 6:2, 70.

Sandrick, K. "Pricing Nursing Services," *Hospitals* 59:22 (November 16, 1985), 75–78.

Wilson, L., Prescott, P. and Aleksantrowicz, L. "Nursing: A Major Hospital Cost Component," *Health Services Research* 22:6 (February, 1988), 773–796.

Status of Accountability and Responsibility for Nursing Practice

12

INTRODUCTION

Throughout the literature on professions and professionalism, the concept of accountability—placing clients' needs above one's own, protecting their rights to receive safe, adequate service, and being answerable for one's professional performance—has received considerable emphasis. Accountability has been defined in terms of holding professionals answerable for the success or failure of their professional practice. The term was rarely used in the 1950s and 1960s, but due to changes in the public's mood, accountability is a key word among present-day citizen groups. Lack of accountability is a battle cry of consumer advocates in the health field. Evidence abounds that consumer groups, having special interests in health-related affairs, are vocally insisting that all health professionals be held accountable for their performance. Since the 1970s, the trend toward greater openness and the public's insistence on being informed about their health status has required professionals to assume accountability for their professional acts.

Several authors, in defining accountability, declared that the time had come for nurses and nursing to accept accountability for the quality of care received by patients. They also declared that patient expectations had not been met by nurses.[1,2] In the late 1970s, this external call for nursing accountability was echoed by many nursing administrators.

Accountability means being answerable for acts carried out in the performance of one's professional role.[3] When one is answerable, it places responsibility for the outcomes of nursing care directly on the practitioner.[4] It is encouraging to learn that bedside nurses are assuming primary responsibility for clinical nursing care.[5] The fact that nurses are showing more concern for their patients and for nursing care goals is a strong indication that accountability is no longer just a byword. Nurses are also becoming more responsible in answering to patients, head nurses, and physicians for the quality of nursing care they provide.

If nurses are sincere in their desire to achieve professional status, then a willingness to be accountable for their actions must be demonstrated. There is no profession that does not call upon its practitioners to assume accountability for their own actions and those of their assistants.[6]

Frequently in literature, accountability is equated with responsibility. In differentiating between responsibility and accountability, the former connotes action, the performance of a task for which one is responsible. Accountability suggests that the outcomes of tasks performed will be judged against outcome criteria. Thus, accountability refers to the results of the actions or tasks performed.

Professional nurses engaged in clinical practice are accountable for their actions as they implement their responsibilities for patient care. Although the ultimate accountability for nursing service delivery rests with nurse administrators, to assure quality delivery they must be convinced that professional workers involved in patient care are meeting their professional responsibilities for outcomes of care. Such accountability can be achieved without exerting excessive controls to "police" professional workers. "To be accountable means to answer to someone for something that one *has done.*"[7]

Without responsibility and authority, autonomy and accountability would be quite ineffective. In order to exercise accountability, one must have authority inherent in the position or role assumed. However, accountability is of little worth unless reinforced by a strong and vigorous autonomy. The two cannot be separated. Nursing accountability has been slow to develop because of the difficulties that arise when nurses, accountable for patient care decisions, lack the authority and freedom to implement them. In these situations, many nurses are forced to lower their standards, settle for inferior nursing care, and be less accountable to the recipients of their care. Unfortunately, many hospitals still support a task-oriented approach for the provision of nursing care.[8] Some nurses believe that nursing care is not recognized or valued. Others feel that accountability means being answerable for tasks and procedures that have little bearing on the professional decisions to be made. "Professional accountability [implying autonomous decision making at the practitioner level] must be integrated to create an environment within which professional nursing practice can take place."[9] Until nursing accountability is required at the practitioner level, with nurses having authority and autonomy to implement their decisions, the dissatisfaction currently experienced by professional nurses will continue and even increase.

MECHANISMS FOR ASSURING ACCOUNTABILITY

Primary Nursing

To understand current modes of nursing care delivery, a review of historical events that have influenced the development of nursing care up to the present period is helpful. During the early decades of this century, graduate nurses had no alternative but to seek private-duty nursing in homes. Undergraduate student nurses provided most of the nursing care to hospitalized patients. Compared to the highly technical, sophisticated nursing care provided to patients in one-to-one relationships today, earlier "private-duty" nursing seems simple and primitive. Yet, patients felt satisfied with the care and concern provided by their nurses.

During and after World War II the shortage of nurses necessitated employment of licensed practical nurses and nurse aides, with registered nurses responsible for making patient assignments, passing medications, charting, and performing treatments for patients. Referred to as functional nursing, such practice exaggerated the splintering of nursing care. Little or no supervision of these workers occurred, and planning for patient care was virtually nonexistent. Moreover, nursing care was task-oriented, with individual patient needs either neglected or treated in a superficial manner.

To remedy this situation, team nursing was introduced. Registered nurses assumed responsibility for the nursing care of team members but rarely gave direct, personalized care to patients. Due to understaffing of units, team leaders lacked knowledge of the diagnosis or medical regimen for patients on these teams, and nursing care plans were never utilized. Patient care was fragmented, with as many as twenty to thirty individuals moving in and out of a patient's room on a daily basis. Frequent pleas to "let the nurse, nurse" were being heard from many sources.

To provide for "my nurse—my patient" and for continuity of care to offset the adverse criticism resulting from functional and team nursing, a new form of nursing care evolved in the late 1960s. Marie Manthey and her colleagues named this new concept "primary nursing" when introducing it at the University of Minnesota hospitals. Designed to establish a one-to-one nurse-patient relationship, primary nursing "embodies an arrangement of nurse and patient that facilitates professional practice and the delivery of nursing care [and] incorporates the strong components of responsibility and accountability into the role of the hospital nurse."[10] "Primary nursing allows the nurse twenty-four hour responsibility for a group of patients, a more satisfying arrangement than supplying various aspects of care to a myriad of different patients."[11, 12] Moreover, "the decentralization of clinical authority and the establishment of systems of reward based on competence, demand that nurses be accountable to and for one another."[13] Above all, nurses must become more willing to assume accountability for the outcomes of their nursing practice.

To facilitate responsibility and accountability, autonomy and a decentralized structure for decision making are required. Furthermore, since primary nurses are responsible over a twenty-four-hour period, seven days a week for planning, implementing, and evaluating nursing care for a small group of patients, they must be given the authority necessary to fulfill their responsibilities. Since the foundation of accountability is based on authority, nurses must strive for the authority needed to function in a professional nursing practice role, just as the medical profession and other health professions function in their practice roles. Above all, nurses should become more willing to assume accountability for the outcomes of their nursing practice. Delegated authority allows nurses to issue directives to those nurses caring for their patients in their absence. Undoubtedly, primary nurses cannot function as true professionals without the three dimensions of autonomy, authority, and accountability. By adopting primary nursing, the nursing profession is self-consciously declaring that patient care is nurses' territory.[14]

As a result of structural changes in delivering nursing care, nursing is becoming more attractive as a profession. Enthusiasm for this type of nursing practice comes from nurses, physicians, and patients. For example, one patient commented that "it's easy to see why a nurse with a chance to do primary work prefers it to dispensing pills all day to people whose names she knows only from the charts at the foot of their beds, and why she prefers to move into a more equal, professional relationship with social workers, dietitians, and even doctors."[15] Primary nursing has been instrumental in promoting professional practice. But it is not a panacea for curing inadequate nursing practice or for changing the attitudes of staff about how much of their time, effort, and concern will be given to patients.[16]

Nursing administrators can foster primary nursing by supporting and trusting their nursing staff to be capable and willing to provide quality care to their patients. Clinical nursing leaders can serve as resources for the staff and head nurses as problems and risks occur from delegating "responsibility and accountability for patient care decisions" to the primary nurse.[17]

Primary nursing, as a means of implementing professional practice through redesigning the delivery system, will promote accountability. However, it will not occur at the practitioner level until the management level demonstrates through role modeling that it values accountability.[18] As a result of restructuring delivery of nursing services, another model of nursing care—case management—is becoming acceptable to nurses. It involves decentralization of accountability for clinical and case—cost outcomes to the staff nurse level.[19]

Models for care management require "administration's relentless focus, openness, and risk-taking, all different approaches to keep while maintaining the usual operations of a department."[20] However, "by establishing case management, accountability—that great divider of professional status—is clarified and assigned to a specific staff primary nurse as case manager."[21] Thus, if nurses do not become the case managers, nursing's work may be carried out by non-nurse providers anxious to take over the business of nursing.[22]

Clinical Career Ladders

For nurses who desire to remain in direct patient care, the creation of the clinical ladder concept has produced a system that rewards clinical competence, knowledge, expertise, and performance. Traditionally, nurses who are competent and skillful in providing quality care were rewarded by promotion to administrative positions offering greater prestige, recognition, and income. The failure to provide for *clinical* advancement caused nurses to seek other options such as teaching or administration in order to acquire status.[23] However, providing a clinical environment that recognizes an individual's competence should permit staff nurses to research "levels of professional excellence," which would provide justification for compensatory rewards that are usually attained by those seeking careers in supervision or administration.[24]

Descriptions of various plans for clinical advancement and how they increase job satisfaction and reduce turnover are well-documented in the literature.[25-27] The concept of rewarding nurses according to their level of competence has been demonstrated in nursing service departments in several health care institutions, including the University of California Health Care Facilities at San Francisco, Los Angeles, and San Diego; Rush Presbyterian-St. Luke's Medical Center, Chicago; Indiana University Hospitals, Indianapolis; and the University of Wisconsin Center for Health Sciences in Madison. "When nurses believe that they are being rewarded according to their corporate worth, the best characteristics of their training will be demonstrated [and] the outcome is improved patient care—the prime objective."[28]

Nursing administrative teams and nurses who will be affected by the new system are assuming responsibility for planning the recognition of the nurse who opts for remaining at the bedside. In collaboration with nursing staff members, "a reward system based on clinical practice behaviors, and a clinically based, behaviorally stated system for evaluation" is being developed in recognition of clinical competence.[29] Originally conceived as horizontal or lateral promotions, a "levels of practice" system of clinical advancement provides movement from one level to the next as professional growth and expertise are recognized.

To qualify for promotion, nurses must demonstrate their achievement of the clinical behaviors required for each level. Advancement to another level is not based on additional education or experience, but on achieving the established criteria. Some institutions form a clinical committee or task force to develop the clinical ladder system. Developing the list of functions and the criteria upon which performance is to be evaluated are the primary responsibilities of this committee.

Since budgetary concerns affect this system, the number of nurses expected to qualify for each level must be determined in advance to assure the necessary positions and funding for them. Salary ranges for the different levels must be defined at the outset. The appointment of a committee to review candidate performance and recommend advancement in the system is another essential step in completing a clinical advancement program. This new system is a reflection of the growing awareness that accountability for quality nursing care provided to consumers is the responsibility of the clinicians.[30]

Nursing Staff Organizations

For several years nurses have eyed the closely knit organizational structure of medical staffs in hospitals and regretted that nursing has lacked a similar type of structure. To remedy this situation, nursing staff organizations (NSO) have been created over the past two decades, similar in design to medical staff organizations, to assure accountability for nursing practice and provide self-governance for the nursing staff.[31] Because groups with common goals planning to organize their members adopt an organizational method of bylaws, nursing departments in several hospitals have begun to use this method of organizing their nursing staff. Bylaws are defined as "rules adopted by an organization to regulate its own local or internal affairs, dealings with others, and the government of its members."[32]

A review of content included in nursing bylaws indicates that it is based on the philosophy of the nursing department and begins with a preamble reflecting the principles upon which the nursing department is organized. For example, one preamble included the following principles:

1. That all patients are entitled to nursing care of the highest quality

2. That such care is enhanced by a democratic environment which recognizes the uniqueness of each individual consumer and provider
3. That the patient can best be served by collaboration with other professions, education programs, and research
4. That the ongoing assessment of nursing and systems is essential to the provision of quality nursing services[33]

Bylaws are usually organized into nine or ten articles:[34,35]

Article I	Name
Article II	Purposes
Article III	Organization of the Nursing Department
Article IV	Categories of Nursing Staff
Article V	Appointment to Staff
Article VI	Advancement Opportunities
Article VII	Continuing Education
Article VIII	Committees
Article IX	Amendments

As a result of this organization, opportunities were increased to interpret and explain to the hospital board of trustees and the medical director the purposes and functions of an organized nursing staff having its own set of bylaws. Moreover, staff nurses expressed satisfaction with the opportunity to become more directly involved in decision making and committee activities. By establishing an NSO, professional nurses can function at their full potential and practice accountability to themselves and their patients for the nursing care they provide.[36]

Code of Ethics

One of the major reasons for having a code of ethics is to specify the obligations of the professional in order to protect a dependent public from exploitation by its members. The code expresses a service orientation in identifying the status of the professional and the client. When made public, clients can judge whether or not professionals are fulfilling the standards of their profession. Concern for the public's welfare ensures their confidence, the granting of privileges, and the right to function as autonomous practitioners.

In response to the trust a client places in the nurse, the American Nurses' Association developed a code of ethics that reflects acceptance of this trust. The need for such a code was first expressed in 1897, and a tentative code, prepared by an ANA Committee on Ethical Standards, was presented to the House of Delegates in 1926.[37] After referral back to this committee, a *Preliminary Code for the Nursing Profession* was completed in 1940. However, subsequent revisions necessitated the creation of a new code, which was adopted officially in 1950 at the ANA Convention. Ten years later, the code was again revised and re-adopted.[38] Since that time, two other revisions have occurred, one in 1968 and one in 1976.

Each revision indicated the changes occurring in society and within nursing itself. For example, the later revisions removed the connotation of dependency on physicians and stressed the nurse's accountability for nursing care. In the 1976 Code, consisting of eleven statements, it is noteworthy that accountability is stressed as having considerable significance for nursing (see the ANA Code of Ethics). The code emphasizes the professional obligations that nurses have to society to promote high standards of nursing care and to challenge the personal integrity of every nurse.

Licensure of Practitioners

Licensing of practitioners involves a legal process that is one of the oldest mechanisms for credentialing practitioners. Professions control entry into their ranks through the process of licensing, thereby demonstrating their accountability to clients and the general public. Licensing represents control of a profession by society, who, in turn, grants autonomy for the profession to accomplish its particular mission. In order to protect the public's health, safety, and welfare, licensing examinations by State Boards of Nursing provide a mechanism for determining minimal safety of practitioners to practice nursing. To be eligible to write this examination a candidate must have graduated from a state-approved school of nursing.

Actually, requirements for licensure simply indicate that a minimum level of competency has been achieved by candidates upon successful completion of a written examination. The degree of competency individual nurses may have acquired beyond this minimum is not measured by the licensing examination. Among the advantages of a national State Board Test Pool Examination available to all the states, licensure by endorsement can be obtained by registered nurses desiring to move from one state to another.[39]

The problem of standardization of state licensure has been solved, but it is evident that the issue of who should be licensed has not.[40] Involved in the licensing debate is the fact that presently all registered nurses are licensed by means of the same examination, which validates technical knowledge, but not professional knowledge.[41] For the past few years, the American Nurses' Association has been conducting surveys on state nurses' associations actions to resolve the entry into practice issue.[42] The efforts of proponents recommending separate licensing examinations for two levels of nursing—professional and technical—have had only limited success. To assure accountability for professional nursing practice requires

American Nurses' Association Code for Nurses (1976)

Preamble

The Code for Nurses is based upon belief about the nature of individuals, nursing, health, and society. Recipients and providers of nursing services are viewed as individuals and groups who possess basic rights and responsibilities, and whose values and circumstances command respect at all times. Nursing encompasses the promotion and restoration of health, the prevention of illness, and the alleviation of suffering. The statements of the Code and their interpretation provide guidance for conduct and relationships in carrying out nursing responsibilities consistent with the ethical obligations of the profession and quality in nursing care.

1. The nurse provides services with respect for human dignity and the uniqueness of the client unrestricted by considerations of social or economic status, personal attributes, or the nature of health problems.
2. The nurse safeguards the client's right to privacy by judiciously protecting information of a confidential nature.
3. The nurse acts to safeguard the client and the public when health care and safety are affected by the incompetent, unethical, or illegal practice of any person.
4. The nurse assumes responsibility and accountability for individual nursing judgments and actions.
5. The nurse maintains competence in nursing.
6. The nurse exercises informed judgment and uses individual competence and qualifications as criteria in seeking consultation, accepting responsibilities, and delegating nursing activities to others.
7. The nurse participates in activities that contribute to the ongoing development of the professions's body of knowledge.
8. The nurse participates in the profession's efforts to implement and improve standards of nursing.
9. The nurse participates in the profession's efforts to establish and maintain conditions of employment conducive to high quality nursing care.
10. The nurse participates in the profession's effort to protect the public from misinformation and misrepresentation and to maintain the integrity of nursing.
11. The nurse collaborates with members of the health professions and other citizens in promoting community and national efforts to meet the health needs of the public.

(From *Code for Nurses with Interpretive Statements*. Kansas City, Mo.: The American Nurses Association, 1976. Reproduced with permission of the publisher.)

"limiting licensure to only one type within the occupation of nursing," with all other nursing personnel registering on a national registry on a voluntary basis.[43] Hinsvark raises the important question of *who* under this plan should be so licensed. Thus far, no specific movement has occurred to facilitate such a plan.

Certification for Specialty Practice

Certification represents another mechanism of credentialing nurses that demonstrates accountability to the public. Originally, certification was intended to provide recognition for professional achievement and for excellence in clinical practice. More recently, however, emphasis is placed on certification for advanced specialty practice. Due to pressures from patients and the public for additional evidence of the competence of nurses to assume greater responsibilities for more complicated equipment, procedures, and levels of care, the ANA developed a certification program in 1973 to give formal recognition for specialty competence in nursing practice. Nurses who successfully complete the certification examination sponsored by the ANA provide evidence to the public that they have acquired advanced education in a specific specialty area and are capable of assuming responsibilities for advanced clinical practice in that area.

Providing external recognition to nurses with advanced specialty preparation should prove to the public that these nurses are qualified to engage in specialty practice. Additional preparation, clinical experience, and the recognition that certification provides can only improve the quality of patient care and serve as a strong motivation for certified nurses to continue to excel.

If autonomy or freedom from outside control is to prevail in nursing, then certification should be one means of acquiring it. As nursing demonstrates continued excellence in clinical practice, autonomy will eventually increase as the public is convinced that quality patient care is nursing's number one priority. However, because there are currently "no uniform standards for entry into specialty nursing practice," and no periodic assessment of specialists' competencies, certification is beset with problems.[44] Frequently nurses express their concerns about the lack of standardized preparation for specialty nursing.

Current issues in the certification of nurse specialists were addressed at a conference on certification held in San Antonio, Texas, in the spring of 1984. Hildegard Peplau, noted nurse leader, spoke on several issues, such as: "ambivalence among nurses about allowing some better educated nurses to be called specialists; the interchangeable use of 'nurse practitioners' and 'specialists' despite major differences in credentials; the interchangeable use of titles—specialists, practitioners, clinician, etc.—for graduates of master's programs."[45] At this same conference, it was asserted that without unity among nurses, too many voices are heard. The public, understandably, is uncertain which voice it should heed.[46]

With voluntary professional credentialing programs becoming more accepted, problems arise when these programs are used to form the basis for employment, advancement, and reimbursement. Associations responsible for these programs will be under close governmental scrutiny to determine how reasonable and procedurally fair they are.[47]

Confusion created by a variety of agencies granting certification led to a proposal for the establishment of a national nursing credentialing center at some future date. Major nursing organizations are exploring the potential for a national board that would standardize and conceivably consolidate the certification criteria and processes for specialty nursing practice.[48]

At a steering committee meeting held in San Antonio in 1989 with over 150 nurses representing fifty-six specialty and certification groups, a need for standardization and a "clearer definition of the nature of specialties in nursing" was unanimously felt among those in attendance.[49] In reporting for the Committee for the National Board of Nursing Specialties, project director, Jeanette Hartshorn stated that the proposed board would provide "a degree of equivalency among nursing certification programs."[50] She pointed out that within nursing, thirty-five certification programs currently exist. Twenty-eight specialty organizations belong to the Federation of Specialty Nursing Organizations (NFSNO) with the ANA providing the largest number of certification programs. Issues yet to be resolved include whether specialty certification by states will be required for specialty practice and whether states will accept certification by voluntary professional associations as part of their state requirements.

A proliferation of certifying agencies and variations of standards among the various states creates confusion for the public and for nursing. Presently, New York, New Jersey, and other states believe that certification should occur only at the master's degree level. Thus, it appears that a trend toward master's degree preparation for the various specialties is rapidly becoming a requirement. Growing distrust on the part of the public requires that nursing should move ahead and take the initiative to address these issues if public trust is to be restored.

In order to qualify for certification at present, individuals must be currently licensed to practice in the United States or its territories. In addition, they must be currently practicing nursing and have the required educational preparation (including a practice component) in the area chosen for this examination. Between 1975 and 1984, over 1,000 nurses became certified in New York State, Massachusetts, and California. Currently, more than 72,000 registered nurses in the country have achieved certification through the ANA certification program.[51] The number of certification examinations offered by the ANA has increased from thirteen specialty areas in 1980 to twenty-one generalist and specialist nursing areas in 1990 (nineteen in nursing practice and two in nursing administration). The following list contains the certification examinations offered:

1. Clinical Specialist in Community Health Nursing
2. Community Health Nurse
3. Adult Nurse Practitioner
4. Family Nurse Practitioner
5. School Nurse
6. School Nurse Practitioner
7. Gerontological Nurse
8. Gerontological Nurse Practitioner
9. Clinical Specialist in Gerontological Nursing
10. Perinatal Nurse
11. Pediatric Nurse
12. Pediatric Nurse Practitioner
13. Medical-Surgical Nurse
14. Clinical Specialist in Medical-Surgical Nursing
15. Psychiatric and Mental Health Nurse
16. Clinical Specialist in Adult Psychiatric and Mental Health Nursing
17. Clinical Specialist in Child and Adolescent Psychiatric and Mental Health Nursing
18. Nursing Administration
19. Nursing Administration, Advanced
20. College Health Nurse
21. General Nursing Practice

The American Nurses Credentialing Center (ANCC) became incorporated and operational on January 1, 1991.[52] "By incorporating as a subsidiary of ANA, the ANCC will move toward meeting nationally accepted credentialing standards to ensure the credibility of the credentialing process, clarify ANA's role in standard setting and promulgation, and act as a better liaison with other nursing organizations and specialty certifying agencies."[53]

COMPONENTS TO MONITOR AND EVALUATE QUALITY NURSING CARE

To ensure quality nursing care within the contemporary health care system, mechanisms for monitoring and evaluating care are under scrutiny. As the level of knowledge increases for a profession, the demand for accountability of its services likewise increases. Individuals within the profession must assume responsibility for their professional actions and be answerable to the recipients of their care. As professions become more interdependent, it appears that the power base will become more balanced, allowing individual practitioners to demonstrate their competence and expertise. Several mechanisms are presented in the following sections to demonstrate effectiveness in monitoring patient care.

Quality Assurance Mechanisms

Quality assurance provides the mechanisms to effectively monitor patient care provided by health care professionals using cost-effective resources. Nursing programs of quality assurance are concerned with the quantitative assessment of nursing care as measured by proven standards of nursing practice. In addition, they motivate practitioners in nursing to strive for excellence in delivering quality care and to be more open and flexible in experimenting with innovative ways to change outmoded systems.

Peer Review

If, "evaluation of one's performance by peers is a hallmark of professionalism" and a mechanism through which the profession is accountable to society, why is it not used more generally by practicing nurses?[54] In order for nurses to control their practice, and become accountable to society, they should be diligent in conducting peer review. However, there are several difficulties associated with this mechanism:

1. Facing the issue of trust
2. Relating professional standards developed by peers to the policies and procedures that govern the settings where nurses practice
3. Closing the gap between actual practice and the boundaries of practice as defined in nursing practice acts
4. Respecting the confidentiality of recipient data, which must be dealt with in peer review in any type of 'audit' procedure
5. Helping nurses to accept the *lack* of anonymity of their performance; individuals must be identifiable if an adequate evaluation of the extent of accountability of a practicing nurse is to be conducted
6. Cost analyzing nursing contributions at differential levels of quality[55]

Traditionally, professions have been perceived as a group of individuals of equal status who are motivated through codes of ethics and regulations to uphold the standards of their profession in the interest of the society they serve. To maintain high standards, peer review has been initiated to carefully review the quality of practice demonstrated by members of a professional group. Peer review is divided into two types. One centers on the recipients of health services by means of auditing the quality of services rendered. The other centers on the health professional by evaluating the quality of individual performance.

Nursing Audit

Documented evidence of nursing practice has become increasingly important since nursing has assumed more responsibility and accountability for nursing care. Now that the Joint Commission on Accreditation of Healthcare Organizations (JCAHO) is concerned with the quality of nursing care, and many nurses throughout the country are evaluating the outcomes of their care, the nursing audit has been developed to help achieve higher quality patient care.

Nursing audit may be defined as a detailed review and evaluation of selected clinical records in order to evaluate the quality of nursing care and performance by comparing it with accepted standards. To be effective a nursing audit must be based on established criteria and a feedback mechanism that provides information to providers on the quality of care delivered. "To evaluate quality nursing care regularly, many staff nurses do indeed welcome opportunity to develop criteria, to review nursing care retrospectively and concurrently, and to discover methods of achieving higher levels of quality nursing care."[56]

The JCAH published a standard on quality assurance in 1980, which emphasized identification of problems and their resolution along with requiring a quality assurance program in each health care institution.[57] Again in 1982 the JCAH established standards for nursing care as measured against written criteria on a quarterly basis. For example, Standard I required that a qualified nurse director be employed to administer the nursing service department.[58] Standard IV stated that "individualized, goal-directed nursing care should be provided to patients through use of the nursing process."[59] The JCAHO standards, which place emphasis on *quality* and the need for continuous review and evaluation of care provided by professional workers, should serve as excellent guidelines for monitoring patient care.

Most hospitals have established committees to develop criteria and review medical records to determine if any inconsistencies or deviations from stated criteria exist. However, to conduct nursing audits because the JCAHO *requires* them may defeat the main purpose—*improvement* and *upgrading of* quality care.

Nursing audit committees establish valid criteria to be utilized prior to implementing the audit. Individual units and nurses within each unit should be informed of audit outcomes in order to rectify any discrepancies or deviations from stated criteria. If medical records indicate that a high level of quality care exists, then nurses responsible should be informed. Positive feedback can be a strong motivator to continue providing excellent care. Likewise, individual nurses can profit from knowledge about any omissions or mistakes made in delivering patient care, and making this information available can assist nurses to improve their performance.

Individual Peer Review

Peer review of the individual's performance is conducted by means of evaluations and judgments that nurses make for each other. Generally, nurses, like other health professionals (e.g., dentists and physicians) are reluctant to "sit in judgment" of their peers. Because individuals cannot claim perfection in their day-to-day activities, they should be willing to admit that mistakes and errors of omission or commission can and do occur. Moreover, their actions and the outcome of the actions are observable and open to evaluation by their colleagues, clients, and other health workers. Individual peer review can add to the data obtained through the nursing audit.

Peer review, if effective, should be formally conducted and based on established standards familiar to the individuals being evaluated. Confidentiality implies *trust* and should be present if a peer review system is to function successfully. Reviewing the individual's performance helps document how certain strategies and techniques affect positive outcomes of nursing care. It also reveals data which are sorely needed if nursing is to be more than a practice based on "intuition." If weaknesses are found in performance, the individual can profit by this knowledge and endeavor to correct the inadequacy.

Above all, if nurses sincerely believe that as professionals they are accountable to their patients, then they should be willing to solicit the opinion of their peers. Honesty with themselves and with one another should prevent any "politicizing" to evaluate incorrectly for fear of incurring the displeasure of those being evaluated. The danger of peer review becoming an "exercise in futility" for the reason just mentioned can be removed by the forthrightness of nurses who recognize the need for accountable practice within their ranks.

ANA Standards of Nursing Practice

Recognizing its responsibility for establishing standards for the nursing profession, the ANA has developed and published standards for nursing practice since the 1930s. Robert Merton, in 1960, reminded the profession that one of its "foremost obligations is to set rigorous standards for the profession and help enforce them."[60] Members of professional asso ciations meet to establish and maintain the highest standards, to educate the public as to what to expect from the profession, and to protect the public from individuals who deviate from professional standards.[61]

In 1973, the ANA Congress on Nursing Practice established *Standards for Nursing Practice,* which "provide a means for determining the quality of nursing that a client/patient receives regardless of whether such services are provided by a professional nurse or by a professional nurse and nonprofessional assistants."[62] During the 1974–1975 biennium, the ANA made its first priority the improvement of nursing practice by implementing the standards for practice established by the Congress for Nursing Practice. These eight standards were:

Standard 1. The collection of data about the health status of the client/patient is systematic and continuous. The data are accessible, communicative, and recorded.

Standard 2. Nursing diagnoses are derived from health status data.

Standard 3. The plan of nursing care includes goals derived from the nursing diagnoses.

Standard 4. The plan of nursing care includes priorities and the prescribed nursing approaches or measures to achieve the goals derived from the nursing diagnoses.

Standard 5. Nursing actions provide for client/patient participation in health promotion, maintenance, and restoration.

Standard 6. Nursing actions assist the client/patient to maximize his health capabilities.

Standard 7. The client's/patient's progress or lack of progress toward goal achievement is determined by the client/patient and the nurse.

Standard 8. The client's/patient's progress or lack of progress toward goal achievement directs reassessment, reordering of priorities, new goal setting, and a revision of the plan of nursing care.[63]

According to data released by the Joint Commission on Accreditation of Healthcare Organizations, nursing outstrips most other hospital services in meeting quality standards. Results of a study distributed in mid-1990 that analyzed the performance of 5,200 hospitals inspected during a three year accreditation cycle, revealed how state and national averages conformed to the accreditation standards.[64] Although these standards do not require any specific numbers of nurses or ancillary workers, each hospital must simply define and meet its need for nursing personnel based on its patient population.[65] This represents the first major revision of nursing standards in the JCAHO Accreditation Manual for Hospitals since

1978. A selected twenty-one member task force in 1989 revised the standards that define how hospital nursing services are accredited. These revised standards had undergone a final review process at JCAHO and became effective in January 1991.[66]

Preceptorships

In addition to facilitating new employee orientation, preceptorships instill a sense of accountability in new graduates, enabling them to provide quality care more effectively. Collaborative programs between education and service are making the transition from student to graduate far easier. Allowing for ample time in which to learn their new role under competent, friendly, supportive supervision, new graduates are experiencing less strain, burnout, and turnover than new nurses oriented in the more traditional systems. Not infrequently, orientation programs add to a new graduate's stress level by imparting an overload of material without sufficient time to absorb it.

Preceptors work on a one-to-one basis with new graduates, providing ample opportunity for meeting their individual needs. Some new graduates adjust more readily to new situations, and thus, learning objectives may be quite different than for those lacking self-confidence and needing greater reinforcement. Although the length of time for each new graduate may vary, preceptors have as a goal to allow the learner to function independently as soon as possible. Increasing their own accountability by serving as role models capable of giving expert nursing care, preceptors are themselves challenged by the opportunities to influence new graduates in their practice. Observing progress made by each learner can be a gratifying and rewarding experience for the preceptor.

COMMITMENT TO GOALS AND ACCOUNTABLE NURSING PRACTICE

Professionalism implies commitment, and commitment, in turn, is an indicator of a high degree of professionalization. Commitment to a calling involves accepting appropriate norms and standards and identifying with the profession and one's peers as a collectivity.[67] Nurses reflect varying degrees of commitment in their professional lives. Some have little association with their peers, believing that nurses have limited power and status. Thus, they seek recognition from other professions having more visible power and authority. Unlike the nurses just described, nurses with a high degree of commitment seem inwardly moved by their conscience to develop their full potential and be visibly active in furthering the goals of the profession. Their commitment reflects "a lifestyle demonstrated by a set of values that stimulate the growth and information of a professional conscience, an inner voice, that guides and monitors behavior."[68]

That some individual practitioners and groups of professionals continue to be unwilling to make and implement commitments to competence in patient care delivery and to further their own professional growth and that of the nursing profession is observable in many health care settings. That a previous imbalance exists between their professional commitment and their personal ambitions is also evident to the observer.[69]

To meet the growing demand for leaders within the profession, the problem of commitment must be addressed by all nurses. To simply say that one is committed to the profession is insufficient to produce the results nursing needs at this stage of its professional development. Nursing needs nurses who are personally committed upon graduation and who become licensed to work continuously for changes to improve nursing care.

If nurses are committed to the improvement of nursing, they will be inwardly motivated to strive for excellence and acquire the knowledge, skill, and experience that will enhance their practice. For many nurses this means additional educational preparation, continuing education, involvement in research, and development of innovative methods to further develop their assessment and diagnostic skills.

Another means of demonstrating commitment is to establish goals for a lifetime career in nursing and then to pursue the means necessary to accomplish these goals. Unlike other health professionals, who choose a career with the understanding that they will be committed to it over many years, a large number of nurses have yet to develop a similar commitment. As a result, marked differences are observed in the professional's depth of commitment and clinical competence and in the extent of effort devoted to controlled improvement.[70]

"The challenge for nursing in the 1990s will be to determine whether nurses can reaffirm their commitment to clinical excellence and demonstrate its importance with sufficient persuasiveness to cause administrators of health care institutions and ambulatory settings to restructure nursing responsibilities in ways that keep pace with nurses' career expectations."[71] To accomplish this task, every nurse should be diligently committed to pursuing the goal of clinical excellence in patient care.

SUMMARY

Accountability requires professional practitioners to be responsible for the actions performed in fulfilling their professional role. To encourage accountability, primary nursing was introduced in the late 1960s to facilitate professional practice and provide a one-to-one nurse-patient relationship.

Autonomy, authority, and accountability are essential in making primary nursing work. Also necessary is a decentralized decision-making structure. Redesigning the organizational structure to implement professional practice through primary nursing has promoted accountability. Moreover, management should demonstrate that it values accountability as an important concept and expects it from professional practitioners.

Recognizing the need to reward clinical competence by means of horizontal promotion and not by moving the individual upward into supervisory or administrative positions, the concept of clinical career ladders was developed to provide status and recognition for bedside nurses. To qualify, nurses must demonstrate the achievement of clinical behaviors required for each level. Such a system places responsibility on the practicing nurse, who is accountable for the quality of nursing care provided to patients.

To provide self-governance for the nursing staff and to increase accountability, nursing staff organizations have been established over the past decade. A set of bylaws or rules are adopted regulating the internal affairs of the organization and governance of its members. Staff nurses have expressed satisfaction with this type of organization. It provides a needed opportunity to become directly involved in decision making and encourages more active involvement in the organization.

Individual performance can be reviewed through peer review by having nurses conduct formal evaluations based on recognized standards well-known to the person being evaluated. Trust and forth-rightness on the part of nurses must be present if peer review is to serve an effective purpose.

The American Nurses' Association has established standards for nursing practice to acquaint the public with expectations for its practitioners, to protect the public from persons deviating from those standards, and to assure that high standards are maintained. Preceptorships have been created to provide ample opportunity for meeting the needs of new graduates in the work environment. The ultimate goal is to allow them to function independently as quickly as possible. Experience with the program indicates that less strain, burnout, and tension result, as compared with the traditional form of orientation.

Commitment to nursing implies that individual nurses are willing to work continuously to improve and upgrade nursing care. In order to further their professional development and enhance their practice, many nurses will have to acquire additional educational preparation and clinical experience. As nurses, individually and collectively, improve their knowledge and skills, nursing itself will profit and advance closer to genuine professionalism. Although, nursing has made tremendous progress in efforts to improve its status with the public and other health providers, the goal of true professionalism can only be reached if nurses continue to strive for it.

REFERENCES

1. Fagin, C. and McClure, M. "Can We Bring Order Out of the Chaos of Nursing?" *American Journal of Nursing* 76:1 (January, 1976), 103.
2. Conway, M. "Accountability and Its Acceptance by Professional Nurses," in M. Batey (ed.), *Communicating Nursing Research Priorities: Choice or Chance.* Boulder, Co.: Western Interstate Commission on Higher Education, 1977, 82.
3. *Ibid.*
4. Christman, L. "The Autonomous Nursing Staff in the Hospital," *Nursing Digest* 6:4 (Summer, 1978), 71.
5. Joel, L. (ed.), "Self-Regulation Protects Nursing's Growing Edge," *American Nurse* 16:2 (February, 1984), 42.
6. Schlotfeldt, R. "Nursing in the Future," *Nursing Outlook* 29:5 (May, 1981), 299.
7. "4.3—Accountability," in *Code for Nurses with Interpretive Statement.* Kansas City, Mo.: American Nurses' Association, 1976, 10.
8. Clifford, J. "Managerial Control Versus Professional Autonomy: A Paradox," *Journal of Nursing Administration* 11:9 (September, 1981), 20.
9. *Ibid.,* 21.
10. Manthey, M., Ciske, K., Robertson, P. "Primary Nursing," *Nursing Forum* 9:1 (1970), 65–66.
11. Beercroft, P. "A Contractual Model for the Department of Nursing" *Journal of Nursing Administration* 18:9 (September, 1988), 20.
12. Joel, L. "Changes in the Hospital as a Place of Practice," in J. McCloskey and Helen Grace (eds.), *Current Issues in Nursing* (3d. ed.), St. Louis: C.V. Mosby, 1990, 179.
13. *Ibid.*
14. Pannell, M. "Teaching Hospitals Build Models for Nursing Organization," *Hospitals* 56:3 (February 1, 1982), 63.
15. Springarn, N. "Primary Nurses Bring Back One-on-One Care," *The New York Times Magazine* (December 26, 1982), 22.
16. Ciske, K. "Primary Nursing: An Organization that Promotes Professional Practice," *Journal of Nursing Administration* 4:1 (January–February, 1974), 31.
17. *Ibid.*
18. Clifford, J. "Managerial Control Versus Professional Autonomy," 20.
19. Zander, K. "Nursing Case Management: Strategic Management of Cost and Quality Outcomes," *Journal of Nursing Administration* 18:5 (May, 1988), 25.
20. *Ibid.*
21. *Ibid.,* 29.
22. *Ibid.,* 30.
23. Zimmer, M. "Rationale for a Ladder for Clinical Advancement in Nursing Practice," *Journal of Nursing Administration* 2:6 (June, 1972), 18–24.
24. Bracken, R. and Christman, L. "An Incentive Program Designed to Develop and Reward Clinical Competence," *Journal of Nursing Administration* 7:6 (December, 1977), 9, 18.
25. Zimmer, M. "Rationale for a Ladder for Clinical Advancement," 18–24.
26. Ulsafer-Van Lanen, J. "Lateral Promotion Keeps Skilled Nurses in Direct Patient Care," *Hospitals* 55:5 (March, 1981), 87–90.

27. Haymor, P. "Career Ladder—Back to the Bedside," *Supervisor Nurse* 9:2 (February, 1978), 33–36.
28. Bracken, R. and Christman, L. "An Incentive Program," 18.
29. Knox, S. "A Clinical Advancement Program," *Journal of Nursing Administration* 10 (July, 1980), 29.
30. Colavecchio, R., Pescher, B. and Scalzi, C. "A Clinical Ladder for Nursing Practice," *Journal of Nursing Administration* 4:5 (September–October, 1974), 54–58.
31. Kimbro, C. and Gifford, A. "The Nursing Staff Organization: A Needed Development," *Nursing Outlook* 28:10 (October, 1980), 610, 616.
32. Carson, F. and Ames, A. "Nursing Staff Bylaws," *American Journal of Nursing* 80:6 (June, 1980), 1130.
33. Sample, S. "Development of Organizational Bylaws," *Nursing Clinics of North America* 13:3 (March, 1978), 95.
34. Carson, F. and Ames, A. "Nursing Staff Bylaws," 1130.
35. Sample, S. "Development of Organizational Bylaws," 95.
36. Beercroft, P. "A Contractual Model for the Department of Nursing," 20.
37. Dock, L. and Stewart, I. *Short History of Nursing.* 3d ed., New York: G. P. Putnam's Sons, 1931.
38. "Code for Professional Nurses," *American Journal of Nursing* 60:9 (September, 1960), 1287.
39. National League for Nursing. "The Origin of the State Board Test Pool Examination Service," *Nursing Outlook* 12 (1964), 55.
40. Hinsvark, I. "Credentialing in Nursing," in J. McCloskey and H. Grace (eds.), *Current Issues in Nursing.* Boston: Blackwell Scientific Publications, 1981, 322.
41. Schlotfeldt, R. "Nursing in the Future," 299.
42. "AJN—Special Report: A National Survey on State Action on Entry into Practice," *American Journal of Nursing* 78 (1978), 535.
43. Hinsvark, I. "Credentialing in Nursing," 322.
44. Schlotfeldt, R. "Nursing in the Future," 299.
45. "Credentialing Serves Public, Profession, says Keynoter," *American Nurse* 16:6 (June, 1984), 7.
46. *Ibid.*
47. *Ibid.*
48. "RN Groups Eye National Certifying Board," *American Journal of Nursing* 89:3 (March, 1989), 414.
49. *Ibid.*
50. "Liaison Forum Hears Vital Issues," *American Nurse* 22:1 (January, 1989), 37.
51. Markway, P. "How to Become Certified in 1990," *American Nurse* 22:2 (February, 1990) 23.
52. "Credentialing Center Set to Incorporate in 1991," *American Nurse* 22:6 (June, 1990), 14.
53. *Ibid.*
54. Passos, J. "Accountability: Myth or Mandate," *Journal of Nursing Administration* 3:3 (May–June, 1973), 18.
55. *Ibid.*

56. Moore, K. "Quality Assurance and Nursing Audit: Are They Effective?" *Nursing Management* 13 (February, 1982), 18.
57. *The QA Guide: A Resource for Hospital Quality Assurance.* Chicago: Joint Commission on Accreditation of Hospitals, 1980, xii.
58. Joint Commission on Accreditation of Hospitals. *Accreditation Manual for Hospitals.* 1983 ed. Chicago: Joint Commission on Accreditation of Hospitals, 1983, 116.
59. *Ibid.,* 118.
60. Merton, R. "The Search for Professional Status," *American Journal of Nursing* 60:5 (May, 1960), 662.
61. Metcalf, H. and Urwick, L. (eds.), *Dynamic Administration: The Collected Papers of Mary Follett.* New York: Harper and Brothers, 1942, 136.
62. *Standards of Nursing Practice.* Kansas City, Mo.: American Nurses' Association, 1973, 2.
63. *Ibid.,* 105.
64. "New JCAHO Data Spotlights Quality Problems," *American Journal of Nursing* 90:5 (May, 1990), 18.
65. Bradley, K. "JCAHO Discussions Set for Fall," *American Nurse* 22:5 (May, 1990), 4.
66. "New JCAHO Data Spotlights Quality Problems," 18.
67. Moore, W. *The Professions: Roles and Rules.* New York: Russell Sage Foundation, 1970, 8.
68. Christman, L. "Leadership in Practice," *Image: The Journal of Nursing Scholarship* 12:2 (June, 1980), 32.
69. Clarke, A. "Candidly Speaking: On Nursing Forum and Professionalism," *Nursing Forum* 7:1 (January, 1968), 12.
70. Christman, L. "Leadership in Practice," 32.
71. Aiken, L. *Nursing in the 1980s: Crises, Opportunities, Challenges.* Philadelphia: J. B. Lippincott, 1982, xvi.

SUGGESTED READINGS

Aleksandrowicz, L. and Dickau, S. "A Clinical Ladder," *Nursing and Health Care* 4:9 (November, 1983), 510–514.

ANA Today. "ANA New Agency Launch Nursing Standards Project," *American Nurse* 22:9 (October, 1990), 11.

Anderson, M. and Denyes, M. "A Ladder for Clinical Advancement in Nursing: Implementation," *Journal of Nursing Administration* 5:2 (February, 1975), 16–22.

Blenkorn, H., D'Amico, M. and Virtu, E. "Primary Nursing and Job Satisfaction," *Nursing Management* 19:4 (April, 1988), 41–42.

Cushing, M. "Expanding the Meaning of Accountability," *American Journal of Nursing* 83:10 (October, 1983), 1472.

Dugan, A. "Nursing Autonomy: Key to Quality Nurturance," *Journal of Nursing Administration* 1:6 (July–August, 1971), 51.

Fickeissen, J. "56 Ways to Get Certified," *American Journal of Nursing* 90:3 (March, 1990), 50–57.

Hegedus, K. and Bourdon, S. "Evaluation Research: A Quality Assurance Program," *Nursing Administrative Quarterly* 5:3 (Spring, 1981), 26–30.

Holmes, A. "Problem-Printed Medical Records, Nursing Audit and Accountability," *Supervisor Nurse* 11:4 (April, 1980), 40.

Isquith, R. "HHS News," U.S. Department of Health and Human Services, (September 20, 1990), 1.

Kaska, M. "Quality—Thy Name is Nursing Care," *Hospitals* 63:3 (February 5, 1989), 32.

Luke, R., Krueger, J., and Modrow, R. (eds.), *Organization and Change in Health Care Quality Assurance.* Rockville, Md.: Aspen Systems Corp., 1983.

McKenna, P. "The Community Nursing Audit . . . How To Make the Audit Work," *Nursing Administrative Quarterly* 4:4 (Summer, 1980), 75–82.

Manthey, M. "Myths that Threaten . . . What Primary Nursing Really Is," *Nursing Management* 19:6 (June, 1988), 54–55.

Morrow, K. *Preceptorships in Nursing Staff Development,* Rockville, Md.: Aspen Systems Corp., 1984.

Mullins, A., Colavecchio, R., and Tescher, B. "Peer Review: A Model for Professional Accountability," *Journal of Nursing Administration* 9:12 (September, 1979), 25–30.

Peplau, H. "Is Nursing's Self-Regulatory Power Being Eroded?" *American Journal of Nursing* 85:2 (February, 1985), 141–143.

Phaneuf, M. and Lang, N. "Standards of Nursing Practice," in R. Piemonte and I. Hirsch. *Issues in Professional Nursing Practice.* (No. 7 in series) Kansas City, Mo.: American Nurses' Association, 1984.

"Project L.I.N.C. (Ladders in Nursing Careers): An Innovative Model of Educational Mobility," *Nursing and Health Care* 10:10 (September, 1989), 398.

Sanford, R. "Clinical Ladders: Do They Serve Their Purpose?" *Journal of Nursing Administration* 17, 34–37.

Schutzenhofer, K., "The Measurement of Professional Autonomy," *Journal of Professional Nursing* 3:5 (September–October, 1987), 278–283.

Schmodl, J. "Quality Assurance: Examination of the Concept," *Nursing Outlook* 27:7 (July, 1979), 462–464.

Tousley, M. "Certification as a Credential: What Are the Issues?" *Perspectives in Psychological Care* 20:1 (January, 1982), 23–26.

STRATEGIES TO ADVANCE PROFESSIONALIZATION, PRESENT AND FUTURE

VI

Power and Motivation: Essential Elements for Professionalism

13

INTRODUCTION

Nursing currently recognizes its need for power and is seeking ways in which to strengthen and obtain additional power for its members. However, there are many nurses who do not understand why nursing needs to build a strong power-base among its practitioners. In fact, the concept of power has been given serious consideration only within the last decade. Nurses must not only understand the nature and meaning of power and its importance in the professionalization process but also how power can provide freedom to act in the best interest of patients. Questions such as "Who are the power holders?" and "How power is acquired?" are rarely asked by practicing nurses.

A sizable number of nurses in the 1990s continue to base their practice on the technical aspects of care, which is highly acceptable to hospital administrators and physicians. "The dull, monotonous grind of taking care of patients by routines, procedures, policies, and rules can hardly be labeled professional practice."[1] To implement nursing care that necessitates the application of knowledge based on research findings in the solution of patients' problems requires an intellectual process on the part of professional practitioners. "There is a clear choice to be made between the role expression of knowledge as innovation, risk taking, and exciting, or as dull, safe, and constrained."[2]

Unfortunately, professional practice, growth of professional practitioners of nursing, and nursing's need for power have never been of prime concern to hospital administrators or physicians. Furthermore, because the majority of professional nurses lack hospital privileges for admitting patients to health care institutions, their power and influence as compared with physicians are extremely limited. Power accrues to professions that are instrumental in providing resources that are highly valued. This power enables such professions to obtain more of those critical resources allocated within the institution. In other words, power obtained from acquiring resources can be used to produce more power—power begets power. Although nurses do not add to the financial base of the hospital by increasing patient census, they do produce substantial revenues through the nursing care provided, a benefit for which little recognition is given. This lack of recognition in most U.S. hospitals should help convince nurses that an attempt to gain power to achieve personal and professional goals is neither inappropriate nor unprofessional.

What strength could be generated if nurses united and as one cohesive group let their voices be heard as they clamor for changes in the health care delivery system and in reimbursement policies for their members. Through acquiring third-party reimbursement (fee-for-service), nurses and their contributions would be recognized and their power to negotiate would be considerably strengthened. To rely on negotiation alone to accomplish professional goals would be futile unless the negotiating groups have equal power. Nursing must acquire such power if nurses' ideals for better health care for all Americans are to be realized. Nursing represents the largest group of health workers in the country, numbering over 2,000,000 registered nurses.

> Nursing's greatest resource is people. For too long nurses have underestimated the power they have in being the largest group of health professionals in the nation. If nurses as a group mobilized for patient advocacy, they could radically change the picture of health care delivery in the United States.[3]

Margaret N. Heckler, former Secretary of Health and Human Services, in addressing the audience during the 1984 ANA convention observed that "there is great power in your numbers . . . and through your representatives in Washington we are obviously aware you have the numbers that will make other's listen."[4]

> It's a different thing to use power in a position of potency. Perhaps it's time we look at our situation anew. If things are really changed, then let's consider how to act from strength rather than from weakness. . . .[n]egotiating from strength may feel a little different than negotiating from weakness. The only way to find out is to put on the new role. We might like it.[5]

Nurses often experience and declare themselves powerless, forgetting the tremendous potential for power within their ranks. Using power to influence others and to utilize knowledge in improving health care will strengthen nursing's determination to assure society the best possible care. Moreover, as nursing's power increases, the push for professionalization will be heightened, also.

One author states that she "doesn't know what it will take to make nurses . . . reach out intellectually and emotionally toward implementing a powerful professional model."[6] She believes that " . . . we need to cultivate our ability to steer our power away from the narrow focus of power in nursing to the broader one of power within the health care system."[7] As reflected at the 1989 NLN Convention in Seattle, there was "[a] shift away from internal, professional concerns toward health issues in the nation and the world."[8] And yet, this change in focus will not necessarily remedy the problems that beset nursing in its efforts to achieve true professionalism nor will it eliminate them in their entirety.

These problems should be addressed. Acquiring *power* in the health arena can move nursing to seek solutions for them. I repeat—*they will not go away!* Moreover, "to the extent that we abrogate our responsibility for professional decision making and fail to collaborate with other nurses in exercising power, we fail our patients, ourselves, and our profession."[9]

Luther Christman, one of the leading proponents for effectively mobilizing nurse power, has repeatedly stated that power, to a great extent, is connected with "the strength of basic preparation and entry into the field," and examining the educational process is crucial to all other issues.[10]

> Unlike all major professional groups, nurses are splintered into opposing camps from the outset of their preparatory programs. The discord which emanates from having such varied educational entries into the field greatly inhibits the development of unity. Cooperation is unlikely when "turf protection" is a primary concern. . . . An esprit de corps is impossible when an atmosphere of petty jealousies dominate our deliberation. . . .
>
> For far too long nurses have focused their attention on the educational preparation of nurses compared to other nurses, instead of looking at nurses compared to significant others in the health care field. . . . Books and articles on nursing as a semiprofession will continue to flourish until nurses make a commitment to full professional education.[11]

Until such time as the difference in educational preparation between nurses and other health professionals is removed, nurses' power will be limited.

CONCEPT OF POWER DEFINED

If power can be acquired by having an occupation's expertise recognized by society and by gaining monopoly over services in which it alone can claim to have expertise, then the process of professionalization can be greatly facilitated by concentrating on such means for acquiring a strong power base. "Public belief in the competence of a profession to educate, evaluate, and socialize its practitioners through lengthy processes is a prerequisite to attaining power."[12]

The discrepancy between nursing's responsibility and authority in health care institutions prevents its practitioners from being accountable, even though employers expect such accountability. Ample evidence attests to this fact. Unless power is valued, since it controls resources needed by professionals, it cannot influence their behavior. Whether power is insufficiently valued by nurses or whether it seems beyond their ability to acquire continues to be an issue.

First, however, the concept of power must be clearly understood and valued before nurses will be willing to exert their collective efforts toward acquiring and increasing power, both individually and as a group. There are many nurses, however, who have ceased to complain about their "powerlessness" and are demonstrating that power can be achieved when competence, skills, and expertise are recognized as needed by the public and other health professionals.

Sociologists and political scientists have attempted to define power for a long time. Taken in its broadest context, power may be defined as the ability to influence and change the behavior of others. As the individual or group's power increases in a given situation, the more effective the influence will be. Power is the source of influence, although influence can be exerted by individuals having little or no power. Several renowned scientists in history, for example, have greatly affected the thinking of other individuals and their findings have altered behavior, but they have had little or no personal power at all. Power implies the vigor or strength to control or command others. It is the "ability to employ force, not its actual employment, the ability to apply sanctions, not the actual application . . . [since it has] the predisposition of prior capacity which makes the application of force possible."[13] Moreover, "it is associated with autonomy, control of practice, and organizational influence."[14]

Health professionals have been "under fire" from consumers, who complain about the excessive costs of health care and the impersonal treatment received. As a result, the power bases of some professions are beginning to show signs of erosion from a weakening of their public image. "Power is also temporary and continually shifting, in accordance with changing pressures and tension [and] there are no guarantees of permanent power, though it may last longer if it is earned or sanctioned as legitimate, leading to acquiescence by the less powerful."[15]

Nurses, for many years, have observed the power plays that the medical profession engages in to increase its power and resources. Physicians continue relentlessly to validate their public image by acquainting the public with new techniques, equipment, and research efforts that will improve the nation's health and keep physicians in great demand. "Physicians have been able to maintain high public visibility through the press, their contributions, and their dominant leadership role in health care issues, decisions, and legislative actions."[16] Consequently, the public continues to believe that the medical profession safeguards their most important commodity—health. Interprofessional relationships can be problematic due to the imbalance of power among the different professions, particularly nursing as it relates to medicine and hospital administration. The fact that nurses as women lack power affects their bargaining power. However, to acquire more power, some power must have been obtained. "Power is not identical with professional label, although some types of professionals seem to have more of it than others and contending for power is a prominent activity in situations involving multiple professions."[17]

> The different types of professionals in an organization each have their own requirements for carrying out their mission. They also are likely to have differing ideas about where the organization is going and what are its conditions for more or less open competition and conflict among distinctive groups within the organization.[18]

In attempting to answer where power comes from, various authors such as French and Raven describe five major sources of power:

> **Reward power**—implies the use of sanctions such as recognition, monetary awards, opportunities for travel, and greater visibility
> **Coercive power**—ability to inflict punishment or withhold rewards for nonacquiescent behavior
> **Legitimate power**—power derived from values and beliefs held; vested in positions accepted by organizational members
> **Referent power**—based on basic attractiveness of the person that others identify with and aim to please
> **Informational power**—arising from the ability to access and share information[19]

Each of these sources has been discussed by sociologists interested in studying power sources. They are each used by nurses in fulfilling their nursing roles.

EXPANSION OF NURSING'S POWER BASE

A review of nursing literature on power reveals that although nursing's power base and potential for increased power is substantial, it has not been used to greatly advance the goal of professionalism. The power of nurse leaders, national professional nursing associations, and the collectivity of nursing to achieve unity and consensus on issues involving education, autonomous practice, and monopoly over practice has not been highly successful.

> . . . groups within nursing often act like separate classes competing with each other for status in the system. A collective class consciousness on the part of the total nursing community is largely noticeable by its absence. As a result, collective action on any national scale is almost unheard of, and the powers of the several groups are scattered in many diverse directions.[20]

In 1973, it was observed that powerful groups making decisions affecting the future of nursing are hardly threatened by nurses representing a health field majority that is, indeed, a silent one.[21] Thus, nursing over the next twenty-five years is faced with the severe challenge of acquiring a "strong resource and power base" in order to move ahead.[22]

In fact, since the beginning of nursing's history, the absence of such a power base has limited nursing's movement in achieving its potential. Economic conditions throughout the remainder of this century will make the achievement of such a base very difficult.[23] Individuals and groups recognized for their expertise and professionalism are generally observed to have power and are accorded privileges by the public because of their expertise. If "power begets power" then a group with limited power that unites will strengthen its power base. However, nursing has yet to reach consensus on what its specific expertise is and how it can be demonstrated in order to obtain recognition from other health professionals and the public.

In previous chapters it was pointed out that loyalty to the institution rather than to nursing, the existence of supervisory personnel over nurses' work, and a strong tradition of acquiescence to authority continue to promote dependency of nurses. These factors also decrease nursing's bases of power. Presently, neither physicians nor hospital administrators are overly concerned about nursing's power, which to date has not been highly visible. As previously mentioned, the power struggle currently experienced between doctors and nurses may alter this situation in the decades ahead.

In order for nursing to achieve greater independence and power it must convince physicians and the public of the legitimate services it has to offer beyond that of "producing that which physicians wish to dispense in the name of health care."[24] If the prevention of illness and emphasis on health or wellness is equally as important as curing disease, then nurses must attain power to have their message of health promotion attended to by society. "Without the capacity to act, we are powerless to carry out our social contract, and thus, are deserving of no one's trust."[25]

POWER—POTENTIAL FOR EFFECTING CHANGE

It has been said that nurses' potential power was negated in the past by the "internal power struggles between cliques." However, the potential for power in nursing is considerable and should make nurses willing to unite to exercise it to the fullest extent.[26] To move nursing closer to authentic professionalism or to effect any significant changes in health care delivery, nurses must use their power to reach agreement on such goals.

Nursing derives its greatest power source from a dynamic professional association that is substantially supported by its members.[27] Many nurses agree with this statement. But as mentioned in previous chapters, only approximately 195,500 nurses are members of the professional nurses association when over 2,000,000 nurses are currently registered. Such a low percentage of membership significantly dilutes this important source of power.

Progress made by the ANA, despite its problems with membership, in accomplishing goals for improved economic security, in upgrading nursing education to a collegiate level, in defining nursing, and in establishing standards for practice, should be acknowledged. Power is what is needed to move these accomplishments beyond the verbalization stage into specific actions. Unless positive movement occurs, written standards, definitions, and other resources become meaningless. It was noted in 1974 that although positions on issues were taken, they were not followed by action.[28] Can it be stated almost two decades later that this is no longer true? As important as action is for reaching these articulated goals, the philosophy of administration in nursing departments is equally crucial to achieving them.

POLITICAL ACTIVISM TO INCREASE NURSE POWER

The need for nurses to become politically active has appeared frequently in nursing literature throughout the 1970s and into the 1980s.[29–33] For nursing to increase its power and have its interests represented it must emerge as a political force. To accomplish this goal, nurses are beginning to be more politically active. In the past, nursing has tended to isolate itself from policy-making groups and not assert its views. In fact, nursing's contribution in discussions aimed at solving the nation's health care problems has been noticeably lacking, with the exception of a few nurse leaders who are serving on boards of directors and national inter-disciplinary health teams. Another problem mentioned many times throughout this book—that nursing's internal strife has given it an image of conflict—has prevented nursing from making any serious impact on health policy decisions.

In reviewing literature on nursing's lack of political involvement, many of the factors discussed in earlier chapters are frequently presented: the predominance of women in nursing, poor self and occupational image, lack of confidence, interest, assertiveness, and fear of confronting other health professionals. Unfortunately, nursing has allowed other health care disciplines to assume responsibility for shaping national and local health policies. However, as the focus in health care gradually changes from illness to wellness, nurses will be in the forefront in shaping health policies for the future. Shaping such policies will occur through the use of *political power* that allows people, organizations, and associations to make sure their concerns are addressed.[34] Furthermore, "nurses have political power because of their numbers, because their organizational structure contains all of the elements necessary to yield influence, and because nurses are informed, active, and dedicated people."[35] However, nurses should become better informed about proposed and existing legislation affecting health care issues and organization and, where possible, enroll in courses that will increase and enlighten them about the political process. "The nurse of tomorrow must understand the nature of power and politics . . . [and] will need to know about political behavior, political processes, and their conse-quences."[36]

Marilyn Goldwater, former Congresswoman and registered nurse from Maryland, observes that "because many health-related issues are decided in state legislatures and Congress, it is important for all of us to consider how we, as nurses, can influence legislative bodies."[37] She offers the following lobbying tips:

1. Work through your professional organizations. They will keep you informed about current issues.
2. Know who your friends are in the state legislature and in Con-gress. Keep in touch with them; support them.
3. Become familiar with the committees that handle health legis-lation. Both at the state and federal level, the real spadework is done in committees. This is where you can be most effective.

4. Get to know your own local representatives. Question their stands on health legislation and let them know where you stand.
5. Increase your influence by supporting candidates in a campaign. Be active in N-CAP and the political action group of your state association. If your state doesn't have one, organize one.
6. Remind candidates that 1 out of every 44 registered women voters is a registered nurse and that registered nurses have families and friends who endorse candidates and contribute to their campaigns.[38]

To assist nurses to improve their political skills, the ANA, as part of their "Nurses: Visible in Politics" program, sponsored workshops in Boston, Miami, Chicago, and San Francisco in 1984–1985. Designed to "help nurses gain recognition as a political force and to get results from their political activities," topics under discussion consisted of lobbying for legislation and how to secure appointments for nurses.[39] In addition, information on political resources and materials and techniques for building influence were provided.

Nursing, through the employment of ANA nurse lobbyists in Washington, is well represented at the national level. Through active and intense lobbying efforts, several bills vital to nursing have been passed. For example, certain nurse practitioners are now receiving third-party reimbursement, due to nurses convincing certain members of Congress that they were well prepared to provide primary care in underserved areas. This reimbursement for nurse-midwives and other types of nurse practitioners has occurred through nurses' successful lobbying efforts. Changes in nurse practice acts throughout the various states, and continuation of the Nurse Training Act over several years, have been the result of nursing's visibility and skillful use of political strategies in achieving these goals.

Senator Daniel Inouye of Hawaii, in writing the Foreword to *Politics of Nursing*, raised four pertinent questions that nurses should consider:

1. Why has not a sufficient number of professional nurses been promoted to nonclinical leadership positions, for example, in the area of developing health policy on both the state and federal levels?
2. Why hasn't the nursing profession utilized the true extent of their potential political power?
3. Do our nations' nurses really want to be true professionals—are they willing to accept and, if necessary, to demand both the responsibility and prerogatives of power and authority?
4. Is there any serious institutional support for the development of a true cadre of professional nurses?[40]

Individually, nurses can evaluate themselves in light of these four questions. Their answers would, undoubtedly, enlighten those interested in the professionalization process. Unless nurses can convert their beliefs into positive actions about what nursing is and what, ideally, it must become it will be impossible to mobilize and empower nurses to reach their full potential in this evolving, powerful profession. "As we look to the future, we must prepare nurses to deal effectively and successfully with power and political behaviors within and outside the nursing profession [since] . . . to carve new pathways, achieve new goals in nursing and enter into true health partnerships, nurses must be politically oriented and goal-directed."[41]

MOTIVATION TO ACHIEVE CLINICAL EXCELLENCE AND PROFESSIONALISM

Over the past decades researchers have found that more successful groups possess a high degree of motivation as evidenced in their commitment to and interest in their work.[42] Since no two people are alike, their needs vary and may even differ within a specific individual from time to time. Some desire status, honors, and prestige; others seek financial gains or opportunities for personal and professional advancement. In most instances, individuals want their contributions and talents recognized. They want to feel that their presence in the organization does make a difference. The challenge for nurse leaders in organizations is to find ways to appeal to these individual motivations.

In many health care institutions, maintaining the status quo prevails, with energy and abilities being controlled rather than being allowed to freely express dynamic action, innovation, and creativity. "There is nothing that stifles motivation and productivity more quickly than not allowing individuals to do what they are prepared to do."[43] Changes in educational preparation, in quality of clinical practice involving increased intellectual knowledge and skills, and in intraprofessional and interprofessional sensitivity and skills are noticeably on the increase as nursing moves closer to true professionalism. With change occurring at a rapid rate, the means must be provided to assist individuals in coping with change and what it demands of them.

I agree that characteristics of professionalism viewed in isolation are insufficient to motivate nurses to achieve societal recognition. However, such characteristics serve to enlighten nursing and nurses as to which of them have yet to be achieved. As a result, the professional association and key nurse groups continue to strive diligently to reach the goal of professionalism. But apparently their efforts have not greatly affected the rank and file of nurses. As mentioned previously, many individuals are convinced that nursing has achieved professionalism. Thus, they see no reason to work toward a goal that they believe has already been accomplished.

What *is* needed to challenge and motivate nurses to become actively engaged in furthering their own professional development, while simultaneously advancing the status of nursing as a profession? Socializing new recruits about nursing's efforts to achieve professional status cannot be the only means to accomplish this goal. Perhaps if nurses in education and practice could address the needs and motives of individual nurses by first satisfying their needs for adequate compensation, etc., change in motivation might occur. To expect behavioral changes without understanding what motivates the behavior is futile. Nor can knowledge of existing needs alone spur individuals on with renewed vigor to embrace the need for change within themselves and within nursing. To arouse newer motivations implies the ability to understand the individuals' motive base and then to work toward mobilizing newer sources of motivational behavior.

Because nurse leaders have not been successful in arousing and elevating the hopes and aspirations of thousands of practicing nurses, a closer look at motivational needs may provide some answers to this failure. Two questions may serve to guide an in-depth look at the concept of motivation: What motivation makes individuals join an organization and remain with it? and What motivates individuals to exert energy and effort to meet the expectations of the organization?

If it could be said that all nurses are achieving the best that is in them, that their potential has been fully tapped, and that they are productive in meeting personal and professional goals, then there would be little need to work for the advancement of nursing. Realistically, the ideal of striving to fulfill one's highest potential is not highly visible among many nurses, nor has it served to inspire and increase enthusiasm for the pursuit of worthwhile goals.

If nursing could unlock talent lying dormant in many nurses, what positive changes would occur! Self-growth and determination to excel would become a "magnificent obsession" or an inner drive that is augmented by new challenges to succeed. "Striving for self-actualization and living up to our highest potential" can be achieved "through an awakening of our consciousness as a profession and as women, allowing us to overturn, overthrow, and reclaim what has been ours throughout time and through the integration of this consciousness into positive goals and gains."[44] Fortunately, nurses are changing their attitudes and goals toward the workplace.

> The new breed of workers will only respond to a participative style, never to edicts. . . . Knowledgeable workers will expect reasons, not 'manage-

ment might' to prevail; intellectual respect and challenge will be management's only real motivators.

Management's success in the 90's will depend on its ability to be that of inspirer and builder of cohesion and loyalty to the organization as opposed to the supervisor of timecards and rituals of the past.[45]

SYSTEMATIC THEORIES OF MOTIVATION

For several years, many theories of what motivates individuals to work and to be productive have been advanced. Theories of motivation attempt to explain the reasons why individuals act the way they do. Circumstances or conditions in work and personal life can be arranged to foster motivation. In a sense, however, people cannot be motivated. No matter how often efforts are expended to do so, people can only *motivate themselves*. And people do become motivated, even though in many instances their personal goals lack congruence with organizational goals. To the extent that organizational goals are in agreement with those of the individual, commitment to joint goals usually follows. The challenge lies in providing a climate or circumstances that will stimulate the inner drive required for motivation.

Hierarchy of Needs Theory

Abraham Maslow, a psychologist, developed an interesting theory of motivation which arranges human needs into a five-level taxonomy placed in a hierarchical order of prepotency (Fig. 13-1). According to this theory, basic human needs that are interdependent and motivate human behavior include the following:

> **Physiological needs**—include essentials such as food, water, housing, sleep, and clothing
>
> **Security or safety needs**—freedom from physical harm and fears involving loss of position, food, shelter, or property
>
> **Affiliation or acceptance needs**—for belonging, association, acceptance by others, giving and receiving love and friendship
>
> **Esteem needs**—for self-confidence, prestige, status, recognition, respect from others
>
> **Self-actualization needs**—for continued self-development, maximizing one's potential, being creative, and becoming all one is capable of becoming

Maslow's needs theory has become one of the most prominent theories of motivation found in the literature.

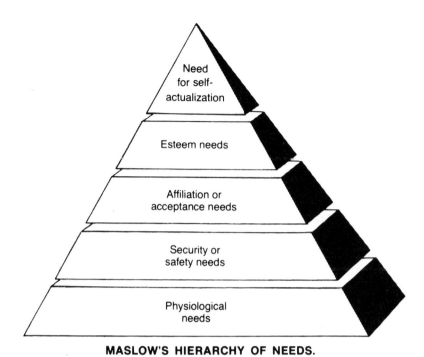

MASLOW'S HIERARCHY OF NEEDS.

Figure 13-1. Maslow's hierarchy of human needs. From Koontz, H. et al.
Essentials of Management, 3rd ed. New York: McGraw-Hill Book Co., 1982,
401. Copyright ©McGraw-Hill Book Co., 1970. *Reproduced with permission of publisher.*

> Maslow utilized the two concepts of deprivation and gratification to pro-
> vide the dynamic forces that linked needs to behavior . . . He postulated
> that deprivation or dissatisfaction of a need of high prepotency will lead to
> the domination of this need over the organism's personality . . . Relative
> gratification of a given need submerges it and "activates" the next higher
> need in the hierarchy. The activated need then dominates and organizes
> the individual's personality and capacities, so that instead of the individ-
> ual being hunger obsessed, he now becomes safety obsessed.
>   This process of deprivation-domination-gratification-activation con-
> tinues until the physiological, safety, affiliation and esteem needs have all
> been gratified and the self-actualization need has been activated.[46]

Since physiological and safety needs for professionals have been
reasonably met in today's society, the need for self-actualization, autonomy, recognition, and respect as competent professionals has increased.
Ordinarily professionals have a high degree of need for achievement and
self-actualization. They tend to be motivated by intrinsic rewards coming
from within the person rather than from external rewards or sanctions.[47]

"[P]rofessionals tend to seek rewards as full utilization of their talents and training; professional status [not necessarily within the organization, but externally with respect to their profession]; and opportunities for development and further learning."[48] In other words, "the 'good place' to work resembles a super-graduate school, alive with dialogue and senior colleagues, where the employee will work not only to satisfy organizational demands, but perhaps primarily, to fulfill self-imposed demands of his profession."[49]

Motivation-Hygiene Theory of Job Satisfaction

In recent years, the theory of motivation that has stimulated considerable research is referred to as the Motivation-Hygiene theory developed by Frederick Herzberg and his colleagues.[50] Presuming that the lower needs of society, as proposed by Maslow, are being met, Herzberg sought in a study of 200 engineers and accountants to find factors that would increase job satisfaction. Conclusions drawn from Herzberg's study reveal that there are conditions of the job that produce dissatisfaction when absent. However, their presence does not motivate employees to produce at higher levels. Ten factors referred to as hygiene factors, or dissatisfiers, are:

1. Company policy and administration
2. Supervision
3. Relationship with supervisor
4. Work conditions
5. Relationship with peers
6. Salary
7. Personal life
8. Relationship with subordinates
9. Status
10. Security

Other job conditions contributed to high levels of motivation and job satisfaction. Their absence, however, did not prove dissatisfying. Six motivational factors or satisfiers described by Herzberg were:

1. Achievement
2. Recognition
3. Advancement
4. Work itself
5. Growth
6. Responsibility

Figure 13-2 shows a comparison of Maslow's needs theory and Herzberg's two-factor theory and their resemblance to each other. Herzberg summarized his findings by stating that "the opposite of job satisfaction is not job dissatisfaction but, rather, no job satisfaction."[51]

Unless individuals find challenge in their work situation, they will lack motivation to strive for a high level of performance. Thus, nurse leaders must not only be aware of the significance of Herzberg's findings but also must endeavor to accentuate the satisfiers in the work content and decrease the dissatisfiers occurring in the context of the workplace. One concludes that satisfiers are dependent on decreasing or even eliminating the dissatisfiers.

Achievement Theory

The question of why some people are consistently more oriented toward achievement than others has been studied frequently by psycholo-

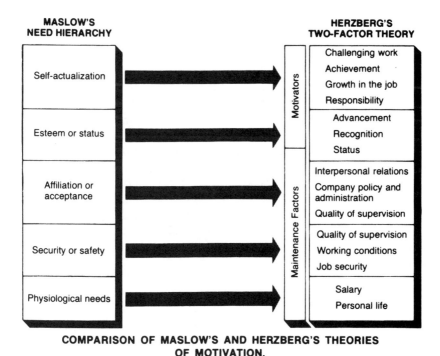

COMPARISON OF MASLOW'S AND HERZBERG'S THEORIES OF MOTIVATION.

Figure 13-2. Comparison of Maslow's and Herzberg's theories of motivation.
From Koontz, H. et al. *Essentials of Management*, 3rd ed. New York: McGraw-Hill Book Co., 1982, 403. Copyright ©McGraw-Hill Book Co., 1970.
Reproduced with permission of publisher.

gists for several years. Some regard it as a basic attitude toward life. Others concur that a strong achievement drive is what motivates certain individuals to demand more of themselves. These individuals delight in winning and in improving their performance, especially when given a challenge to do so. Not unduly concerned with monetary rewards, these individuals use money as a means to measure their progress rather than as a source of economic security. To foster goal-directed behavior, the need for achievement is essential if organizations and individuals within them are to succeed in achieving their goals.

David McClelland's Achievement Theory is one of the most interesting modern theories of motivation.[52] He identified three types of motivation needs: power, affiliation, and achievement. McClelland and colleagues have conducted considerable research on motivation, particularly on the achievement motive. His theory on achievement states that a person's desire to perform better is the result of a specific achievement motive that can be acquired through training and is not genetically produced.

Moreover, environmental factors can contribute and encourage the development of this motive. McClelland asserts that "most people in this world, psychologically, can be divided into two broad groups [because] there is that minority which is challenged by opportunity and willing to work hard to achieve something and the majority which really does not care all that much."[53] He believes that persons high in the achievement motive (an Ach motive) possess a specific type of human motivation and strongly prefer work situations where feedback can be readily obtained. Also, these individuals are given frequent raises and promotions since they constantly seek ways in which to improve their jobs. It appears that as the achievement motive increases so does the likelihood that the individual will achieve positions of greater power and responsibility.

Achievement motivation can be aroused in the workplace by allowing individuals to take calculated risks and be innovative, by providing recognition and reward for excellent performance, and by convincing them that they are part of a successful team.[54]

Value-Expectancy Theory

Another approach to understanding how individuals are motivated to act the way they do is the Value-Expectancy theory. Victor H. Vroom, a leader among the various psychologists providing explanations of this theory, asserts that individuals will be motivated to seek goals if they are convinced that the goals have value for them and that their performance will enable them to achieve them.[55] Of course, it is presumed that individuals possess the necessary ability and skills needed to perform the behavior and that they will work diligently to achieve the goal. Vroom's theory may be stated as:

$$\text{Motivational Force} = \text{value to be derived} \times \text{expectancy of receiving value}$$

Individuals must decide what values are of greater significance to themselves. Maslow's hierarchy of needs gives an understanding of human values, such as money and its importance to particular individuals. Herzberg's findings reveal that values of an intrinsic nature, such as pride or satisfaction in work accomplishment, can be far more potent in motivating people than any extrinsic values. However, the worth of Vroom's theory lies in the fact that it recognizes the individual motives and needs of each person. It shows how values for one individual can be very different from those of other persons. Thus, it seems to reflect reality more so than Maslow's and Herzberg's theories. It is quite logical to believe that an individual will "choose certain behaviors on the basis of the satisfactions he perceives as connected with the outcomes of such behavior and on the probability that his behavior will result in such outcomes."[56]

ONE MORE TIME: WILL NURSES BE MOTIVATED TO EXCEL AND ADVANCE NURSING AS A PROFESSION?

Perhaps one of the reasons nurses are not highly motivated to exert time, effort, and energy in excelling in their role or in advancing nursing is that, for many, nursing has lost some of its value. If the value attached to performance is not great, then little effort will be expended in seeking to acquire it. For nurses to behave as professionals, there must be a strong motivating force within them that convinces them of nursing's value and the rewards to be acquired by pursuing it.

> . . . nurses graduate, start practice and continue practice, seeing nursing as nothing more than a collection of knowledge and skills and finding nothing or no one in their environments to stimulate them to a broader perspective. The profession must . . . renew its efforts to reach them, but I question whether this can be done on the basis of national programs and goals. We have to start where *they* are, moving through a sort of professional adaptation of Maslow's hierarchy of needs.[57]

Motivation strengthens commitment and can be activated daily by individuals as they conscientiously strive for professionalism. According to Herzberg, when nurses have their own generator, they will need no outside stimulation, as they will *want* to perform and advance themselves.[58] How such a generator can be developed is a significant question in motivation theory.

If nurses are not motivated to improve their status through advanced educational preparation and autonomous practice, then what factors are needed to change this situation? What can nurse leaders do to assist other nurses in increasing their motivation and improving and advancing their status? I believe that nurses can be made to feel important as persons and be recognized as competent, respected professionals. Furthermore, I believe they must be given opportunities to realize their own potential, to continue self-development, and to engage in creative experiences as they desire.

However, many nurses are constantly struggling and diverting their energies to meet lower-level needs (job security, salary, etc.) and, as a result, their needs for self-fulfillment or self-actualization are rarely perceived. In order to obtain satisfaction from work, one's energies must not be depleted by unsatisfactory conditions in the work situation.

Moving from esteem needs to autonomy and ultimately to self-actualization will enable nurses to become self-motivated and require little or no supervision. For the collectivity of nurses to reach this goal, many changes in commitment, in level of educational preparation, and in organizational climate must first take place. Explicit trust in the ability and dedication of fellow nurses can enhance and encourage nurses to further their talents and increase their potential.

> . . . those of us who are in the grips of the vision of nursing as a social force dominating and reforming the health scene are like anxious, self-important diamond cutters, circling a giant uncut stone. We argue as to where the cleavage must be made to release its greatest brilliance; hesitant to act lest, through misstroke, the gem be shattered into dull bits of glass, swept into history's dustbin of unfilled promise.
>
> The fallacy in this drama is that there is no giant stone—only myriad smaller ones. It is in each of these—in each of us—that the radiance must be developed through each facet.[59]

SUMMARY

Power is an essential element in the professionalization process. However, the concept of power, its nature and meaning, has been given serious consideration by nurses only since the early 1970s. If power is generated by providing resources that society highly values, nursing must concentrate its efforts on convincing the public of the significance of its services. As power obtains greater resources within institutions, additional power is generated, and thus power begets more power.

Nursing outnumbers all other groups of health workers in the United States, with over 2,000,000 registered nurses providing health care services in the nation. The power of such numbers gives nursing the potential to make legislators and other health professionals listen. But greater unity among nurses must be realized. The quest for power will advance professionalization of nursing and ultimately, will assist in improving the quality of health care provided to society.

Interestingly, many nurses have ceased complaining about their lack of power and are demonstrating that power can be gained when nurses' competence and expertise are recognized as important commodities needed by the public. The imbalance of power among the different health professions and particularly nurses' lack of power, has hurt nursing's ability to negotiate with other health professions. Undoubtedly, the absence of a strong power base has severely limited nursing's ability to achieve full professionalism.

In order to increase its power, nursing should become more politically active and emerge as a powerful political force. Lack of political involvement has been attributed to the predominance of women in nursing, poor self-image, and fear of confrontation with other health professionals. As the focus of health care changes from illness to wellness, nurses need to be in the forefront in shaping future health policies.

To achieve increased power, clinical excellence, and professionalism, nurses will have to be strongly motivated to work toward their accomplishment. Several theories of motivation—Maslow's Needs Theory, Herzberg's Motivation-Hygiene Theory of job satisfaction, McClelland's Achievement Theory, and Vroom's Value-Expectancy Theory—describe the inner drives that propel people to pursue goals. Because individuals cannot be motivated by others, but only through their own efforts, an environment conducive to the pursuit of organizational goals is desirable. If nurses realize their own worth as persons and as professionals, no outside stimulation should be required, as they will want to improve their performance, advance their status, and continue their efforts to achieve self-development and self-actualization.

REFERENCES

1. Christman, L. "Effective Mobilization of Power," *Nursing Digest* 6:4 (Summer, 1978), 25.
2. *Ibid.*
3. Bowman, R. and Culpepper, R. "Power: Rx for Change," *American Journal of Nursing* 74:6 (June, 1974), 1056.
4. "A.N.A. '84, Challenging the Choices," *American Journal of Nursing* 84:7 (July, 1984), 917.

5. Barnum, B. "Power: We Love to Talk About It," *Nursing and Health Care* 10:10 (December, 1989), 531.
6. Smith, G. "More Power to You," *American Journal of Nursing* 89:3 (March, 1989), 358.
7. *Ibid.*
8. "Convention '89," *Nursing and Health Care* 10:7 (September, 1989), 370.
9. Boyle, K. "Power in Nursing: A Collaborative Approach," *Nursing Outlook* 32:3 (May–June, 1984), 164.
10. Christman, L. "Effective Mobilization of Power," 24.
11. *Ibid.*
12. Cabinet on Nursing Education. *Education for Nursing Practice in the Context of the 1980s,* (Pub. No.: NE-115M 4183). Kansas City, Mo.: American Nurses' Association, 1983, 4.
13. Bierstedt, R. "An Analysis of Social Power," *American Sociological Review* 15 (December, 1950), 733.
14. Cabinet on Nursing Education, *Education for Nursing Practice in the Context of the 1980's,* 4.
15. Leininger, M. "Political Nursing: Essential for Health Service and Education Systems of Tomorrow," *Nursing Administrative Quarterly* 2:2 (February, 1978), 2–3.
16. McFarland, D. and Shiflett, N. "The Role of Power in the Nursing Profession," *Nursing Dimensions* 7:2 (Summer, 1979), 3.
17. Bucher R, and Stelling, J. "Characteristics of Professional Organization," *Journal of Health and Social Behavior* 10:1 (March, 1969), 12.
18. *Ibid.*
19. French, J., Jr. and Raven, B. "The Bases of Social Power," in D. Cartwright (ed.), *Studies in Social Power.* Ann Arbor, Mich.: Institute of Social Research, University of Michigan, 1959, 150–167.
20. Ashley, J. "This I Believe About Power in Nursing," *Nursing Outlook* 21:10 (October, 1973), 640.
21. *Ibid.*
22. Kalisch, B. "The Promise of Power," *Nursing Outlook* 26:1 (January, 1978), 43.
23. *Ibid.*
24. Ashley, J. "This I Believe," 641.
25. "Work Hazards, Economic Value of Care Discussed," *American Nurse* 14:8 (September, 1982), 3.
26. Bowman, R. and Culpepper, R. "Power," 1056.
27. "Power, Professionalism Discussed," *A.N.A. Convention News* June 28, 1982, 3.
28. Bowman, R. and Culpepper, R. "Power," 1056.
29. Ashley, J. *Hospitals, Paternalism and the Role of the Nurse.* New York: Teacher's College, Columbia University Press, 1976, 21.
30. Kalisch, B. and Kalisch, P. *Politics of Nursing.* Philadelphia: J. B. Lippincott, 1982.
31. Lawrence, J. "Confronting Nurses' Political Apathy," *Nursing Forum* 15:4 (1976), 363.
32. Powell, J. "Nursing and Politics: The Struggle Outside Nursing's Body Politic," *Nursing Forum* 15 (1976), 341–362.

33. Archer, S. and Goehner, P. *Nurses: A Political Force*. North Scituate, Mass.: Wadsworth Health Sciences Division, 1982.
34. *'82–'84: Expanding Our Influence*. Kansas City, Mo.: American Nurses' Association, 1984.
35. *Ibid.*
36. Leininger, M. "Political Nursing," 3.
37. Goldwater, M. "From Legislator: View on Third-Party Reimbursement for Nurses," *American Journal of Nursing* 82:3 (March, 1982), 414.
38. *Ibid.*
39. "100 Nurses Learn Political Skills, Savvy at A.N.A Workshop," *American Nurse* 16:2 (February, 1984), 26.
40. Inouye, D. Foreword in B. Kalisch and P. Kalisch. *Politics of Nursing*. Philadelphia: J. B. Lippincott, 1982, x.
41. Leininger, M. "Political Nursing," 15.
42. Chopra, A. "Motivation in Task-Oriented Groups," in S. Stone, M. Berger, D. Elhart, S. Firsich and S. Jordan (eds.), *Management for Nurses: A Multidisciplinary Approach*. St. Louis: C. V. Mosby, 1976, 155.
43. Moraldo, P., "The Nineties: A Decade in Search of Meaning," *Nursing and Health Care* 11:1 (January, 1990), 13.
44. Watson, J. "Professional Identity Crisis—Is Nursing Finally Growing Up?" *American Journal of Nursing* 81:8 (August, 1981), 1490.
45. Moraldo, P., "The Nineties: A Decade in Search of Meaning," 13.
46. Maslow, A. *Motivation and Personality*. New York: Harper & Row, 1954, 38.
47. Wahba, M. and Bridwell, L. "Maslow Reconsidered: A Review of Research on the Need Hierarchy Theory," *Organizational Behavior and Human Performance*, Vol. 15:2 (April, 1976), 213.
48. Bennis, W. "New Patterns of Leadership for Tomorrow's Organizations," in S. Stone *et al.* (eds.), *Management for Nurses: A Multidisciplinary Approach*. St. Louis: C. V. Mosby, 1976, 119.
49. *Ibid.*
50. Herzberg, F., Mausner, B., and Snyderman, B. *The Motivation to Work*, 2d ed., New York: McGraw-Hill, 1972.
51. Herzberg, F. "One More Time: How Do You Motivate Employees?" *Harvard Business Review* 46:1 (January–February, 1968), 56.
52. McClelland, D., Atkinson, J., Clark, R. and Lowell, E. *The Achievement Motive*. New York: Appleton-Century-Crofts, 1953.
53. McClelland, D. "That Urge to Achieve," *Think* 32:6 (November–December, 1966), 19.
54. Litwin, G. and Stringer, R., Jr. *Motivation and Organizational Climate*. Boston: Division of Research, Graduate School of Business Administration, Harvard University, 1968, 189.
55. Vroom, V. *Work and Motivation*. New York: John Wiley & Sons, 1964.
56. Moloney, M. *Leadership in Nursing: Theory, Strategies, Action*. St. Louis: C. V. Mosby, 1979, 62.
57. Lewis, E. "The Professionally Uncommitted," *Nursing Outlook* 27:5 (May, 1979), 323.
58. Herzberg, F. "One More Time," 55.
59. Styles, M. *On Nursing: Toward a New Endowment*. St. Louis: C. V. Mosby, 1982, 113.

SUGGESTED READINGS

Bagwell, M. and Clements, S. *A Political Handbook for Health Professionals.* Boston: Little, Brown & Co. 1984.

Beck, C. "The Conceptualization of Power," *Advances in Nursing Science* 4:1 (January, 1982), 1–17.

Chaney, H. and Knebel, E. "Health Care Agencies and Power," in K. Stevens (ed.), *Power and Influence: A Source Book for Nurses.* New York: John Wiley & Sons, 1983.

Gordon, G. "Motivating Staff: A Look at Assumptions," *Journal of Nursing Administration* 12:11 (November, 1982), 27–29.

Hendricks, D. "The Power Problem," *Nursing Management* 13:10 (October, 1982), 23–24.

Howe, F. (ed.), *Women and the Power to Change.* New York: McGraw-Hill, 1975.

Janik, A. "Power Base of Nursing in Bargaining Relationships," *Image: The Journal of Nursing Scholarship* 16:3 (Summer, 1984), 93–96.

Kelly, L. "The Power of Powerlessness," *Nursing Outlook* 26:7 (July, 1978), 468.

Kennedy, M. *Powerbase: How to Build It—How To Keep It.* New York: Macmillan, 1984.

Larsen, J. "Nurse Power for the 80s," *Nursing Administrative Quarterly* 6:4 (Summer, 1982), 74–82.

"Nurses, Political Participation, and Attitudes Toward Reforms in the Health Care System," *Nursing and Health Care* 4:9 (November, 1983), 504–507.

Morris, L., "The War Between Doctors and Nurses," *Good Housekeeping* (July, 1983), 93–94; 169–172.

Moses, E. and Roth, A. "Nurse Power: What Do Statistics Reveal About the Nation's Nurses?" *American Journal of Nursing* 79:10 (October, 1979), 1745–1746.

Wieczorek, E. *Power, Politics and Policy in Nursing.* New York: Springer Publishing Co., 1984.

Futuristic View of Nursing in the 1990s and Beyond

14

INTRODUCTION

Any attempt to envision what nursing may become by the end of this century can only be speculative. Yet a vision of what could be is brought closer to reality by nurses who boldly dream of a future in which nursing is recognized as a scientific primary health profession. Such a vision creates optimism, encourages the faint-hearted, and motivates nurses to work unceasingly for the professionalization of nursing.

Nurses should be concerned about future directions for nursing. As the twenty-first century approaches, opportunities abound to facilitate movement toward the goal of full professional status. Whether nursing will have a bright, new professional image depends on how conscientious and industrious nurses are in their efforts to achieve professionalism. If nursing is to fulfill its social mandate for providing optimum health care for society, then nurses should be responsible and committed to this endeavor. In order for nursing to become a recognized, scientific profession, dynamic action is required, especially on the part of those referred to as professionals.

Nursing will be recognized as a science if nurse researchers and nurse scientists identify and study phenomena of unique concern to nursing. By studying concepts related to such phenomena and their derived hypotheses, nurse researchers and nurse practitioners will, ultimately, establish nursing as a scientific field serving society with expert knowledge, compassion, and competence.

PERSPECTIVES ON THE HEALTH CARE SYSTEM OF THE FUTURE

Some major health policy issues facing the U.S. in the 1990s that demand resolution revolve around health care costs, access to care, and changes in the health care delivery system. Public expectations for health care delivery have changed. Citizens not only are frustrated with the present health delivery system but also are demanding that radical changes occur in the foreseeable future.

No other country allocates as much of its resources—over $600 billion annually to health care, as does the United States.[1-3] And yet, in the last decade of this century, 37 million Americans have no access to health care since they lack health insurance or cannot afford care for themselves and their families. "The demand for health coverage for the uninsured and underinsured will continue as will the demand for coverage of long-term care for the elderly."[4] Most nurses agree that economic conditions can be conducive to creating needed changes in nursing. Moreover, the excessive cost of health care should allow nursing to move adroitly in capitalizing on its unlimited potential for providing more economical health care delivery.[5] For example, as health promotion and wellness become a national priority, the public can anticipate staying well and will seek alternative, noninstitutional settings for health care, such as community health centers or their own homes. Earlier discharge of patients from acute care settings is already creating a substantial decline in hospital in-patient census. In fact, significant changes in health care reimbursement have drastically altered the number of admissions in many hospitals.

Health Maintenance Organizations (HMO) and Preferred Provider Organizations (PPO) are affecting hospital census in addition to the Prospective Payment System (PPS) that encourages early hospital discharge. As a result, the trend toward more closures of community-based hospitals will hinder access to care while depriving local areas of the income generated by employment in these institutions. "Health care services must be made available to the unemployed, the indigent, the homeless, the well and the sick and to vulnerable populations like the elderly, children, the mentally ill, persons with HIV infection, and individuals with chronic diseases, if we really believe that health care is a right for all persons and not a privilege for only those who can afford it."[6] In a tightened economy, nursing will continue to have difficulty implementing future goals. However, "adversity need not be an impossible obstacle to progress."[7]

"Control over the labor supply coupled with monopolization of a socially significant function seems to be the *sine qua non* of a professional."[8] If the supply of nurses cannot be controlled by nursing, and if other health workers can be substituted to replace nursing personnel, then monopoly over nursing practice and the social significance of its services cannot be assured. Until nursing is recognized as the sole provider of services that society considers indispensable, efforts to achieve professional status will fail. Lobbying efforts with Congressional leaders to assure nursing's legitimate right to these services must continue until success is achieved. Strategic planning by individual nurses to accomplish long-range goals can be helpful, but unless a national plan of action acceptable to the majority of nurses can be agreed upon, nursing will continue to progress at a relatively slow rate.

The approach of the next century should remind nurses that their struggle to achieve professionalism has continued for over a century. Progress has been made—but the goal of full professional status has yet to be achieved. How practicing nurses respond to the plans and recommendations over the next fifteen to twenty years will determine nursing's future. Only nurses can implement the changes required to advance nursing from an evolving profession to a genuine, true profession.

Thus, nurses should direct nursing's future course of action and not allow other health professions to determine its direction. Disinterestedness and negative attitudes can be overcome. Now is the time to change fragmented, diversified views into positive, meaningful action that only a united group can achieve.

NATIONAL HEALTH OBJECTIVES

Efforts of the U.S. Public Health Service under the auspices of the Institute of Medicine to determine strategies to upgrade the nation's health for the twenty-first century, resulted in publication in 1990 of the National Health Prevention Objectives for the year 2000.[9] On October 31 and November 1, 1989, a meeting was held for approximately 300 "consortium member organizations to provide representatives . . . with an opportunity to respond to the public comment draft" of these objectives.[10]

Two authors in particular, Salmon and Viadro, feel strongly that a national nursing agenda "should reflect the framework and approach of the objectives for the Nation, and describe a corollary set of objectives for nursing with an outline of potential nursing health promotion disease prevention measures supportive of and derived from the national health agenda."[11]

The basic tenet of a health care model for the future should be that of proactive primary health care focused on prevention rather than reactive acute medical care.[12] In such a model, "community involvement and decision-making is critical to the planning and implementation of health care policy and program."[13] Certainly nurses can become more active and influential in reshaping this type of health care system.

> For nurses the opportunity is enormous. Who is more qualified to seize the moment and to rescue health care than the immediate, constant, hands-on providers? Nurses are on-the-line professionals—the first guard—who have seen it all and are the most knowledgeable.[14]

Despite problems resulting from the acute nursing shortage that dominated the 1980s and extends into the 1990s, excellent media coverage has made the public more aware of nursing's role and contribution to the health care system. However, more effort by nurses is necessary to acquaint society with nursing's cost-saving abilities in primary care and long-term care delivery and its concern for quality care to clients.

NEW FORMS OF HEALTH CARE

" . . . The health care system has been moving towards 'corporatization' through amalgamation of health care entities into larger multi-agency 'systems' and increased competitiveness through a variety of choices in health insurance and the ways in which health services are delivered and by whom, such as the growth of prepaid and capitated insurance programs."[15]

> In the new value conscious care climate of the 90s, nurses will be well positioned to compete with other providers to offer the best package of services at the best price. Community nursing centers, nurse-run HMOs, school HMOs and community clinics will become the preferred arrangement in the managed care environment of the 90s.[16]

The role of case manager and a managed care environment have emerged as competition among various health providers. Other options such as nurse managed home visits and community nursing centers are additional means of strengthening an ailing health care system.

Third party payors and policy makers under pressure to reduce health care costs have begun to consider the possibility of new nurse-managed options for improved health care delivery. As a result, nurses should be leaders in facilitating growth in managed care and case management programs.

Case Managed Care

In seeking solutions to the insidious problems of access, quality, and escalating costs of health care, several alternative health care delivery options have been available. A major shift from an in-patient hospital-based delivery system to a community-oriented managed care system based on prevention, has placed nursing in a favorable position to effect changes in health care delivery. Managed care is an option that provides health care services to specific groups of patients at a competitive price. This new option is an opportunity for nursing to demonstrate its potential for cost-effectiveness and its right to become *the* health provider in the 90s. Moreover, with an upsurge in recognition of nurses by the general public, some have predicted that the 1990s will turn out to be the decade of the nurse.

According to Zander, one of a nursing group operating a free-standing consulting company in New England, "Case management is a patient-centered system that unites the nurse's clinical and management skills in providing or arranging for whatever health care a person needs."[17] A primary nurse in the hospital can arrange for home care services for a patient. This service can also be provided by case managers employed by insurance companies or "case management companies whom clients call or who get referrals from hospitals or HMOs."[18]

RESTRUCTURING THE HEALTH CARE SYSTEM

Perspectives on the evolving health care system provide insight into nursing's future as this present century draws to a close. According to several health futurists, provision of health care services for all of the nation's citizens through a national, comprehensive health plan will gradually occur, with maternal-child care being among the first services to become available.

Health promotion and health maintenance will become a top priority, with ambulatory health clinics absorbing heavier caseloads than the acute care settings. Community and university health centers will continue to play an even greater role than at present because many of them will be closely associated with specialty hospitals and assume responsibility for patients after early hospital discharge.

Health assessments and health histories already are being performed within these various centers or in clients' homes. Undoubtedly, "the quality of our healthcare system depends on a national health plan which reduces the inordinate and costly bias toward expensive inpatient care and places the emphasis on less expensive alternatives, reducing unnecessary procedures and the use of costly technology."[19]

National Nursing Health Plan

Due to significant shifts in health care, nurse leaders are convinced that a national nursing-sponsored health plan is appropriate to remedy the many problems already existing in this system. To accomplish this goal, ANA appointed a Board of Director's Task Force on Health Policy in support of access, quality and cost-efficiency, chaired by Gloria Hope, Ph.D., RN, to produce a health policy plan. The NLN Board also produced a proposal for a new health policy agenda.[20]

At the National Commission on Nursing Implementation Project (NCNIP) 1990 spring conference in Palm Springs, California, key nursing spokespersons provided nursing solutions for the nation's ailing health care system. They stressed that nursing care cuts costs and improves access and quality.[21] During this meeting, representatives of the Tri-Council discussed next steps in shaping nursing's national health plan.

League representatives presented key principles endorsed by the NLN Board that appeared congruent with ANAs approach to a national health proposal. Principles such as reasonable health services costs, public-private financing, reimbursement of services by nurses, and a restructured delivery system were among those proposed.

It was anticipated that after ANA and NLN had developed their proposals based on these principles that agreement would occur. Then with Tri-Council approval, ultimately a proposal for a national nursing health plan would be introduced into legislation.[22] The American Association of Retired Persons (AARP) Legislative Council has also been active in calling for a fairer system of health care delivery and a comprehensive national health plan assuring needed health care and long-term care to all Americans.[23]

ECONOMIC REFORMS FOR NURSING

Undoubtedly, nursing is in need of major economic reforms in order to assume a more effective role in health care delivery.[24] Economic reform and restructuring nursing practice in the workplace would make nursing more attractive due to acquiring a higher degree of professional autonomy. "Social workers, psychologists, physical therapists and the like have achieved considerable gains in acquiring third party payment and establishing fee for service and group practices in all types of settings."[25] According to Mauksch, "nurses should quit being employees," incorporate as PAs (professional associates), and contract with health care facilities and individuals for their services.[26]

Since social workers and psychologists have acquired reimbursement under Medicare, why then has nursing not been eligible? As mentioned previously, the government and certain providers have not recognized nursing's professional status. Medicine and the medical model along with hospital administrators remain firmly in control of the health care arena. Several health professions already require graduate professional preparation for entry into practice, have achieved a distinct body of knowledge, an autonomous practice, and an accountability system for patient care that the public fully accepts.

Nursing cannot afford to prolong its efforts to achieve similar goals. It becomes abundantly clear that even if nursing was successful in accomplishing all of these goals, it must demonstrate their relevance for the public agenda on improved health care. Nurses should remain in the forefront to convince the public that the ills affecting Americans such as AIDS, homelessness, illegal drug control, alcohol abuse, and care of the elderly and indigent, can be remedied by a national health plan that promotes accessible, quality health care for all its citizens.

Corporations Involved in Health Care

In addition to clinics and community health centers, new corporate structures for hospitals are developing, with corporations operating multihospitals and extensions into home care. A new medical-industrial complex is creating a booming business in health care. This ongoing development, which has begun to revamp the delivery of health care, has been described by a health economist as "one of the greatest achievements of America's government and private sectors."[27] Dr. Arnold Relman, director of the New England Journal of Medicine, refers to it as "an unprecedented phenomenon with broad and potentially troubling implications."[28]

The movement away from non-profit hospitals to corporate-owned hospitals, home health-care services, and retirement homes is rapidly producing fierce competition for the available health care dollars. Some fear that doctors in these corporations will succumb to pressures and with less control over their practice, reduce the quality of care rendered.

Trends in Out-Patient Care

Another new form of health care development involves the walk-in medical clinic, often located in shopping malls or near busy highways. Figures indicated that there were 950 free-standing emergency centers and 4,000 more were predicted by 1990.[29] One-day surgical units are another booming industry. Predictions are that profits soon will total one billion dollars a year, with over 500 such units in operation.[30] With approximately seventy percent of hospitals providing out-patient surgery, some reduction in costs resulting from competition from free-standing emergency centers is occurring. If this trend continues, a new face in medical care delivery should soon become a permanent mode for the future. According to a study released by Arthur Andersen and Company and the American College of Hospital Administrators, "for profit" hospitals will double over the next decade and Health Maintenance Organizations will be five times more numerous.[31]

It has long been recognized that hospitals and medical care represent one of the largest industries in the United States, and recent efforts to control health care costs have produced severe competition. Hospitals are exerting every effort to make their services more attractive and have resorted to the media to advertise their benefits and services. Profit from the prospective payment system (PPS) as an incentive for hospitals to encourage early patient discharge is resulting in reduced costs and reimbursement from the government for hospitals that manage their institutions more economically.

Biomedical technology continues at a rapid pace, and researchers predict that between now and the year 2000 several new innovative technologies will appear. Artificial transplants (lung, liver, heart) and other natural organ transplants, even artificial ears and implants (bone, lens, teeth), are becoming available for individuals in need of such surgery.

Technologic devices, such as telemetry for physiological monitoring and rehabilitative devices, are already on the market and drastically altering the speed with which patients recover. Even joint reconstructive surgery and artificial joint replacements are undergoing change as human bone replaces the metal or synthetic material previously used.

Breakthroughs in cancer research will alter or perhaps eliminate the growth of cancer cells through discovery of their cause and remedial action to prevent their occurrence. New knowledge of chromosomes, genes, and the positive effects of vitamin and mineral therapy that are aiding in the possible elimination of cancerous growths are creating optimism for the future. The list of new technologies and preventive medicine that is becoming available indicates that the health care scene fifteen to twenty years from now will present a vastly different picture than the one currently existing.

Progress presents moral and ethical dilemmas as health professionals are confronted with decisions that severely affect the lives and welfare of people needing new, innovative therapies. As progress in the health field continues, numerous varieties of health care personnel representing various health disciplines are assisting individuals in their pursuit of health. Greater involvement of people in securing a healthier state of well-being will result in a definite decline of patients seeking facilities for illness care, as alternative health services and health providers become readily available.

Nursing's Changing Health Care Role

As nursing's transition from an illness-care orientation to health promotion and health maintenance increases, and as future health needs begin to surface, new perspectives are needed. A changing health care system requires that nursing meet its societal responsibility by orienting nurses to their evolving health care role.

As identified in the definition of nursing addressed in the ANA's Social Policy Statement, "Nursing is the diagnosis and treatment of human responses to actual or potential health problems." Once nurses accept this social mission, they should be able to articulate what contributions nursing makes to the health care of individuals, regardless of their health state.[32] If nurses demonstrate that these human responses are the main focus of nursing practice and if they define a specific, theoretical knowledge base to support this claim, then nursing will have justified its assertion of being a socially significant profession deserving of full professional status.

To assume responsibility for assessing the health status of people within society will require a greater nursing knowledge and more skillful nursing practice than previously possessed by practicing nurses. Negotiations with multidisciplinary team members for collaboration and cooperation in providing health care will, of necessity, require skill in developing sound interpersonal relationships in order to communicate effectively with other health disciplines. Referrals between nurses and other health professionals will increase as nurses demonstrate their knowledge, competence, and skills, calling for a greater level of trust and respect among professionals as competition among them increases.

Nursing is beginning to witness a trend toward professional nurses functioning in private practice as primary health care providers. If they obtain admitting privileges in hospitals they will be responsible for planning the total care of their patients over a twenty-four-hour period. Nurse technicians will implement the nursing care plan with reinforcement from the professional nurse. Although the percentage of nurses employed in hospitals in 1980 was sixty-eight percent, this number is changing as professional nurses opt for other practice settings. Some estimates indicate that only twenty-five percent of professional nurses will choose to remain in hospital nursing in the future. Approximately seventy-five percent of technical nurses will provide direct care under the supervision of more qualified professional nurses. For those professional nurses involved in multidisciplinary health teams, leadership in coordinating health services for patients will be nurses's responsibility.

Independent, autonomous nursing practice will characterize nurses' future roles in fulfilling their responsibilities to patients and society. As independent practitioners, professional nurses of the future will, as the patient's needs require, work collaboratively with physicians and other health care personnel to restore health, provide necessary life-supporting therapies, or prepare the patient for death with dignity. As healthy clients seek assistance in maintaining health, future professional nurses will be well qualified to provide independent health maintenance services. By urging clients to modify their lifestyles and health behavior and by screening for early detection of abnormalities, professional nurses can contribute substantially to keeping people well.

The challenge to nurses will be to translate nursing's specific knowledge base into innovative ways to provide nursing care in promoting and maintaining health. It is anticipated that specialization in nursing will undergo many changes, as new specialty areas are developed from nursing diagnostic classifications, such as anxiety, pain, oncological, burn, chronicity, cardiovascular, and respiratory categories.[33,34]

The increase of chronic illnesses and an aging population will lead to greater involvement of future professional nurses in long-term care of the elderly in various stages of health. Nurses will care for clients in their homes, ambulatory health clinics, nursing homes, hospitals, HMOs, day care, wellness centers, and other extended care facilities. An increase in the number of home health care agencies in the 1980s represented a trend that is likely to continue over the next two decades, particularly if funding for long-term care in homes becomes available.

Impact of Nursing Research on Future Nursing Practice

Perhaps in another two decades the impact of nursing research on nursing as a profession will become more evident. Nurse scientists and nurse researchers are painstakingly pursuing the development of new knowledge in order to establish a scientific base for nursing. With the development of new technologies for prolonging life, demands for sophisticated, knowledgeable nursing care to provide support and assistance to individuals as they cope and adapt to new forms of therapy will be more essential than ever before.

Nursing research is essential to produce a specific theoretical knowledge base that professional nurses can use to provide quality nursing care for individuals with critical or chronic illnesses or for people seeking health promotion and health maintenance services. To date, the degree of consensus regarding nursing's specific knowledge base remains questionable, but the horizon brightens as nurse researchers unfold their scientific research and reveal new insights about nursing's unique body of knowledge.

The quantity of nursing research required to strengthen and enrich nursing practice has grown substantially over the past few years. However, when comparing the research productivity of nursing with that of other disciplines, nursing research still lags behind. With the limited number of nurses holding earned doctorates (2.6%), several of whom are not actively involved in nursing research, such findings are not unusual.[35] The fact that a sizable number of nurses earned their doctoral degree in a discipline other than nursing is another reason for fewer nursing studies, particularly clinical research studies.

Now that forty-eight doctoral programs in nursing are available throughout the country, the amount of nursing research is increasing.[36] Research development programs in service agencies, continued federal support for nurse researchers and for pre- and postdoctoral fellowships, involvement on multidisciplinary research teams, creation of research centers of excellence in schools of nursing, and a climate supporting nurse researchers will all have a positive effect on the amount of nursing research generated over the next decade. Efforts of the ANA Council of Nurse Researchers to support and encourage the development of nursing research is also commendable.

Another interesting development in funding for nursing research is the shift from supporting the research process itself to that of support for the phenomena of concern to nursing.[37] Over the next two decades, nursing research will continue to generate new knowledge and nurse researchers will increase their efforts to apply research findings to nursing practice. As nurse researchers and nurse clinicians interact and collaborate with one another, research findings will be utilized, and nursing practice will be greatly improved.

Reflecting on the future of nursing science and nursing research, Susan Gortner, Professor of Nursing at the University of California, San Francisco, made the following observation: "Were we to dream about the vitality and credibility of our science 10 years hence, it would be that a number of well-defined programmatic areas of research could be identified as on-going, each containing not one or two, but a dozen or more investigators with national reputations and impressive track records of productivity in the area."[38]

EFFECTS OF COMPUTERIZED TECHNOLOGY ON NURSING'S FUTURE

The decade of the 1990s has ushered in a technological revolution attributed to computers that continues to change communication patterns among health professionals.[39] Having moved from the post-industrial age to a technological age, new information will be readily available to the public in the 1990s, when it is estimated that 80 percent of American homes will have their own personal computers. Also, people will be able to remain at home and learn via computer systems.

Within the health care environment, computer equipment, once cumbersome to manage, has been reduced in size to the form of mini- or microcomputers. A variety of computer systems are available, such as the hospital medical information system, the management information system, and the nursing information system. Computer assisted instructional materials (CAI) for practicing nurses and nurse educators are increasing as microcomputer software is further developed and refined. Learning how to select appropriate CAI material, match it to the best format, and write, edit, and review using CAI are steps that should be learned by nurses in the foreseeable future.[40] In some hospitals, nurses already are expected to master computer literacy programs in order to use computers effectively in documenting patient care and in utilizing computerized care plans.

Computer terminals located in nursing units in hospitals are revolutionizing nursing functions and reducing the time needed to order medications and supplies from pharmacy, to transcribe and implement medical regimens, and as mentioned previously, to develop and use computerized care plans. Computers located in patient units in hospitals are providing easy access for caregivers in decision-making and in acquiring more effective communication. Computer networking for nurse administrators can save time, with interoffice memoranda computerized and transmitted to other offices within hospitals or university campuses, thus providing the capability for receiving feedback in far less time than in previous systems.

Although computer-assisted nursing practice is in the beginning stages, great strides are being made by nurses knowledgeable about computer hardware and software.[41] Nursing practice in the future will become highly sophisticated as a result of advances in computer technology. Despite the progress made in computers, the missing parameter continues to be trained personnel required to monitor data bases. With approximately 2.8 million computers on the market, and predictions of double that amount by the 1990s, knowledgeable computer personnel will be in great demand.

There is excitement and challenge as a new world of technological advances opens up vistas heretofore unheard of. For example, who would have believed that a paraplegic college student at Wright State University in Dayton, Ohio, permanently paralyzed from a serious auto accident, would be able to stand and walk up to receive her baccalaureate degree at the 1983 commencement? By means of a very small computer programmed to allow the brain to reactivate impaired muscles, this student, confined to a wheelchair, executed a spectacular performance and raised the hopes of paralyzed individuals nationwide. Nurses providing support services will be called upon to assist clients experiencing the therapeutic effects of computerized technology. "High tech" will require new knowledge and commitment to "caring," and "high touch" will be evident as nurses carry out their societal mission.

EDUCATION OF FUTURE PRACTITIONERS FOR A CHANGING HEALTH CARE SYSTEM

Nurse educators responsible for preparing tomorrow's nurses for professional nursing practice must prepare them for a future that can only be vaguely envisioned in this present decade. Professional nurses are assuming more complex responsibilities for health care than ever before. The speed of this changing pattern will continue at an accelerated pace into the next century.

The burden on nurse educators to predict health care needs and to prepare nurses for a world of nursing vastly different from that of the present period challenges them to be risk takers and leaders if they are to move nursing forward with vision and confidence. Social forces in the environment will not allow delay of this important mission. Fortunately, many nurse educators and nurse leaders in the United States are in agreement about nursing's future role in health care. *It is no longer a debatable issue.* However, if nursing continues to limp along, perpetuating patterns of nursing education that are not only unsatisfactory but are also incapable of providing the quality of preparation needed for a changing health care system, society will be deprived. Nursing will remain subservient to other health professions.

Unequal education preparation for entry into practice continues to present obstacles in nursing's attempt to acquire reimbursement and control over its practice. Requiring a baccalaureate degree for entry by 1990, which ANA had proposed in 1965, has yet to be accomplished. However, North Dakota is the first state to establish educational levels for entry into practice. According to Karen Macdonald, R.N., Executive Director of the North Dakota Board of Nursing, only baccalaureate graduates are admitted for the National Council Licensure Examination–RN (NCLEX-RN) examination, since anyone completing a diploma or associate degree RN program at this time would have entered the program after January 1, 1987. North Dakota's administrative rules require that anyone entering the nursing program after January 1, 1987 that applies for licensure must have completed a baccalaureate program in order to be eligible for RN licensure (endorsement or examination) or an associate degree practical nurse program to be eligible for LPN licensure (endorsement or examination).[42] In reviewing the history of North Dakota's struggle, it is apparent that strong leadership and innumerable hours of hard work and effort were required in accomplishing this goal.

Trends Affecting L.P.N. Educational Programs

Changes in health care delivery are seriously affecting licensed practical nurses in many states across the country. The replacement of licensed practical nurses by registered nurses in hospital nursing departments is becoming a serious problem for the former category of nursing personnel. Such action is the result of declining hospital patient census and an increase in the acuity level of illness among patients.

LPNs lack the additional knowledge and skill required for the acutely ill patient in today's hospitals. Concerned about the job security of LPNs, the National Federation of Licensed Practical Nurses, at its August 1984 House of Delegates meeting, endorsed expanding LPN/VN nursing education programs to at least eighteen months.[43] By acquiring an associate degree in nursing, graduates would meet the requirements for practical nurse licensure. ANA's goal of two levels of nursing—professional for the baccalaureate nurse and technical for the associate degree nurse—is consistent with this resolution.

It is anticipated that by 2005, anti-intellectual dissent will have abated and a standardized pattern of nursing education will have been universally accepted by all practicing nurses. Some nurse educators question whether or not a baccalaureate degree is adequate preparation for entry into professional practice. If it is not, should the baccalaureate nursing degree be a degree for technical nursing? Should the entry level for professional nursing be at the master's level by 2005 and at the doctoral level by the year 2025 or shortly thereafter? The turn of the century will occur in less than 10 years. Can nurses take a stand now and declare, once and for all, what they believe preparation for professional nursing should be and move this belief forward to a creative plan for standardizing nursing education for the future?

The admonitions and views of knowledgeable, visionary nurses, who have worked strenuously over the years to advance nursing and provide society with a socially significant service, should be listened to and acted on. What are some of the views prominent nurses are repeating over and over again to the vast body of nurses in today's nursing world? The following is a brief list of quotes worthy of consideration:

- Because of the tremendous rate at which scientific knowledge is accumulating, it is not risky to predict that the clinical doctorate will become the entry level requirement.[44]
- Nurses' education in general is still not equivalent to that of physician's and other health professionals whose minimum is education at a post-baccalaureate level.[45]
- . . . the future pathway to nursing on the professional level is not the BSN . . . (but) the professional nurse educated at the specialist post baccalaureate (liberal arts and science) level.[46]

- By the year 2000 all new nursing professionals will enjoy education that will prepare them to fulfill their potential in improving the health status of the nation.[47]

Predictions for Educational Distribution of RNs for the Future

Predictions for educational distribution of registered nurses of the future are noted in Table 14-1. A review of the data shows a decline in A.D. and Diploma RNs from 1,027,700 in 1990 to 698,400 in 2020, due to the aging of nurses and severe decline of diploma nursing programs. If diploma program enrollments continue to rise as evidenced recently, these trends may be reversed. A slight increase of RNs with baccalaureate degrees is observed from 535,500 (30.5 percent) in 1990 to 627,000 (37.8 percent) in 2020. Nurses with master's or doctoral degrees rise from 124,000 (7.3 percent) in 1990 to 317,500 (18.8 percent) in 2020. This latter figure indicates the greatest increase during the entire thirty year period under consideration.[48]

While numbers and changing characteristics of students are pressuring nurse educators, so too, the movement to restructure nursing care delivery systems is creating pressure. As nursing practice requires change, nurse educators must be prepared to meet these new expectations. "Nurses of the future will need to be prepared to practice in community settings and in a variety of health care institutions, in joint and independent practice, and in new organizational and practice arrangements that meet the needs of an aging population and assist in controlling health care costs."[49]

Table 14-1. Highest educational preparation of registered nurse supply: 1990–2020

Year	Total	A.D. & diploma	Baccalaureate	Master's & doctorate
1990	1,687,100	1,027,700	535,500	124,000
1995	1,813,300	1,028,200	624,600	160,400
2000	1,912,600	1,011,000	695,600	206,100
2005	1,947,600	965,100	734,600	247,900
2010	1,900,100	885,600	733,900	280,600
2015	1,780,400	784,100	693,800	302,500
2020	1,642,900	698,400	627,000	317,500

From *Seventh Report to the President and Congress on the Status of Health Personnel in the United States.* U.S. Dept. of Health and Human Services, Division of Nursing, Public Health Service, Health Resources & Services Administration, Bureau of Health Professions, Washington, DC, March 9, 1990, VIII-28.

COLLABORATION BETWEEN NURSING
AND CONSUMER INTEREST GROUPS
FOR IMPROVED HEALTH CARE

If present trends indicating a rise in the interest level of consumers in health care delivery continue, future health care systems will include even more active consumer participation. Nursing enjoys a reputation for "caring" for people and their health needs, even though the scientific knowledge and clinical expertise of many nurses are frequently not recognized. Consumers respect the advocacy role of nursing in meeting their health needs because they believe that nurses care.

With more intense interest and activism in health care demonstrated by consumer groups, nurses should avail themselves of every opportunity to foster strong links between the consumers of health care services and themselves. In so doing, nursing will win public support for its efforts to upgrade health care delivery in this country. Nurses should be knowledgeable of consumer health needs, fully aware of nursing's ability to meet these needs, and informed of the economic benefits to be achieved from nursing practice. "In any future major reform of national health policies, nurses and consumers must be integrally involved in defining quality in its various dimensions and aspects."[50]

Since consumers and the business community continue to be concerned over the high cost and quality of health care delivery, they are looking to preferred providers and alternative health care options for solutions to these problems. "Consumers, businesses, private and public insurers, and administrators of health care organizations need to know that nursing, as a responsible profession, is concerned with quality and cost issues . . . (and) how current changes in nursing practice and education affect them personally, organizationally, and as a community."[51] "Identifying outcomes of care will gain application and acceptance, . . . as consumers increasingly take health matters into their own hands . . . and demand greater knowledge of health care issues and indicators with which to judge the *value*—cost and quality—of the services they are purchasing."[52]

Nurses and consumers have similar values about consumer health needs. Fortunately, consumers are now beginning to recognize nursing's value in promoting their health and well-being.[53] Thus, the importance of nurses demonstrating, through patient outcome data, that both quality and cost-effectiveness can be achieved through nursing practice. The consumer movement is here to stay, and nursing has an opportunity to increase the advantage it presently enjoys of being trusted and viewed favorably by the public.

Several reasons for the heightened interest of consumers and their demands for adequate health care are found in nursing literature.[54, 55] A more enlightened public resulting from increased public education, insurance companies insulating health care costs, and deductions in income tax for medical expenses are some of the reasons cited.[56]

How skillful nursing becomes in developing creative partnerships and interaction with consumers will affect the rapidity with which nursing develops as a full profession. To develop interaction, consumers should be kept informed about nursing's contribution to health care, the social significance of its services, and how it has been categorized as a semiprofession, despite its long struggle to achieve professionalism. Moreover, consumers should be convinced that nursing can meet their health care needs and therefore, is deserving of autonomy, professional status, and the public's support.

Nurses should be aware that "the health care consumer is no longer a captive in a world he does not understand."[57] Nurses, along with other health professionals, are being held accountable for the health services they provide. The formation of citizen boards and active consumer involvement in Health Maintenance Organizations, hospital boards, and community health center activities has provided an atmosphere for consumers to express their concerns about health care delivery.

To assist consumers in obtaining noninstitutional health care at reduced costs, nurses should be willing to change their perspective from solely that of a "sick care" role to one emphasizing health and wellness. Many professional nurses have accepted this responsibility to provide wellness care. But it will take time to prepare future nurses for this new role.

Consumers will play a key role in deciding whether nurse practitioners will continue to function in the future. In states where consumers have played an active role in protecting the rights of NPs to practice, nurses have won the battle.[58] Consumers, supportive of certified nurse-midwives in Nebraska, drafted their own bill and through strenuous lobbying efforts and communication, achieved a successful outcome with the legislators— "consumer sophistication . . . at the grass roots."[59]

Alvin Toffler, a well-known futurist, offers worthwhile advice in *The Third Wave*:

> the responsibility for change . . . lies with us. We must begin with ourselves, teaching ourselves not to close our minds prematurely to the novel, the surprising, the seemingly radical. This means fighting off [those] who rush forward to kill any new suggestion on grounds of its impracticality, while defending whatever now exists as practical, no matter how . . . unworkable it may be.[60]

Applying his words to nursing education indicates that the traditional patterns of nurse preparation of the past should give way to new modes of preparation. Achieving consensus on a standardized plan of nursing education is the key to adequately preparing future nurses to fulfill society's health needs in the decades ahead.

Whether society will prefer a nursing model of health care or continue to support a medical model remains to be seen. Evidence of the public's preference for and the value of alternative models of health care is currently on the increase. Nursing leaders agree that "the time has come to restructure nursing in a way that ensures that there is a more direct relationship between the consumer of nursing services and the providers of nursing services."[61] According to Grace "a revolution of the citizenry is the only force to create change in a democracy [and] nursing has the capacity to educate the consumer to create such changes."[62]

In becoming consumer advocates, nursing's major challenge is to join U.S. health consumers in supporting a national nursing health plan that supports a professional model of nursing practice emphasizing health, wellness and disease prevention through quality, affordable nursing care delivery.

ADDITIONAL PERSPECTIVES

Unlike any other time in its history, nursing now has an agenda for its future development, which, if agreed and acted upon by its members, will allow it to achieve its mission of optimum health care for all citizens. Health maintenance and health promotion can be claimed as nursing's primary function. The challenge rests in convincing the public, other health professions, and all nurses that this role is nursing's exclusive right. When nursing's primary function is understood by all these various groups, especially the medical profession, attitudes of resistance, claims of nurses illegally practicing medicine, and fears that nursing will usurp medicine's "turf" will eventually disappear. By the year 2000 it is hoped that all health professions will have achieved equality and such attitudes will rapidly become nonexistent.

Meanwhile, physicians need a clearer explanation of nursing's mission to allay their concerns about nurses providing "watered down" medical care. The trend for citizens to assume responsibility for their own health and to seek medical care from physicians when required does not present a problem. However, if the medical profession accepts the fact that nurses provide services to clients to promote their health and wellness and by so doing, reduce the cost of health care, then competition from nursing should not affect them. Patients requiring illness care and physician care know how to obtain it and when to seek it.

Another interesting development is the fact that nursing's primary function can be achieved in noninstitutional settings as well as in hospitals. For those professional nurses desiring to remain in institutional nursing, greater emphasis on accountability, quality assurance, and control of nursing practice is already happening in many of the nation's hospitals. However, opportunities for admitting patients to hospitals will bring changes long overdue for professional nurses functioning in these institutions. Time cards, hourly wages, and the lack of a written contractual agreement between qualified professional nurses and their employers should be eliminated in the foreseeable future if nursing is to be considered a profession, independent in its own right.

Regardless of the setting, nursing should entrust health care delivery to its most capable practitioners—professional nurses equipped with the education and experience to provide this care. Nurse technicians can supply traditional nursing care, but professional nurses are needed to fulfill nursing's primary mission of health promotion. The time is fast approaching when the ANA should give serious consideration to its future membership and decide whether or not to become an association representing only *professional* nurses, exclusive of technical level practitioners. A proposal submitted by a State Nurses' Association to the ANA House of Delegates in 1984 contained a similar message. The future holds the answer to this issue. If and when two levels of nursing are accepted by the profession—professional and technical—changes may be made in the membership of ANA, nursing's professional association.

Social forces are slowly convincing nurses that the present multitiered system of nursing education should be changed in order to standardize nursing education and align it with the educational base of other professions by the twenty-first century. This burden rests on present nurse educators as they prepare nursing personnel for the future.

Knowledge about health care systems and the needs of specific groups of clients, rather than traditional nursing knowledge, will characterize the future professional nurse. The demand for these knowledgeable professionals can only be imagined in the 1990s, but future nurses will be well-informed about the social consequences of their role, its economic worth, and the legitimacy of nursing as a recognized, full-fledged profession.

Increasing educational requirements is not the sole way to professionalize, although improved education and research will advance professional expertise and improve the health care provided. Demonstrating expertise and informing the public of how essential, indispensable, and socially significant its services are will help nursing achieve a monopoly over them. Lobbying efforts to achieve this monopoly should be ongoing.

Finally, nursing should be able to control the numbers of future professional nurses so that supply will not exceed demand. Nursing should address the number of professional and technical nurses needed in the future to implement its social mission. Efforts should continue to convince hospital administrators that employment of less prepared nursing personnel is not economically sound.

Now that nursing's agenda, as advocated by many nurse leaders and educators, has been presented, the decision to effect change is up to nursing itself. Further delays in resolving the recurrent issues presented throughout this book will prevent the professionalization of nursing. It is readily apparent that, in light of future predictions for nursing, the path to professionalism may seem remote and unattainable. And yet, if nursing will use the power, courage, strength, commitment, and leadership that nurses possess, the goal of professionalization will be reached, and quality health care will result.

SUMMARY

As health promotion and wellness become a national priority, nursing has begun to confidently enunciate its specific focus and mission. Perspectives on future health care delivery indicate that nursing's traditional role in hospital nursing will be substantially altered. Now that the public is beginning to seek alternative, noninstitutional settings for health care, the potential for nursing, particularly in community health centers, nursing homes, and home health care, far exceeds what was envisioned ten or fifteen years ago.

New, innovative types of health care, such as the walk-in medical clinic, corporate owned for-profit hospitals, and home health care services, are increasing. As nursing moves from illness care to health promotion and health maintenance, still newer perspectives are needed. Moreover, greater knowledge and skills will be required to assess the health status of individuals within society. Independent, autonomous nursing practice will characterize the role of future professional nurses.

Nurse researchers over the next two decades will generate new knowledge derived from studying phenomena of concern to nursing and applying this knowledge to nursing practice. Moreover, collaboration between nurse researchers and nurse clinicians will greatly improve and advance the status of nursing practice.

New technology and computers are revolutionizing the health care field. Technology is changing and improving communication patterns among health professionals. As a result, the speed at which professional nurses can assume more complex responsibilities will accelerate in the next decade.

Nurse educators have the responsibility to prepare nurses for a nursing world very different from the present scene. Since nursing's future role in health care delivery is no longer a debatable issue, it is anticipated that by the year 2005, anti-intellectual dissent will have ceased. A regularized nursing education system will have been universally accepted by all practicing nurses.

Now that consumer interest groups are actively concerned with health and health-related matters, nurses should endeavor to foster strong linkages with consumers in order to elicit the public's support for upgrading health care delivery. Consumers need to be informed about nursing's mission, focus, and the social significance of nursing's services. The path to professionalism may seem rather remote and unattainable, but if nursing uses the power, strength, and commitment of nurses, the goal of professionalization will be reached, and quality health care will result.

As noted at the beginning of this chapter, peering *into the future* is a risky enterprise. However, if nurses keep well informed and knowledgeable both about trends and movements already underway and about those on the horizon, perhaps they can move forthrightly in meeting the challenges facing nursing as the next century approaches. Who knows what major changes in health delivery and in nursing can occur, if the strong voices of nursing can unite to bring about a whole new world of health opportunities for all of society?

It is my hope that this book may serve to challenge and motivate nurses to revitalize health care delivery by making quality health care readily available for the nation's citizens. Striving for the professionalization of nursing will, inevitably, make it happen. Individual nurses can meet this challenge, by resolving first to improve their own personal and professional development. Ultimately, they should join with all nurses to achieve full professional status for nursing and thus assure society of the very best that health care services can provide.

REFERENCES

1. Deets, H. "Access to Care Needs to be a Basic Right," *American Association of Retired Persons* XXX:8 (September, 1989), 3.
2. Sorian, R. (ed.), *Medicine and Health*. Washington, D.C.: McGraw-Hill Co., 1988.
3. Pearson, C. "National Health Expenditures 1986–2000," *Health Care Financing Review* 8:4 (April, 1987).
4. Smith, G. "Using the Public Agenda to Shape PHN Practice," *Nursing Outlook* 37:2 (March–April, 1989), 73.
5. Ginzberg, E. "The Economics of Health Care and the Future of Nursing," 32.
6. Shekleton, M. "INA Testimony to the Health Summit," *CHART* 87:2 (February, 1990), 4.
7. Ginzberg, E. "The Economics of Health Care and the Future of Nursing," *Nurse Educator* 6:3 (May–June, 1981), 32.
8. Levi, M. "Functional Redundancy and the Process of Professionalization," in E. Hein and M. Nicholson (eds.), *Contemporary Leadership Behavior*. Boston: Little, Brown & Co., 1982, 379.

9. U.S.P.H.S. "The 1990 Health Objectives for the Nation: A Midcourse Review," Washington, D.C.: Office of Disease Prevention & Health Promotion, 1986.

10. "Academy Responds to Year 2000 National Health Objectives," (Academy News) *Nursing Outlook* 38:3 (May–June, 1990), 112.

11. Salmon, M. and Viadro, C. "Objectives for the Nation: A National Agenda for Nursing Education, Research and Practice," *Nursing Outlook* 37:3 (May–June, 1989), 111.

12. Shekleton, M. "INA Testimony to the Health Summit," 4.

13. *Ibid.*

14. Ahern, J. "Nurses' Influence Projected to Grow During Nineties," *American Nurse.* 22:3 (March, 1990), 9.

15. *Seventh Report to the President and Congress on the Status of Health Personnel in the United States.* U.S. Department of Health & Human Services, Division of Nursing, Public Health Service, Health Resources and Services Administration, Bureau of Health Professions, March, 1990, p. 3.

16. Moraldo, P. "The Nineties: A Decade in Search of Meaning," *Nursing and Health Care* 11:1 (January, 1990), 12.

17. Schoor, T. "Case Management Companies Run By Nurses?" *American Journal of Nursing* 90:10 (October, 1990), 71.

18. *Ibid.*

19. Pretziosi, P. "Developing a National Health Plan: 'Why Now? Why Nurses?' " NLN *Public Policy Bulletin* (Fall, 1989), 1.

20. "Task Force Tackles Health Policy," *American Nurse.* 22:4 (April, 1990), 13.

21. Moraldo, P. NLN *Executive Director Wire* (Spring, 1990), 1.

22. *Ibid.*, 3.

23. "A Fairer System: AARP Council Seeks National Health Plan," *AARP Bulletin* 31:3 (March, 1990), 1.

24. Moraldo, P. NLN *Executive Director Wire* (Spring, 1990), 1.

25. *Ibid.*

26. Mauksch, I. "Will Nurses Contract Their Services?" *American Journal of Nursing* 90:10 (October, 1990), 39.

27. Dentzen, S., Haggar, M., Zuckerman, S. and Relman, A. "The Big Business of Medicine," *Newsweek* 102:18 (October 31, 1983), 62.

28. *Ibid.*

29. Schiffres, M. "Behind the Surge of Walk-In Medical Clinics," *U.S. News and World Report* 95:23 (December 5, 1983), 75.

30. *Ibid.*

31. American College of Hospital Administrators. *Health Care in the 1990s: Trends and Strategies.* Chicago: Arthur Andersen & Co., 1984.

32. Barnard, K. (editorial), "Social Policy Statement Can Move Nursing Ahead," *American Nurse* 15:1 (January, 1983), 4.

33. Roy C. "The Impact of Nursing Diagnosis," *Nursing Digest* 4:4 (Summer, 1976), 68.

34. Leininger, M. "Futurology of Nursing: Goals and Challenges for Tomorrow," in N. Chaska (ed.), *The Nursing Profession: Views Through the Mist.* New York: McGraw Hill, 1978, 39.

35. *Facts About Nursing, 1982–83.* Kansas City, Mo.: American Nurses' Association, 1983.

36. Council of Baccalaureate and Higher Degree Programs. *Doctoral Programs in Nursing, 1983–84.* (Pub. No.: 15–1448). New York: National League for Nursing, 1983.
37. Barnard, K. "Knowledge for Practice: Directions for the Future," *Nursing Research* 29:4 (July, 1980), 208.
38. Gortner, S. "Nursing Research: Out of the Past and Into the Future," *Nursing Research* 29:4 (July–August, 1980), 206.
39. Brose, C. "Computer Technology in Nursing: Revolution or Renaissance?" *Nursing and Health Care* 5:10 (December, 1984), 515.
40. Felton, B. "Planning and Implementing Computer Learning in Departments of Nursing," *Nursing and Health Care* 5:10 (December, 1984), 549–553.
41. Edmunds, L. "Computer Assisted Nursing Care," *American Journal of Nursing* 82:7 (July, 1982), 1076–1079.
42. Phone Conversation with Karen MacDonald, Executive Director, North Dakota Board of Nursing, Bismark, N.D., June, 1990.
43. "LPNs Endorse Two Levels of Nursing, Education," *American Nurse* 16:10 (November–December, 1984), 1, 23.
44. Christman, L. "The Future of the Nursing Profession," *Nursing Administrative Quarterly* 11:2 (Winter, 1987), 2.
45. Roberts, J. "Uncovering Hidden Caring," *Nursing Outlook* 38:2 (March–April, 1990), 68.
46. Welch-Conway, C. "Turning Points in Nursing Education," in N. Chaska (ed.), *The Nursing Profession: Turning Points.* St. Louis: C.V. Mosby, 1990, 573.
47. Schlotfeldt, R. "Nursing in the Future," *Nursing Outlook* 29:5 (May, 1981), 299.
48. *Seventh Report to the President and Congress on the Status of Health Personnel in the United States.* (March, 1990) VIII-28, VIII-29.
49. Waite, R. "The Driving Forces for Change," in *Nursing's Vital Signs: Shaping the Profession for the 1990's.* Battle Creek, Michigan: W.K. Kellogg Foundation, 1989, 21.
50. Pretziosi, P. "Building a Public Policy Agenda," *NLN Public Policy Bulletin* (Summer, 1989), 2.
51. Waite, R. "The Driving Forces for Change," 21–22.
52. Moraldo, P. "The Nineties: A Decade in Search of Meaning," 12.
53. Aaronson, L. "Nurse-Midwives and Obstetricians: Alternative Models of Care and Client 'Fit,' " *Research in Nursing and Health* 10:8 (August, 1987), 217–226.
54. Rothman, D. and Rothman, N. *The Professional Nurse and the Law.* Boston: Little, Brown & Co., 1977.
55. Nixon, J. "The Right to Health Care: Reflections and Implications for Nursing Administrators," *Nursing Administrative Quarterly* 6:4 (Summer, 1982).
56. *Ibid.,* 3.
57. Rothman D. and Rothman N. *The Professional Nurse and the Law,* 84.
58. "Consumers Will Decide Future for NPs, Fagin Tells 'Today,' " *American Nurse* 15:8 (September, 1983), 14.
59. Mallison, M. "Grass Roots Consumerism," *American Journal of Nursing* 84:9 (September, 1984), 1079.
60. Toffler, A. *The Third Wave.* New York: William Morrow Co., 1980, 459.

61. Porter-O'Grady, T. "Restructuring the Nursing Organization for a Consumer-Driven Marketplace," *Nursing Administrative Quarterly* 12:3 (Spring, 1988), 62.
62. Grace, H. "Can Health Care Costs Be Contained?" *Nursing and Health Care* 11:3 (March, 1990), 129.

SUGGESTED READINGS

Andreoli, K. and Musser, L. "Computers in Nursing Care: The State of the Art," *Nursing Outlook* 33:1 (January–February, 1985), 16–21.
Andreoli, K. and Musser, L. "RNs and the Future," *Nursing and Health Care* 6:1 (January, 1985), 47–51.
Ball, M. and Hannah, K. *Using Computers in Nursing.* Reston, Va.: Reston, 1984.
Christensen, W. and Stearns, E. *Microcomputers in Health Care Management.* Rockville, Md.: Aspen Systems Corp., 1984.
Copp, L. "Health Promotion and Disease Prevention: A Data-Based Approach to Curriculum," *Nursing and Health Care* 5:5 (May, 1984), 257–261.
Curtin, L. (ed.), "The Decade Ahead: Five Major Issues," *Nursing Management* 14:10 (October 14, 1983), 9–10.
Edmunds, L. "Teaching Nurses to Use Computers," *Nurse Educator* 7:5 (Autumn, 1982), 32–38.
"Ethical Dilemmas in Health Care Explored at Forum," *American Nurse* 16:10 (November–December, 1984), 9.
Ginzberg, E. "Health Reform: The Outlook for the 1980s," *Inquiry* 15 (December, 1978), 311–326.
"Health Care Reform Report Out for Review," *American Nurse* 22:10 (November–December, 1990), 3.
Healthy People: The Surgeon General's Report on Health Promotion and Disease Prevention (PHS Pub. No.: 79–55071 A). Washington, D.C.: U.S. Government Printing Office, 1979.
Koeppin, C. "Nursing Wins Reimbursement Funding Victories," *American Nurse* 22:10 (November–December, 1990), 1.
Kohnke, M. "The Nurses' Responsibility to the Consumer," *American Journal of Nursing* 78:3 (March, 1978), 440.
Marin, S. "The Computer's Place in Nursing Education," *Nursing and Health Care* 2:9 (November, 1982), 500–506.
Naisbitt, J. *Megatrends: Ten New Directions Transforming Our Lives.* New York: Warner Books, 1982.
Robinson, B. "A Study of Consumer Perspectives Related to Nursing," *Nursing Leadership* 1:2 (June, 1978), 14–18.
Smith, J. *The Idea of Health: Implications for the Nursing Professional.* New York: Teachers College Press, Teachers College, Columbia University, 1983.
Ziemer, M. "Issues of Computer Literacy in Nursing Education," *Nursing and Health Care* 5:10 (December, 1984), 537–542.

Index

Numbers followed by an *f* indicate a figure; *t* following a page number indicates tabular material.